Contemporary Trends in Health Development: A Lifespan Perspective

Contemporary Trends in Health Development: A Lifespan Perspective

Edited by Hardy Lopez

STATES
ACADEMIC PRESS
www.statesacademicpress.com

States Academic Press,
109 South 5th Street,
Brooklyn, NY 11249, USA

Visit us on the World Wide Web at:
www.statesacademicpress.com

ISBN: 978-1-63989-126-9

Cataloging-in-Publication Data

Contemporary trends in health development : a lifespan perspective / edited by Hardy Lopez.
p. cm.
Includes bibliographical references and index.
ISBN 978-1-63989-126-9
1. Health. 2. Medical care. 3. Life cycle, Human. 4. Public health. I. Lopez, Hardy.
RA776 .C66 2022
613--dc23

Table of Contents

Preface VII

Chapter 1 **Early Childhood Health and the Life Course: The State of the Science and Proposed Research Priorities** 1
W. Thomas Boyce and Clyde Hertzman

Chapter 2 **Middle Childhood: An Evolutionary-Developmental Synthesis** 34
Marco DelGiudice

Chapter 3 **Adolescent Health Development: A Relational Developmental Systems Perspective** 47
Richard M. Lerner, Claire D. Brindis, Milena Batanova and Robert Wm. Blum

Chapter 4 **Emerging Adulthood as a Critical Stage in the Life Course** 60
David Wood, Tara Crapnell, Lynette Lau, Ashley Bennett, Debra Lotstein, Maria Ferris and Alice Kuo

Chapter 5 **A Life Course Health Development Perspective on Oral Health** 81
James J. Crall and Christopher B. Forrest

Chapter 6 **Life Course Health Development Outcomes After Prematurity: Developing a Community, Clinical, and Translational Research Agenda to Optimize Health, Behavior, and Functioning** 103
Michael E. Msall, Sarah A. Sobotka, Amelia Dmowska, Dennis Hogan and Mary Sullivan

Chapter 7 **Early in the Life Course: Time for Obesity Prevention** 131
Summer Sherburne Hawkins, Emily Oken and Matthew W. Gillman

Chapter 8 **Using the Fragile Families and Child Wellbeing Study (FFCWS) in Life Course Health Development Research** 159
Amanda Geller, Kate Jaeger and Garrett Pace

Chapter 9 **The Emerging Theoretical Framework of Life Course Health Development** 179
Neal Halfon and Christopher B. Forrest

Chapter 10 **Preconception and Prenatal Factors and Metabolic Risk** 204
Guoying Wang, Tami R. Bartell and Xiaobin Wang

Permissions

List of Contributors

Index

Preface

The continuous and progressive improvement in the health status of a population is termed as health development. It involves borrowing concepts from economics and social development studies, and applying them to health systems. Life course health development is a framework which deals with several fields and organizes their research in order to show how population and individual health develops. It also portrays the ways in which interactions among biological and environmental factors during the lifetime determine developmental trajectories. This approach helps in understanding the impact of experiences in early years of an individual on the functional status and health conditions in later life. It analyzes the connection between the biology of development and the experiences, and helps in understanding furthering knowledge of how diseases occur. This book includes some of the vital pieces of work being conducted across the world, on various topics related to health development from a lifespan perspective. It will also provide interesting topics for research which interested readers can take up. This book will serve as a reference to a broad spectrum of readers.

This book unites the global concepts and researches in an organized manner for a comprehensive understanding of the subject. It is a ripe text for all researchers, students, scientists or anyone else who is interested in acquiring a better knowledge of this dynamic field.

I extend my sincere thanks to the contributors for such eloquent research chapters. Finally, I thank my family for being a source of support and help.

Editor

1

Early Childhood Health and the Life Course: The State of the Science and Proposed Research Priorities

W. Thomas Boyce and Clyde Hertzman

But Laura lay awake a little while, listening to Pa's fiddle softly playing and to the lonely sound of the wind in the Big Woods. She looked at Pa sitting on the bench by the hearth, the firelight gleaming on his brown hair and beard and glistening on the honey-brown fiddle. She looked at Ma, gently rocking and knitting.
She thought to herself, 'This is now.'
She was glad that the cozy house, and Pa and Ma and the firelight and the music, were now. They could not be forgotten, she thought, because now is now. It can never be a long time ago.

Little House in the Big Woods
Laura Ingalls Wilder (1932)

1 Introduction: What's So Special About the Early Years?

In these lines from the *Little House* book series recalling her early years in a nineteenth-century pioneer family, Laura Ingalls Wilder evoked what we deem a timeless and evocative, if modestly sentimental, image of childhood: children's dependency upon the reliable and protective presence of parents, children's uniquely vulnerable and consequential sensibilities, their openness to the character and "feel" of the physical and social worlds, and their singular immersion in the present, the moment at hand. The overarching goals of this chapter are to survey extant literature examining evidence for these special susceptibilities of children to social-environmental conditions, to show how variation in life course health development is attributable to interactive differences in constitutional susceptibility and contextual exposure, and to summarize lacunae in our collective vision of how early adversity becomes biologically embedded in the course of individual health development.

Wilder's portrait of early childhood is the same image promulgated in the eighteenth century writings of Jean Jacque Rousseau, who affirmed children's inherent goodness and receptivity to the social world and educational institutions' responsibility never to impede children's natural independence and curiosity (see *Émile, or Treatise*

W. Thomas Boyce (✉)
Departments of Pediatrics and Psychiatry, University of California San Francisco, San Francisco, CA, USA
e-mail: istom.boyce@ucsf.edu

C. Hertzman
Human Early Learning Partnership, School of Population and Public Health, University of British Columbia, Vancouver, BC, Canada

on Education). Such an image of childhood is also wholly commensurate with twenty-first century visions of youth as a season of special vulnerability within the human life course health development—a developmental discontinuity from the less susceptible, more defended reaches of adulthood and life in an adult society. Some historians of childhood have claimed that these visions of children's special sentience and fragility are social constructions—products of the temporal and cultural epoch in which we now live. Philippe Ariès in his *Centuries of Childhood* (Ariès 1962) and Edward Shorter in *The Making of the Modern Family* (Shorter 1975) argued, for example, that prior to the seventeenth and eighteenth centuries, fewer distinctions were made between children and their adult counterparts in their needs, capacities, and proclivities. They further held that, as a consequence of the extraordinary rates of infant mortality at the time (25–50%; King 2007), parents were less likely to make strong emotional investments in children. Other scholars have judged such claims hyperbolic, however, discerning evidence for qualitative differentiation between children and adults in ancient Egyptian songs ("Hast thou come to kiss the child?/ I will not let thee kiss him!/ Hast thou come to silence him?/ I will not let thee set silence over him!" (Hrdy 1999)), in the writings of Renaissance Italy and Reformation Germany (King 2007) and in the plays of Shakespeare ("Those that do teach young babes/ Do it with gentle means and easy tasks/ He might ha' chid me so; for, in good faith,/ I am a child to chiding." *Romeo and Juliet*) (Chedgzoy et al. 2007). Cultural historian Peter Stearns (Stearns 2011) thus maintained that a special affection for and attentiveness to children and children's vulnerability are no inventions or fabrications of modernity.

Nonetheless, ethnogeographer Jared Diamond points to the dramatic variation that exists, even in the contemporary world, among parenting practices emanating from this differentiated and particular view of childhood (Diamond 2012). Both Stearns and Diamond cite, for example, the historical and contemporary practice of swaddling infants as an iconic parenting act that is grounded in deep cultural beliefs about the nature of infancy and childhood, about the relationship of children to parents, and about the fundamental nature of the human child. Hrdy shows how extraordinary differences in mothering behavior have occurred, historically and contemporaneously, as a consequence of sociocultural and economic conditions, despite strong, evolutionarily conserved commonalities in innate maternal responses (Hrdy 1999). Further, Barr et al. (1991) demonstrate that developmental and temporal patterns of infant crying are invariant between North American and !Kung San infants, but parental responses to such crying are highly divergent. Though parenting practices come and go and beliefs regarding the consequences of such practices vary by geography and cultural era, most historical and present human societies have attributed to young children a special susceptibility to the character of the social and physical contexts in which they are reared.

There have also been abiding cultural convictions—crossing geography and time—that the special sensibilities of young children, when exposed to psychological and physical adversities, can produce forms of morbidity extending well beyond the exposure itself, into the domain of adult life. We have strongly held beliefs in the continuities—for better and for worse—between childhood and adulthood. John Milton (1608–1674) wrote in *Paradise Regained* that "The childhood shews the man/ As morning shews the day" and William Wordsworth (1770–1850) observed, in *My Heart Leaps Up When I Behold*, that "The Child is father of the Man." Marcel Proust (1871–1922) described, in *Remembrance of Things Past*, the sudden, flooding and vivid awareness of a childhood memory in an ordinary moment of adult life:

> When from a long distant past nothing subsists, after the people are dead, after the things are broken and scattered, taste and smell alone, more fragile but enduring, more unsubstantial, more persistent, more faithful, remain poised a long time, like souls, remembering, waiting, hoping, amid the ruins of all the rest.

In the early and mid-twentieth century, these long held beliefs about childhood's capacity for intrusion into the experiences of adult life began to find their way into the borderlands of emerging science. Freud famously asserted that neurotic behavior and obsessions manifesting in mid-adulthood were often linked, without conscious awareness, to experiences of trauma sustained decades before, in very early life (Freud 1940). Biologist and scholar René Dubos invoked "biological Freudianism" to argue that the adverse exposures of childhood can produce lasting *neurobiological* predispositions that persist even when such exposures are later abated or gone (Dubos et al. 1966). Jerome Kagan (e.g., Brim and Kagan 1980) observed the ways in which human health development is characterized by *both* constancy *and* sometimes remarkable discontinuity across developmental periods. Though the experiences of childhood may not overdetermine or dominate the strengths and liabilities of adult life, our cultural heritage avows not only a child's special receptivity to the provisions and predations of its early world but the lifelong echoes of that receptivity, as well.

2 Susceptibility and Continuity: The Echoes of Childhood

The now thriving science of how early social experience influences lifelong health and development might be legitimately portrayed as building a scientific foundation for these two longstanding tenets of cultural belief. These are the claims (a) that childhood is imbued with a distinctive susceptibility to the character of the social and physical world and (b) that, partially as a consequence of the former, the exposures of early life—those both damaging and sustaining—continue to exert their effects on health and well-being long beyond the childhood years. John Bowlby thus concluded that the infants of all primate species show an evolutionarily conserved predisposition to form powerful emotional attachments to their mothers, striving to stay close to her side at all times and thereby reducing the risks of abandonment or endangerment (Bowlby 1969). Harlow, Suomi, and colleagues, in the nonhuman primate equivalent of Bowlby's work with human children, showed that the drive toward early attachment is so strong that, in the mother's absence, an infant macaque will physically and emotionally bond to an inanimate surrogate but with subsequent behavioral aberrations that extend through the infant's lifetime (Harlow et al. 1971). Over the last two decades, Barker and colleagues produced a large body of findings suggesting that chronic, life-threatening cardiovascular disease in mid- to late life is derived from nutritional deficits and impaired growth occurring in very early, even prenatal life (see, e.g., Barker 1990; Barker and Bagby 2005; Bock and Whelan 1991). Kuh and Ben-Shlomo (2004) outlined a "life course approach" to chronic disease epidemiology, assembling convergent evidence for temporally distant relations between markers of childhood deprivation and compromise and indices of chronic morbidity in adult life. The Human Development Program of the Canadian Institute for Advanced Research (CIFAR) showed how population health and developmental science coincide to reveal powerful societal effects on child development and health and how such effects are transcribed into lifetimes of socially partitioned differences in adult disease (Keating and Hertzman 1999). The American Academy of Pediatrics has recently called public attention to the issue of significant, "toxic" stress and adversity in the lives of young children and asserted that many of the chronic disorders of adult life should now be regarded as "developmental disorders," stemming as they do from adverse childhood experiences and events. Abstracting these and other programs of research, three major reports—in the USA (Shonkoff and Phillips 2000), the UK (Marmot 2010), and Canada (Boivin and Hertzman 2012)—have sought and achieved a multidisciplinary consensus that the experiences of early life, dramatically partitioned by aspects of socioeconomic status (SES) and social position, result in societies with widely divergent developmental and health outcomes. Such societies produce visibly and persistently disadvantaged social groups whose children follow blighted developmental trajectories, acquire chronic disease and disability more frequently and severely, learn and achieve less well, and live substantially shorter, less adaptive lives.

3 Constitution, Context, and the Nonrandom Distribution of Morbidity

Although strong, multinational consensus has been reached on the power and pervasiveness of epidemiologic findings in linking early experience to lifelong disparities in health development and health, urgent and challenging new research questions remain. Among these are the following:

- What is the source of the extensive variability in associations between early adversity and health? Why are some children profoundly affected by early stressors and disadvantage, while others appear to thrive in the face of great risk?
- *How* does it happen? That is, what are mechanisms and mediators by which early exposures become biologically embedded in development, yielding lifelong differences in health? How does adversity "get into the body," altering long-term pathogenic processes that predispose to disease and disorder?
- What role, if any, do constitutional differences in vulnerability—genetic variation, neurobiological response biases, or enduring temperamental attributes—play in the consequences of early life adversity?
- Does the timing, frequency, and persistence of exposure matter? That is, is there unevenness in the effects of adversity by the age of the child or by the intensity and duration of the exposure?
- Are there transgenerational effects of early social adversity? Are the "iniquities of the father visited upon their children, to the second and third generation" (Exodus 34:7)? Are the traumas of a single generation transmitted into the lives of the next?

Such questions are not just scientifically compelling; they do not simply appeal to our twenty-first century zeal to understand nuance, contingency, and mechanism. Conceiving and implementing effective societal interventions to mitigate health disparities will be necessarily conditional upon clear and instructive answers. As an organizational approach to these and other life course health development questions, we propose a useful convergence of *two fundamental principles* emerging from this new science of early childhood experience and development. These are:

Principle 1: Most developmental and health endpoints in human populations are derived from causal interactions between contextual and constitutional factors.

Principle 2: Disordered development and health are nonrandomly distributed by population, space, and time.

Principle 1 affirms a now broadly accepted refutation of earlier claims that maladaptive outcomes are principally genetically or environmentally determined. Incontrovertible evidence now rejects both environmental and genetic determinism and views the genesis of disease as involving a dynamic interplay between environments and genes. Even the simple partitioning of developmental variance into environmental and genetic components falls short of a truly interactive view of the conjoint operation of nurture and nature (Boyce et al. 2012b; Meaney 2010). Importantly, our assertion that causal interactions between contextual and constitutional differences will predominate in the pathogenesis of human morbidities does not entail a claim that no main effects of such differences will be found. Far more research is needed to conclude confidently that gene-environment interplay predominates in the pathogenesis of most human diseases, but such interactive processes appear almost certainly more prevalent and common that was imagined even a decade ago (Dunn et al. 2011; Wright and Christiani 2010). Principle 2 contends, as did Bronfenbrenner's bioecological model (e.g., Bronfenbrenner and Morris 2006), that disorders of health and development are neither evenly nor stochastically distributed within human populations and that such disorders are instead informatively clustered by population (both within and across populations), space (both geography and jurisdiction), and time (both developmental and historical). The maldistribution of disorder within human populations signals important and reliable differences in susceptibility to various forms of morbidity and their causal agents. The aggregation of morbidities by space and time extends beyond conventional understandings of epidemicity to include geographic and mobility effects on morbidity and critical periodicity in developmental processes.

A cross-referencing of these Principles 1 and 2 produces the table below, which divides supportive evidential territory into six domains of research: I. social stratification, poverty, and subordination; II. vulnerability, resilience, and neurobiological susceptibility; III. the topography of vulnerability; IV. marginalization and scapegoating; V. history and affliction; and VI. critical periodicity. These six domains codify the *contextual and constitutional sources of disease maldistribution*, aggregated by population, space, and time. In the sections that follow, we abstract and review each of these arenas of research, which together serve to summarize current and emerging findings on the lifetime effects of early childhood exposures. The crosscutting, confluent cell below the six domains designates a section on interactions between context and constitution, in the form of gene-environment interplay, and their role in the biological embedding of early social adversities and the emergence of what has been called "the social brain." Finally, as indicated in table's bottom cell, we conclude with a specification of missing areas of study, unaddressed questions, and an agenda for future work on the developmental origins of life morbidities (Table 1).

4 Six Domains of Early Developmental Research

4.1 Social Stratification, Poverty, and Subordination

Among the most well-replicated, population-level findings in all of the child health services research is illustrated in Fig. 1. Within childhood populations from a broad diversity of settings, cultures, and societies, a subgroup of 15–20% sustain over half of the populations' morbidities, both biomedical and psychiatric, and are responsible for over half of the health-care utilization (Boyce 1985; Diaz et al. 1986). The public health implications of this finding are self-evident: if we could explain and address the disproportionate morbidity carried by this small subgroup of childhood populations, we might prevent over half of the population's diseases, injuries, and disorders.

The search for an explanation for this highly nonrandom distribution of human morbidity begins and ends with the phenomenon of *social stratification*, that is, the hierarchical social organization that characterizes much of invertebrate to

Table 1 Domains of existing, anticipated, and needed research, organized by Principles 1 and 2

		Principle 1: Developmental and health outcomes stem from interactions between	
		Context	**Constitution**
Principle 2: Disordered outcomes are nonrandomly distributed by	**Population**	I. Social stratification, poverty, and subordination	II. Vulnerability, resilience, and neurobiological susceptibility
	Space	III. The topography of vulnerability	IV. Marginalization and scapegoating
	Time	V. History and affliction	VI. Critical periodicity
		Interactions between context and constitution, gene-environment interplay	
		An Agenda for Future Research	

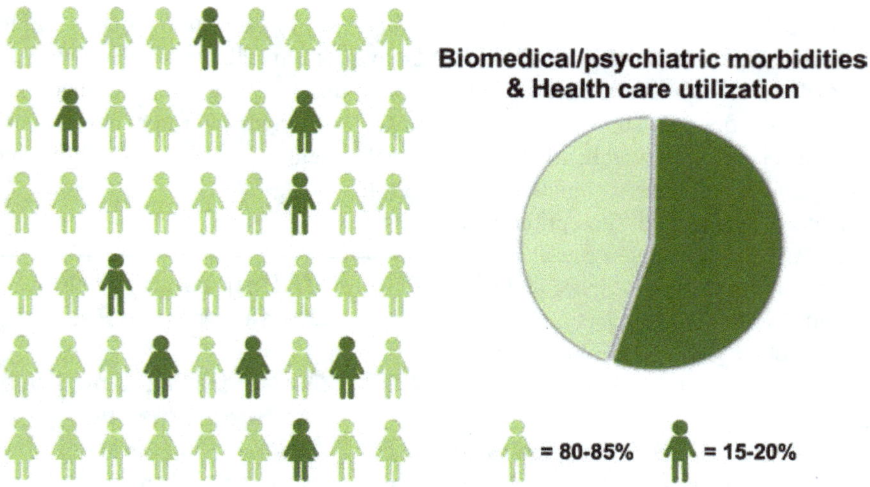

Fig. 1 The nonrandom distribution of biomedical and psychiatric morbidities in child populations

vertebrate phylogeny and manifests as SES within human societies. SES constitutes the single, most powerful epidemiologic determinant of virtually all forms of morbidity, a predictor so potent that we question the authenticity of other associations failing to adjust for SES (Adler et al. 1993, 1994). Beginning early in life, impoverished children and families sustain higher rates of virtually every form of human malady: from low birth weight (Blumenshine et al. 2010) to traumatic injury (Brown 2010), from infectious disease (Dowd et al. 2009) to dental caries (Boyce et al. 2010), and from developmental disability (Msall et al. 1998) to poorer academic achievement (Kawachi et al. 2010). Socioeconomic stratification of developmental psychopathology, moreover, which often emerges in preclinical form in the middle childhood years, exerts lasting influences on academic achievement, employment success, interpersonal relationships, and lifelong well-being (Offord 1995; U.S. Department of Health and Human Services 2011). Figures 2 and 3 show how poor and neglected populations bear disproportionate burdens of disease and disorder throughout the life span (see Marmot 2010)—Fig. 2 showing the graded association between SES and socioemotional adjustment from middle childhood through adolescence and Fig. 3 revealing the same relation with chronic disease at each stage of the life course.

Despite this universality and potency of societal disparities in health, it is only recently that SES has become itself a focus of serious scientific study (Syme 2008). New studies of the SES antecedents of population morbidities have recognized the extended influence of childhood social status on adult disease, even after controlling for SES in adulthood (Cohen et al. 2010; Galobardes et al. 2004; Lawlor et al. 2006). Such evidence for lifelong effects of early disadvantage is rendered still more compelling by research documenting the developmental origins of adult health and disease (Gluckman et al. 2005, 2009) and by epidemiologic work revealing systematic differences in nutrition (Khan and Bhutta 2010), access to medical care (Houweling and Kunst 2010), and physical environmental exposures (Gump et al. 2007) among children of differing social classes.

Although these and other material factors undoubtedly play roles in the origins of health disparities (Hackman et al. 2010), another prominent and increasingly persuasive explanation for such disparities is the SES-stratified differences in early exposures to family adversities and stressors (Brown et al. 2009; Hillis et al. 2004; Wadsworth et al. 2008). Low-SES children live with significantly more family chaos (Evans et al. 2005), sustain more frequent and severe psychological stressors (Evans 2004; Evans and Kim

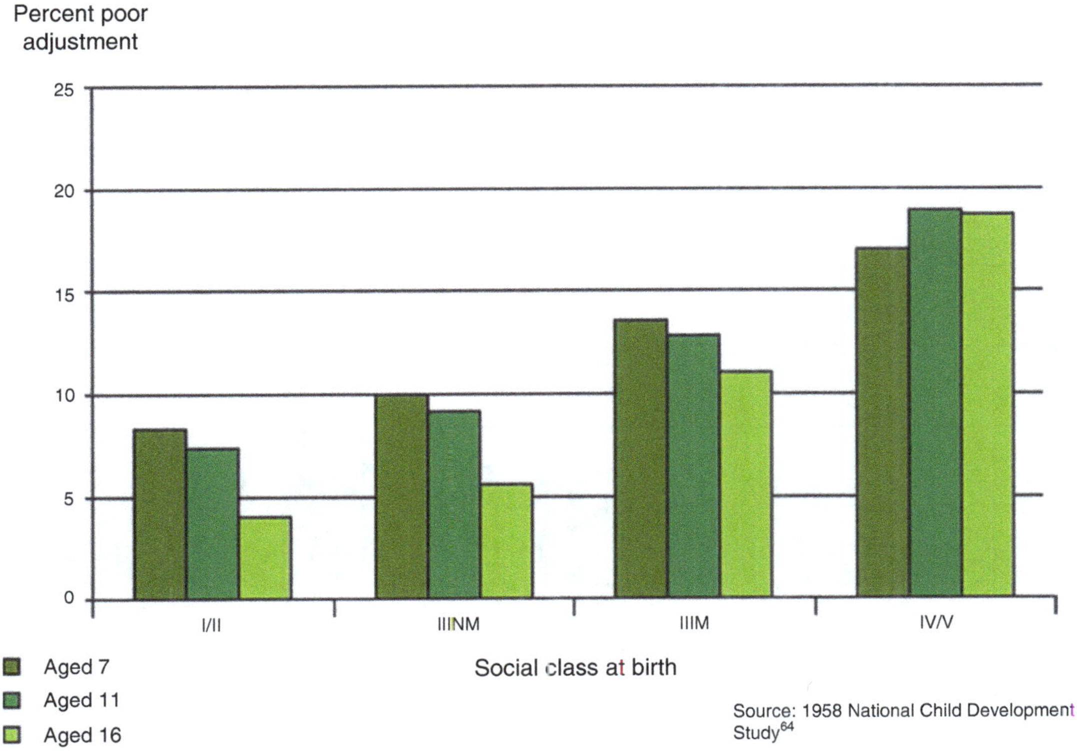

Fig. 2 Rates of poor social/emotional adjustment at ages 7, 11, and 17, by father's social class at birth (Marmot 2010)

2007), and experience fewer supportive parent-child communications (Hart and Risley 1995), relative to their higher SES peers. Low SES children also show greater neurobiological sensitivity to aversive social contexts, in the form of heightened reactivity within the stress-responsive, neuroendocrine pathways, i.e., the hypothalamic-pituitary-adrenocortical (HPA) axis and the autonomic nervous system (ANS) (Boyce et al. 2010; Evans and Kim 2007; Lupien et al. 2001; Steptoe et al. 2002). Further, the exaggerated reactivity of these peripheral stress response systems among disadvantaged youth is subserved by socially partitioned differences in central neural circuits, which also have profound influences on health development, cognitive function, and educational attainment (Curley et al. 2011; Cushing and Kramer 2005; Gianaros and Manuck 2010; Hackman and Farah 2009; MacDonald and Roskams 2009; McEwen and Gianaros 2010).

Influences of childhood SES on health and neurobiological endpoints extend beyond concurrent effects on health and responsivity during childhood to longer-term relations with health status in adult life. Adverse experiences in early childhood, for example, may carry risk effects for coronary artery disease in adult life before the age of 50 years and effects mediated by some form of biological embedding (Kittleson et al. 2006). One important set of candidate mechanisms for such temporally distant effects is the constellation of pro-inflammatory changes that have been shown associated with childhood disadvantage. Programs of work by Miller and Chen (Miller et al. 2009a; Miller et al. 2009b), Cole (Cole 2009; Cole et al. 2007) and others (Danese et al. 2008; McDade 2012), for example, have demonstrated systematic differences in cytokine signaling pathways, transcriptional control, and risk for inflammation- and immune-mediated disease. These studies suggest that changes in immune responsivity and the molecular processes involved in inflammation may be one category of mediating events linking childhood social adversity to adult disease.

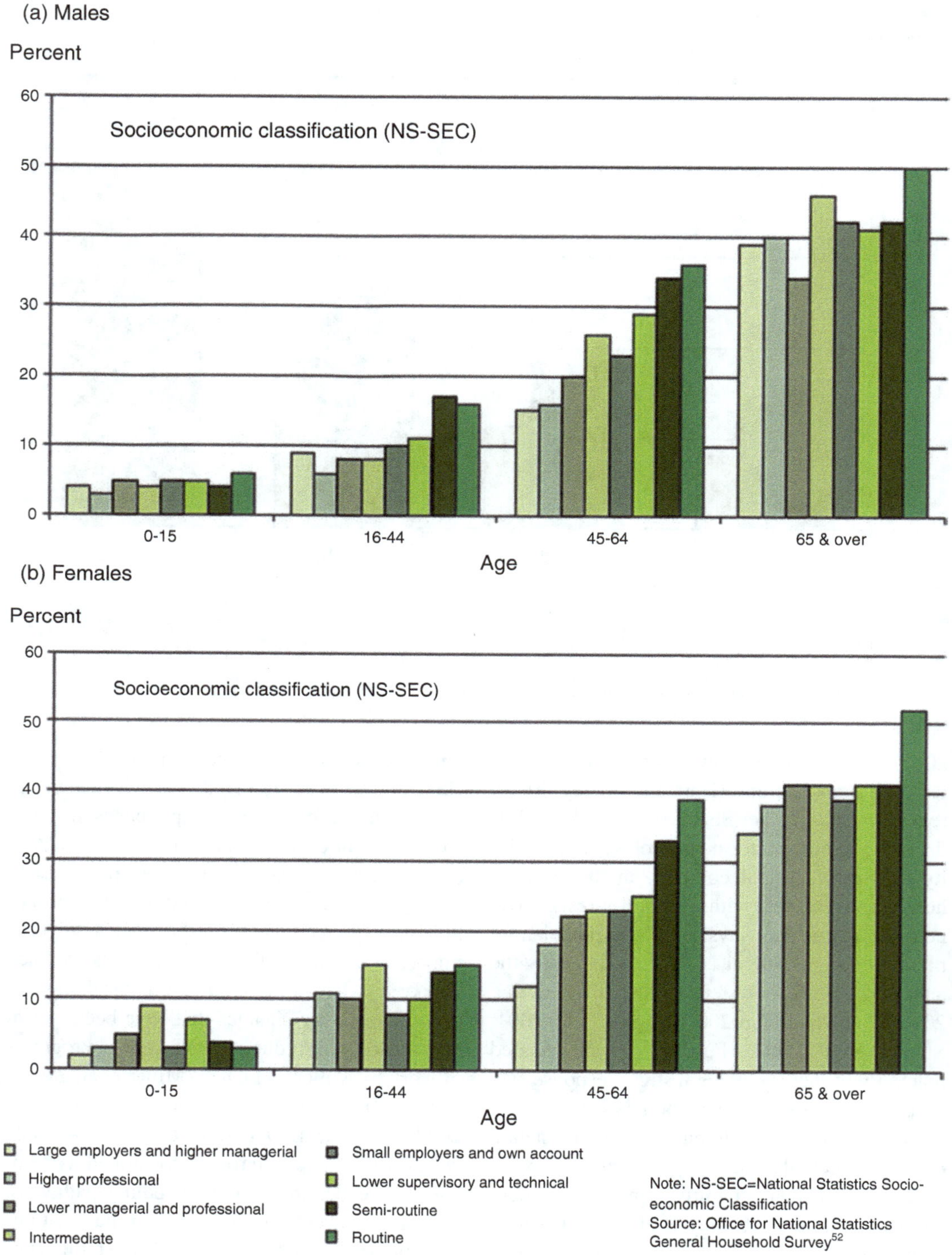

Fig. 3 Percentage of males and females with limiting long-term illness, by age and socioeconomic classification (Marmot 2010)

Finally, there is emerging evidence that experiences of social subordination per se, themselves prevalent sources of human adversity (Keltner et al. 2003), may be related to disorders of mental and physical health, educational failure, and maladaptive behavior, especially in the young. The works of Pellegrini (Pellegrini et al. 2007, 2010), Hawley (Hawley 1999), and Fehr (Fehr et al. 2008) and their colleagues, describing the developmental emergence, behavioral signs, and socioemotional sequelae of childhood dominance and egalitarianism, have offered important "down payments" on such a research agenda. More recently, we have examined linkages between subordination and maladaptive health outcomes in a socioeconomically and ethnically diverse sample of kindergarten children, assessing associations between experiences of dominance-subordination and patterns of maladaptive behavior (Boyce et al. 2012a). As shown in Fig. 4, we found that indicators of mental health in 5-year-old children were stratified within classroom hierarchies in a manner parallel to that seen in larger, adult societies. Children occupying subordinate positions within their classrooms had more depressive symptoms, more frequent episodes of inattention, fewer positive peer relationships, and less evidence of prosocial behavior. Further, we found that the children most likely to show low or diminishing health status were those occupying subordinate social positions who also came from low SES families, and those least likely to show a diminution in health came from classrooms with teachers highly invested in learner-centered pedagogical practices (LCPs). Indeed, as shown in Fig. 4, the link between rank and behavior nearly disappeared in classrooms with strong teacher LCPs, suggesting that classrooms with egalitarian, student-centered "cultures" produced diminished mental health effects of hierarchical social ranks.

Such findings—that social subordination is associated with decrements in mental health, even within hierarchical, early childhood groups—are commensurate, moreover, with prior findings that *subjective* estimates of social class may be a stronger predictor of health outcomes than objective indicators, such as job status, income, or wealth (Adler et al. 2000; Goodman et al. 2003; Ostrove et al. 2000), and that dominance status in *primate* social hierarchies is similarly associated with health, even among captive animals with equal access to food, open environments, and veterinary care (Abbott et al. 2003; Cohen et al. 1997; Kaplan et al. 1982; Sapolsky 2005).

A growing body of research thus demonstrates powerful, graded effects of childhood social stratification and SES on development and health, both in children and their adult counter-

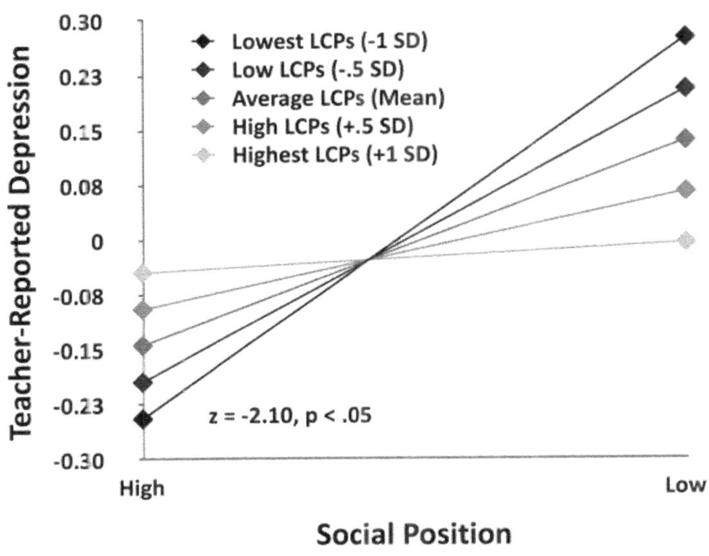

Fig. 4 Depression by social position and learner-centered pedagogical practices (LCPs) at half-SD increments from the mean (−1, −0.5, mean, +0.5, +1 SD) (Boyce et al. 2012a)

parts. Such effects may account, at least in part, for the strikingly uneven distribution of morbidities within human populations. Nonetheless, as noted by Kessler, Duncan, and colleagues (e.g., Kessler et al. 2014), results of large-scale human experiments challenge assumptions that simply augmenting financial resources or moving children out of high-poverty neighborhoods will have salutary effects on health development. Childhood SES effects are likely mediated by a broad array of factors that include diet, exposures to toxic environmental agents, differences in parenting, and access to health care, but substantial evidence also now implicates differential exposures to stress and adversity as a major mechanism of SES influence. Acquired differences in neurobiological reactivity to stressors and pro-inflammatory shifts in immune signaling pathways may also play an important mediating role in SES-health relations. Lastly, research has also begun to document effects of social subordination per se on childhood health outcomes, independent of family or neighborhood SES. Thus, relations between social position within classroom peer hierarchies and subsequent health outcomes show the same graded associations with morbidity found in studies of nations and large human populations.

4.2 Vulnerability, Resilience, and Neurobiological Susceptibility

The aggregation of ill health within human populations appears also attributable to *constitutional* differences underlying a remarkable variation in susceptibility to social-environmental influence. There is now growing evidence for a generalized sensitivity to social contexts within a human subgroups, i.e., highly sensitive or environmentally "permeable" individuals showing maladaptive outcomes in conditions of adversity but unusually positive outcomes in settings characterized by support, predictability, and protection (see, e.g., Aron et al. 2012; Belsky et al. 2007; Boyce 2016; Boyce and Ellis 2005; Ellis et al. 2011a). Such individuals thus show either the least or most adaptive outcomes within the population, depending upon the character of the proximal social contexts in which they are reared. Studies demonstrating this greater susceptibility of neurobiologically responsive children to both positive and negative aspects of their environments have implicated a wide variety of:

- *Stressors and adversities*, including paternal depression (Cummings et al. 2007), marital conflict (El-Sheikh 2005; El-Sheikh et al. 2007), parental psychopathology (Shannon et al. 2007), and overall family distress (Obradovic et al. 2010)
- *Positive environmental features*, including parental warmth (Ellis et al. 1999), beneficial experiences and exposures (Pluess and Belsky 2013), and supportive interventions (Bakermans-Kranenburg et al. 2008a)
- *Defining biological parameters*, including physiological reactivity (e.g., Alkon et al. 2006; Boyce et al. 1995), differences in brain circuitry (Whittle et al. 2010), and gene polymorphisms (Bakermans-Kranenburg et al. 2008b; Knafo et al. 2011; Manuck et al. 2011)

Most importantly, highly susceptible children (and adults) show bidirectional effects on outcomes in contrasting highly supportive and highly stressful settings—not simply an attenuation of negative effects in low stress circumstances.

Such differences in neurobiological sensitivity—likely based, in part, on genetic and epigenetic variation (Boyce and Kobor 2015)—are figuring prominently in the field's exploration of the biological embedding of early stress. Findings suggesting differential susceptibility have been replicated in many samples of children, a troop of rhesus macaques (Boyce et al. 1998), and in a series of randomized controlled trials of socially supportive interventions (Bakermans-Kranenburg and Van Ijzendoorn 2015; Quas et al. 2004). Neurobiological sensitivity has also been the focus of a ten-paper special section of *Development and Psychopathology*

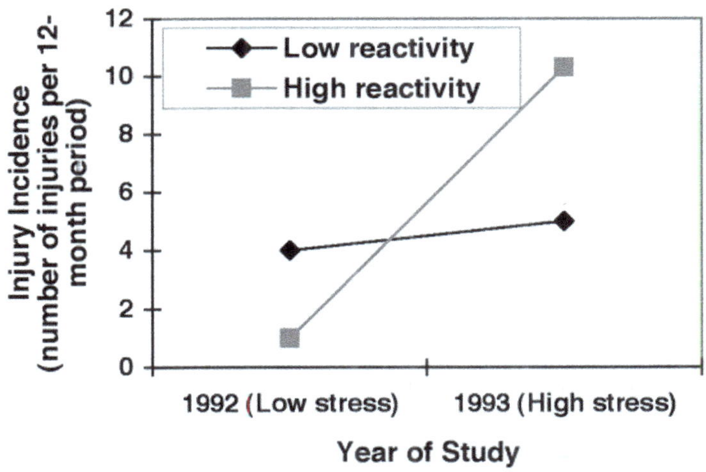

Fig. 5 Incidence of violent injuries in free ranging macaques by confinement stress and reactivity status (Boyce et al. 1998)

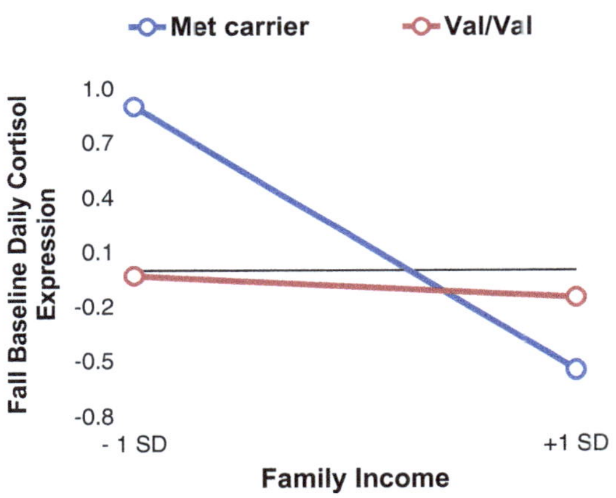

Fig. 6 Daily baseline cortisol expression by family SES and BDNF polymorphism (N. Bush, personal communication, unpublished data, 2017)

(see Ellis et al. 2011a). As shown in the accompanying Figs. 5 and 6, examples have included the differential rates of violent injuries among high and low reactivity rhesus macaques before and during a prolonged period of confinement stress (Fig. 5) and the level of HPA activation among kindergartners by allelic variants in the BDNF gene and family income (Fig. 6). In both cases, the "risky endophenotype" (i.e., high reactivity status or being a Met carrier in the BDNF polymorphism) showed high levels of maladaptive outcomes (injuries or basal cortisol secretion) under stressful conditions but remarkably low levels (lower even than their low-risk counterparts) in positive, low stress settings.

Importantly, strong evolutionary arguments have been made, albeit not without dissension (e.g., Bateson and Gluckman 2011; Overton and Lerner 2014; West-Eberhard 2003) for the conservation of environmental sensitivity within rearing environments of evolutionary adaptedness. Slavich and Cole, for example, have summarized recent evidence on how social-environmental exposures can regulate gene expression, thereby calibrating individual sensitivity to social context (Slavich and Cole 2013). Such sensitivity appears to influence not only the rates and severity of morbidity but also the timing and pace of important developmental transitions, such as puberty (Ellis et al. 2011b). This characteristic, which probably becomes increasingly trait-like over the course of development, appears to emerge as a conditional adaptation, garnering signals from the early social environment about the inherent levels of threat, adversity, support, and nurturance that the growing child is likely to encounter and calibrating stress-responsive biological systems to optimize survival, health, and developmental well-being (Ellis et al. 2006, 2011a; Hane and Fox 2006). Understanding phenotypic variation in environmental susceptibility might logically also play a role in the conceptualization and development of newly individualized approaches to "precision medicine" (Committee on a Framework for Development a New Taxonomy of Disease 2011).

4.3 The Topography of Vulnerability

In addition to their aggregation within *population* subgroups, developmental vulnerability and ill health are also clustered by spatial geography. It is well known, for example, that of the more than 7 million of the world's children less than 5 years of age that die each year, the majority live in the regions of sub-Saharan Africa and South Asia (Liu et al. 2012). Equally familiar is the epidemiologic, small area clustering of neurodevelopmental disorders such as autism spectrum disorder (Mazumdar et al. 2010). Less well known, but equally compelling, are the dramatic differences in developmental vulnerability at primary school entry—differences with major implications for learning and academic success—that are found within major national jurisdictions, such as the Canadian province of British Columbia (see Fig. 7).

Between 2000 and 2011, the provincial BC government, with the assistance and oversight of the Human Early Learning Partnership at UBC Vancouver, completed four population-based assessments of developmental health. Assessments were completed during the kindergarten year, and developmental health was measured using the Early Development Instrument (EDI), a kindergarten teacher-completed checklist for each child based on five scaled measures of development: physical well-being, social competence, emotional maturity, language and cognitive development, and communication and general knowledge (Janus and Offord 2000). The EDI yields, for each child and each scale, a score as "vulnerable" or "not vulnerable." The designation as "vulnerable" is not given directly to the family, however; rather, rates of EDI vulnerability are computed and mapped according to residential neighborhoods where children live. Mapping is done by neighborhoods because local geography defines unique combinations of factors that support or undermine early child development.

Across Canadian neighborhoods, vulnerability rates on one or more of the EDI scales range from

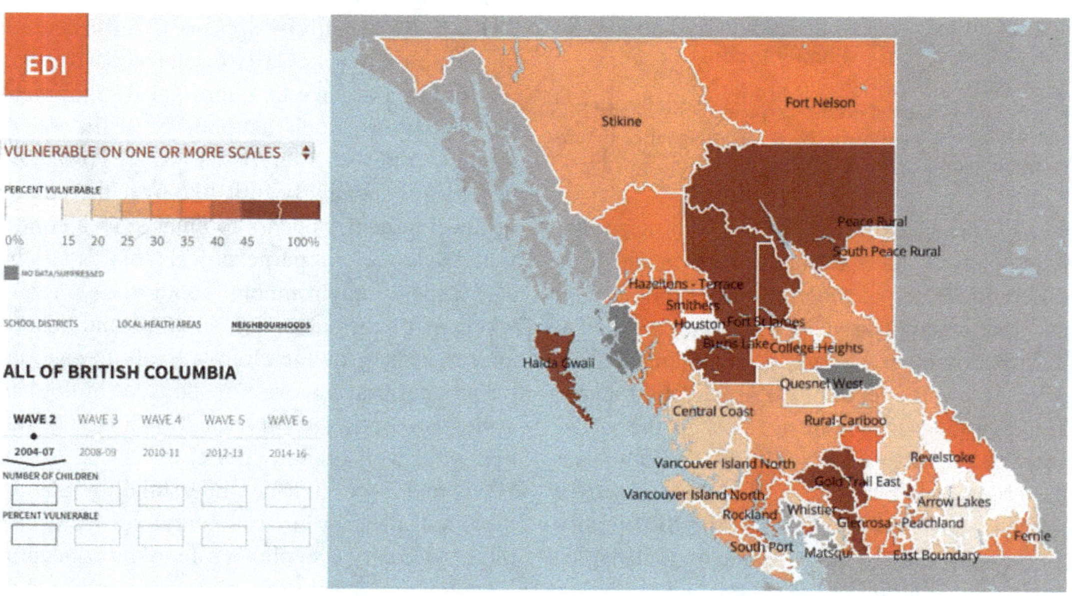

Fig. 7 Neighborhood variation in developmental vulnerability in British Columbia on the early development instrument (http://earlylearning.ubc.ca/interactive-map/)

as low as 4% to as high as 69%, such that there is a more than 17-fold inequality in developmental vulnerability in Canada at the level of the neighborhood. This range is much larger than would be predicted on the basis of random sample surveys of child development, which rarely demonstrate social gradients larger than threefold. Neighborhoods aggregate family environments, reflect broader environments, and have emergent properties, such as safety and social cohesion, that influence developing children. They tend to include families of similar socioeconomic status, unique mixes of relational characteristics (i.e., the factors that shape a family's social identity), and similar levels of access or barriers to programs and services. For analytical purposes, random sample surveys aggregate children from different geographical locales into statistical (rather than real) neighborhoods according to a small number of grouping factors (e.g., median family income or proportion of adults with high school graduation). Such "neighborhood effect" analyses from random sample surveys do not capture the unique circumstances of real neighborhoods. Thus, the 17-fold variation in EDI-estimated developmental health validates this spatial geographic approach to local differences, since only this tactic captures the circumstances of real neighborhoods (Hertzman 2010; Kershaw et al. 2009). Such an approach has been used, for example, to reveal that optimal, area level EDI scores occur within neighborhoods with *mixed*, rather than uniformly affluent, SES representation, i.e., those with relatively equal proportions of affluent and disadvantaged families (Carpiano et al. 2009). Adopted on an even larger scale, such methods are capable of offering social ecological perspectives on the physical, socioeconomic, and social political conditions of children on a global scale (Panter-Brick et al. 2012).

4.4 Marginalization and Scapegoating

Interpersonal marginalization and scapegoating can also contribute to uneven distributions of morbidity and maladaptive development, often based on targeting by individual, constitutional characteristics. Victimization is a well-represented and elemental human behavior, even within groups of very young children. Described by Lord Byron as "the longest pleasure" (*Don Juan*, 13th Canto: "Now hatred is by far the longest pleasure; Men love in haste but they detest at leisure."), hatred and stigmatization have remained, for all of history, a sadly defining feature of human societies. Family systems theory has regarded scapegoating and the designation of an "identified patient" as an effective if personally costly means of securing family solidarity (Vogel and Bell 1961), much as the vilification of Simon in William Golding's *Lord of the Flies* served the cohesion of a marooned band of lost school boys. Behavioral vulnerability stemming from physical weakness, anxiety, poor social skills, or chronic illness has been shown to engender victimization in groups of children (Egan and Perry 1998; Sentenac et al. 2012), and within nonhuman primate troops, the active targeting of highly reactive, more sensitive members has been described during periods of intensive group stress (Boyce et al. 1998). Far from restricted to Western, individualist societies, bullying and victimization are also highly prevalent in more collectivist cultures (Kim et al. 2004). Among human children and youth, such victimization can undermine mental health and lead to poor academic performance (Glew et al. 2005), psychosomatic disorders (Arseneault et al. 2006; Gini and Pozzoli 2009), suicidal ideation behavior (Kim et al. 2009; Turner et al. 2012), and later criminality (Sourander et al. 2007). Among the survivors of population-level genocide, specific genetic variants have been linked to traumatic memory retention and the level of risk for post-traumatic stress disorder (PTSD) (de Quervain et al. 2012). Abusive experiences in children, whether at the hands of family or peers, become itself a social determinant of adult mental and physical health (Greenfield 2010), resulting in the sequestering of morbidities within both perpetrators and their victims.

4.5 History and Affliction

As Kuzawa and Thayer noted (Kuzawa and Thayer 2011), human adaptation to environmental conditions takes place at a variety of timescales, ranging from homeostatic changes that can occur over seconds or minutes to developmental plasticity emerging over months or years to conserved genetic changes that operate on a timescale of millennia. Thus, historical contexts can also concentrate and skew distributions of disease and disorder over epochs of time. For example, prenatal exposures to a natural disaster, such as the 1998 Québec Ice Storm, can contribute to the risk for childhood obesity, even after adjustment for breastfeeding, SES, obstetrical complications, and smoking during pregnancy (Dancause et al. 2012). During historical periods of war, elevated lifetime risks for PTSD are found among children exposed to violent or traumatic events (Javidi and Yadollahie 2012). Researchers have also studied how early life exposures to famine can influence adult health, using historical cohort data from the Finnish crop failure famine of 1866–1868, the Dutch Hunger Winter of 1944–1945, the Siege of Leningrad in 1944, the seasonal famines in the Gambia between 1949 and 1994, and the Chinese Great Leap Forward famine of 1959–1961. Outcomes examined have included adult height and weight, glucose metabolism, blood pressure, lipid profiles, metabolic syndrome, cardiovascular outcomes, self-reported health, mental performance and cognition, mental disorders, and adult mortality (Falconi et al. 2017; Lumey et al. 2011). Exposure episodes related to war, such as the 1944–1945 Dutch Famine of World War II, resulted in elevated odds of developing coronary heart disease in adult life (Painter et al. 2005; Roseboom et al. 2000) and in systematic differences in the epigenetic modification of genes such as insulin-like growth factor (IGF-2) (Heijmans et al. 2008) and aspects of risk that appear capable of crossing into unexposed generations (Painter et al. 2008). Genocide, whether historical in the case of the Holocaust or contemporary, as in the Rwandan atrocities, exerts powerful, lasting damage on children's prospects for health and well-being, both contemporaneous and longitudinal (Hazani and Shasha 2008; Oberg 2008). Each of these examples illustrates how time, in the form of historical period, and context, in the form of broad socioenvironmental perturbations and assaults, converge to influence and bias life course health development.

4.6 Critical Periodicity

Finally, events and exposures within developmental time, rather than historical time, also create constraints and opportunities for healthy development and the avoidance of disorder. The function of neuronal circuits in the brain is guided by experiences in postnatal life that regulate the maturation of inhibitory connections and interneurons (Hensch 2005). Critical periods exist, for example, for the acquisition of language and discrimination of speech sounds in human infants (Weikum et al. 2012), and exposure to music can change auditory preferences in young mice through changes in prelimbic and infralimbic medial prefrontal cortex during an early critical period (Yang et al. 2012). Adult brain plasticity appears to become restricted by structural and functional developmental "brakes," such as perineuronal nets and myelin that inhibit neurite growth and the balance between excitatory and inhibitory circuitries (Bavelier et al. 2010). Genetic, pharmacological, and environmental influences can alter such plasticity, suggesting future opportunities for reopening closed critical periods, such as those for language acquisition or vision, or enhancing recovery from traumatic or cerebrovascular brain injury.

5 Interactions Between Context and Constitution: The Biological Embedding of Early Adversity

These arenas of research, defining the contextual and constitutional origins of disease maldistribution by population, space, and time, converge in a new and growing body of work examining the interplay between genes and environments in determining developmental and health endpoints over the life course. Such research comprises studies of (a) true gene-environment interactions, in which allelic variation moderates primary associations between environmental factors and outcomes, and (b) epigenetic processes, in which exposure-related chemical/structural modifications of chromatin up- or downregulate the transcriptional expression of functionally salient genes. Together, such studies and larger territories of research have begun to advance serious answers, at a variety of analytic levels, to the questions surrounding how socially partitioned early experience "gets under the skin," affecting broad life course trajectories of development and health (Evans et al. 2012; Hertzman and Boyce 2010; Slavich and Cole 2013).

5.1 Chromatin Modification and the Molecular Biology of Epigenesis

As shown in Fig. 8, chromatin is the structural packaging of DNA and its associated proteins into nucleosomes: strands of DNA wrapped around histone protein octamers, like thread around a spool. Nucleosomes in turn form a loosely or tightly wound chromatin "necklace," arrayed like beads on a string. Epigenetics has been defined as a functional modification of DNA that does not involve an alteration of sequence (Meaney 2010). The differentiation of embryonic stem cells into specific tissue lineages, for example, is epigenetically guided by patterns of downregulation and activation of lineage-specific genes (Wu and Sun 2006). Figure 9 shows how DNA methylation changes with development throughout the sequential ontogeny of germ cell development, fertilization, and embryogenesis. The more general processes of gene-environment interplay involve important functional distinctions between gene sequence, epigenetic modifications, and gene expression—variations in each of which may influence individual responses to environmental exposures. Gene sequence variation, for example, has been linked to vulnerability to a variety of maladaptive or disordered health outcomes (Caspi et al. 2002, 2003).

Differences in gene expression have also been associated with disease susceptibility (Liew et al. 2006; Mohr and Liew 2007) and are, in turn, related to a variety of epigenetic, molecular processes, which include DNA methylation, histone modification, production of noncoding microRNAs, presence of various transcription factors, and nucleosome remodeling (Gilbert and Epel 2009). Given the complexities of these chemical mechanisms, however, it is important to understand that (a) DNA methylation is only one form of epigenetic mark, (b) DNA methylation is not the equivalent of gene expression, and (c) it is sometimes unclear whether DNA methylation is a precursor of gene silencing or a marker of such silencing. For purposes of simplicity, the discussion here

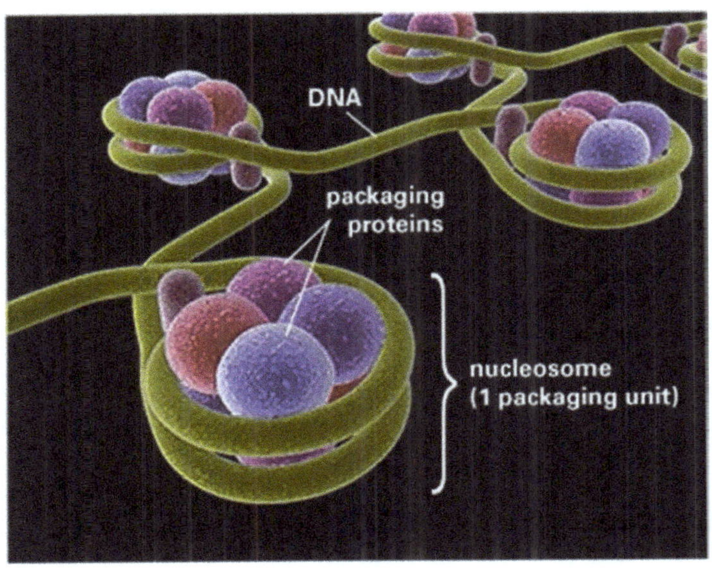

Fig. 8 Chromatin and nucleosome structure (Courtesy of Joseph Roland© 2003 – www.cytographica.com)

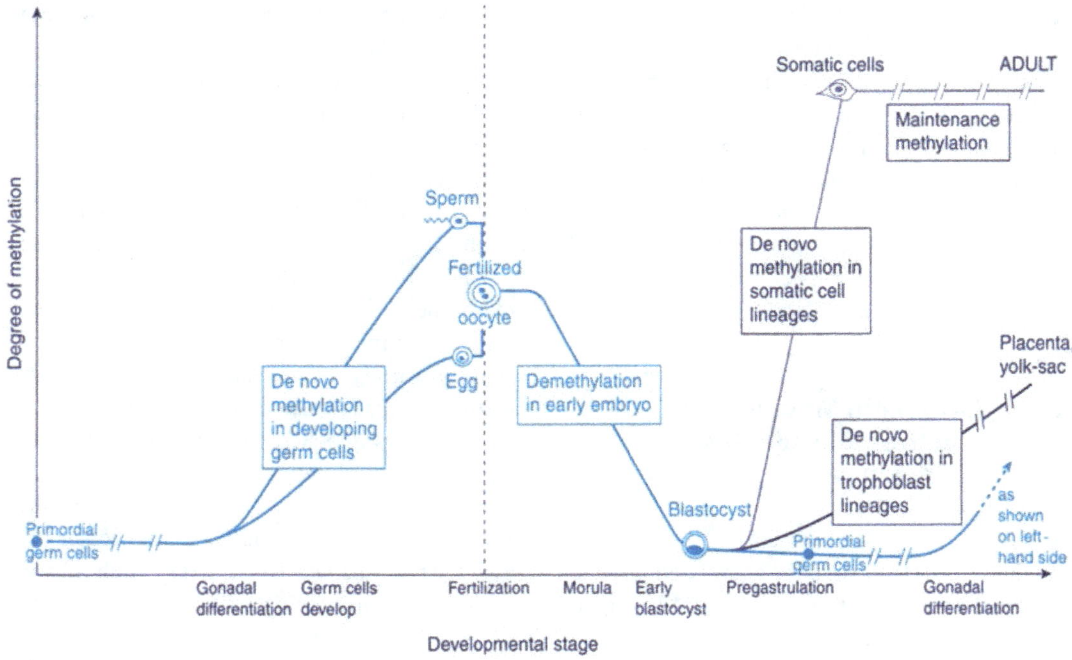

Fig. 9 Epigenetic methylation events in early human gestation (Russo et al. 1999)

focuses primarily upon true gene-environment interactions and a single form of epigenetic modification, the methylation of cytosine-phosphate-guanine (CpG) dinucleotide sites in DNA. The relative stability of DNA methylation suggests that, among epigenetic marks, it may be responsible for longer-term, more developmentally important changes in gene expression.

As shown in Fig. 10, genes have both promoter and coding regions, with the latter demarcated by start and stop sequences recognized by RNA polymerase. RNA polymerase, in association with facilitating transcription factors (i.e., a "transcription complex"), *transcribes* the DNA coding region into messenger RNA, which in turn undergoes ribosomal *translation* into proteins that alter cellular function. Social experiences can result in epigenetic marks, such as CpG methylation, within a gene's promoter region, and the degree of such methylation regulates gene expression, like a dimmer switch regulates light in a room. Transcription start sites and promoters are known to be enriched with CpG sites (areas called "CpG islands") (Turner et al. 2008), and experience-induced methylation of these sites is known to tighten chromatin structure, rendering transcription factor binding sites physically less accessible and interfering with RNA polymerase attachment to the coding start sequence. Thus, the experience-induced methylation of a promoter CpG can effectively silence the gene, altering cellular function and changing physiological processes ranging from neurotransmitter reuptake in neuronal synapses to blood glucose regulation and sympathetic nervous system reactivity.

5.2 The Epigenetics of Social Adversity

Although the study of epigenetics began in the field of cancer biology, research has more recently begun to explore epigenetic processes by which socially stratified exposures to early adversities may condition long-term risks to development and health (Gluckman et al. 2007; Jirtle and Skinner 2007; Tsankova et al. 2007). There is evidence for DNA methylation-associated regulation of adversity-responsive genes in both

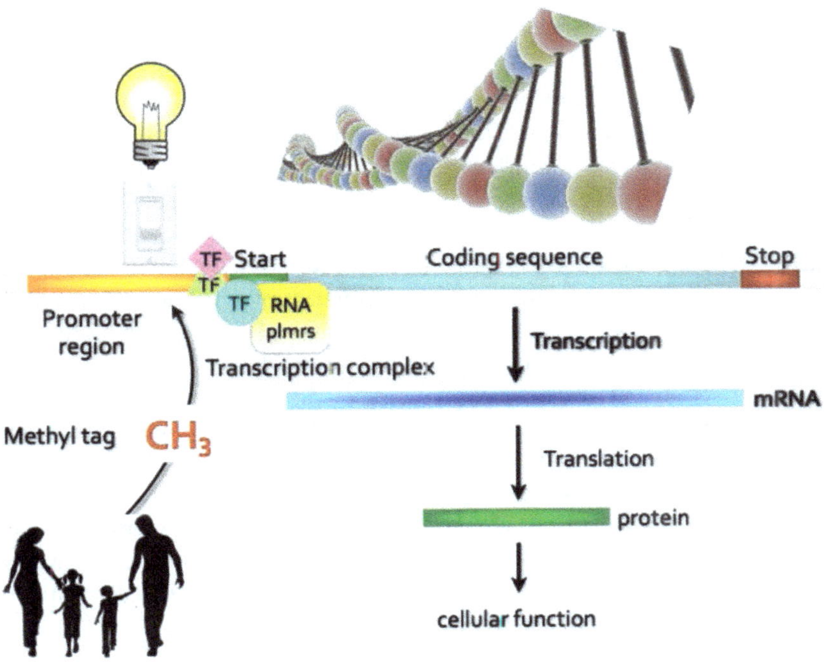

Fig. 10 Simplified representation of epigenetic modification and transcription regulation. *CH_3* methyl group, *Tag* TF transcription factor, *RNA plmrs* RNA polymerase, *mRNA* messenger RNA

laboratory animals (McGowan et al. 2008) and human infants (Oberlander et al. 2008) and for stressor-associated differences in mRNA expression in human subjects (Cole et al. 2007; Morita et al. 2005). Further, the biochemical "markings" of genomic DNA and its associated, nucleosomal histone proteins are the epigenetic mechanisms by which the expression of neuroregulatory genes is controlled (Isles and Wilkinson 2008; Meaney and Ferguson-Smith 2010; Mehler 2008). Epigenetic marks are capable, through this governing of neuroregulatory gene expression, of guiding both neurodevelopment and the function of peripheral and central neural pathways (Liu et al. 2008; MacDonald and Roskams 2009).

The work of Meaney, Szyf, and colleagues (Szyf et al. 2008; Weaver 2009; Weaver et al. 2004; Zhang and Meaney 2010), for example, has demonstrated in the rat pup how maternal licking and grooming in the first several days of life downregulate pups' long-term HPA reactivity through increases in hippocampal glucocorticoid receptor (GR, *NR3C1*) expression and serotonergic tone. Licking and grooming triggers increases in serotonin in the hippocampus, and activation of the 5-HT receptor induces expression of a transcription factor, nerve growth factor-inducible protein-A (NGFI-A). Licking and grooming also facilitates NGFI-A's association with the exon 1_7 GR gene promoter by demethylating a CpG site located in the NGFI-A binding region of this exon. The resulting increased expression of GR results in a downregulation of corticotropin-releasing hormone (CRH) and diminished activation of the HPA axis. Readers are referred to (Hackman et al. 2010) for more detailed description of these molecular events. Other work in rat models of early infant maltreatment has demonstrated enduring methylation of the gene coding for brain-derived neurotrophic factor (BDNF), reduced BDNF expression, and extension of both epigenetic marks and maltreatment of young into a subsequent generation (Roth et al. 2009). Because BDNF is a key mediator of neural plasticity in brain regions such as the prefrontal cortex and hippocampus, such findings might present a legitimate model of the neurocognitive sequelae of transgenerational neglect and abuse of human children. Champagne and colleagues (Champagne et al. 2006) have also shown, in the same model, that the increased estrogen receptor-α (ER-α) expression that occurs in the medial preoptic area of high licking and grooming mothers is associated with cytosine methylation of the ER-α gene promoter.

Nonhuman primate work by Kinnally et al. (Kinnally et al. 2010a, 2010b, 2011) has explored, in infant macaques, interrelations among early stressors (social group vs. nursery rearing and variable foraging vs. control conditions), allelic variation in the *5-HTT* serotonin transporter gene promoter, and both genome-wide and 5-HTT-specific differential methylation in peripheral blood mononuclear cells (PBMCs). Among their findings with direct relevance to the research considered here are the following:

- Higher *5-HTT* CpG methylation, but not sequence variation in the serotonin transporter promoter region, exacerbates the effects of early life stress on behavioral stress reactivity.
- Both greater *5-HTT* and whole-genome methylation level (i.e., 5-methylcytosine content) is associated with enhanced stress reactivity across the subsequent life span.
- When brain tissue is unavailable for methylation analysis, peripheral blood methylation levels may serve as useful surrogates (see also Cupello et al. 2009; Uebelhack et al. 2006).

The Meaney-Szyf research group has also recently advanced evidence, in the postmortem hippocampi of human suicide victims, for hypermethylation of the ribosomal RNA gene and *NR3C1* gene promoters and epigenetic marks suggesting dysregulation in cellular protein synthesis machinery and HPA responsivity (McGowan et al. 2008, 2009). Further, two prospective human studies have now documented differential patterns of DNA methylation conditional upon various aspects of early childhood adversity. First, genome-wide, blood DNA methylation analysis in low- and high-SES subjects from the 1958 British Birth Cohort revealed a cluster of probes obtained from the 500 most variable promoters that was enriched with high-SES individuals, confirming that SES differences contributed to overall epigenetic variation. Methylation levels for 1,252 gene promoters were associated with childhood SES versus 545 promoters for adulthood SES (Borghol et al. 2012). Second, in a subsample of adolescents from the Wisconsin Study of Family and Work birth cohort, Essex et al. (Essex et al. 2013) found differential methylation in 170 CpG sites among participants whose parents reported high levels of stress during their children's early lives. Maternal stressors in infancy and paternal stressors in the preschool years were most strongly predictive of differential methylation, and the patterning of such epigenetic marks varied by children's gender. Both birth cohort studies suggest that epigenetic signatures detectable in adolescence to mid-life are related to early experiences with stressful environments. Other human research has documented:

- Altered DNA methylation of the insulin-like growth factor gene (IGF2) in individuals exposed prenatally to the Dutch Famine of 1944–1945 (Heijmans et al. 2008)
- Increased NR3C1 methylation at an NGFI-A binding site in newborns exposed to mothers' depressed mood in the third trimester of pregnancy (Oberlander et al. 2008)
- Highly variable methylation patterns within the five GR promoters activated in PBMCs, possibly reflecting epigenetic fine-tuning of GR expression by early life experiences (Turner et al. 2008)
- Pro-inflammatory shifts in cytokine expression among young adults with low-SES childhood histories, via transcriptional signaling changes in adrenergic and adrenocortical pathways (Chen et al. 2011; Miller et al. 2009a)
- Both between-tissue and between-individual discordance in epigenetic marks at the insulin-like growth factor, IGF2/H19, locus in multiple tissues at birth, even among monozygotic twins (Ollikainen et al. 2010)
- Differences in risk for psychopathology related to concurrent allelic and epigenetic

variation, such that trauma-related 5-HTT promoter methylation operates as a moderator of the association between the 5-HTT polymorphism and psychological problems (van IJzendoorn et al. 2010)

Taken together, these observations offer evidence for social-environmental regulation of mammalian and human gene expression, at the levels of both whole-genome and candidate gene methylation (Cole 2009). The findings also suggest that divergences in methylation and gene expression begin early in development, even during intrauterine life, and that socially partitioned stress and adversity may be transmuted into mental health risks through molecular modifications of the epigenome. Differential exposures to environmental events may explain, for example, the diverging trajectories of epigenetic profiles found among monozygotic twins over time (Fraga et al. 2005). More broadly, epigenetic remodeling in response to developmentally potent environmental events may serve as a mechanism for neural plasticity and the conditional production of individual differences in attributes and risks for psychopathology (Bagot and Meaney 2010).

5.3 Gene-Environment Interplay in Brain Development

Indeed, there is already emerging evidence that brain processes and neural plasticity may function as key mediators in the linkages between G-E interplay and developmental and health endpoints. Bush et al., for example, have recently shown that the BDNF Val66Met polymorphism confers an increased neuroendocrine sensitivity to socioeconomic context, with Met carriers having the highest and lowest cortisol expression levels, depending on SES (N. Bush, personal communication, unpublished data, 2017). Other findings in the nascent science of "imaging genomics"—a field merging high-throughput genotyping with new brain imaging technologies—are revealing how variations in DNA sequence are associated with structural and functional connectivity in specific brain regions (Thompson et al. 2010). Recent fMRI studies, for example, have demonstrated the heritability of patterns of task-related brain region activation and shown how the COMT val108/158met functional polymorphism is associated with systematic differences in prefrontal cortical physiology and function (Egan et al. 2001). Consistent with the same general hypothesis, Hariri and colleagues (Hariri et al. 2005; Hariri and Weinberger 2003) have found that subjects carrying the less efficient short allele of the 5-HTT gene promoter had an increased amygdalar response to fearful stimuli in comparison with subjects homozygous for the long allele. Even more to the point in regard to the development of brain structures subserving socioemotional development, Alexander et al. (Alexander et al. 2012) recently reported a significant GxE interaction effect on neural response patterns and functional amygdala-hypothalamus connectivity—circuitry that appears closely tied to emotional control and the interpretation of social processes (Blakemore 2010; Norman et al. 2012). Such findings begin to reveal possible neural substrates for previously observed, epidemiological observations linking functional polymorphisms, early stressful events, and vulnerability to psychopathology (Caspi et al. 2003; Moffitt et al. 2005).

Also coming into view through the work of a range of investigators (Adolphs 2009; Blakemore 2010, 2012; Lesch 2007; Norman et al. 2012; Robinson et al. 2005, 2008) is a new corpus of research describing and exploring the *social brain*. Such work has begun to address a neurogenomic basis for complex social cognitions, including the capacities for inferences about others' thoughts and emotions (a cognitive ability referred to in the child development literature as "theory of mind"), recognition of self, processing of facial information, differentiation of social opportunities and challenges, and control of socially evoked emotion. The substrates for these capacities are already known to lie, at the neural circuit level, in functional connectivity between limbic structures, such as the amygdala, hippocampus, and basal ganglia, and prefrontal cortical regions, including the dorsolateral and orbitofrontal cortex, the anterior cingulate and the posterior superior temporal sulcus at the temporoparietal junction. At the molecular level, there is evidence for perturbations in the functionality of such circuits related to allelic and epigenetic variation in genes such as those coding for the serotonin transporter (Lesch 2007), oxytocin (Norman et al. 2012), and endorphins (Keverne et al. 1989). There is to date no single definition of the social brain, but a consensus appears to be forming that a subset of autonomic, neuroendocrine, neural, and genomic processes influence and are influenced by aspects of social cognition and behavior (see Robinson et al. 2005, 2008). Although it will be important to avoid a simplistic attribution of complex cognitive and perceptual events to discrete neural, endocrine, or cellular structures (Norman et al. 2012), there is clearly much to be learned about the nature of sociality, the mechanisms that underpin it, the degree to which these mechanisms are conserved in animal phylogeny, and the implications of perturbations in its development.

In sum, a burgeoning research enterprise is producing evidence, in both animal models and human studies, that many if not most human morbidities have their points of origin in early childhood (Shonkoff and Garner 2012), are the products of gene-environment interplay (Rutter 2006), and influence developing neural circuits that are directly linked to long-term trajectories of health, disease, and life achievement. Although the fields of social epigenetics and developmental neuroscience are yet in their relative infancies, promising advances in both suggest a scientific frontier in which functional interactions among social environments, genetic and epigenetic variation, and the functionality of neural circuits will offer compelling new knowledge of how developmental variation emerges.

6 Summary: What We Know and What We Don't

Deep cultural traditions affirming the special sensibilities of children and the echoing of childhood difficulties and stress into the decades of adult life are becoming now powerfully grounded in a new science describing the biological embedding of early social adversity (Boivin and Hertzman 2012; Boyce et al. 2012a; Hertzman and Boyce 2010). No longer relegated to categories of either unsupported belief or speculative hypothesis, the science of early child development has become a multidisciplinary landscape of novel findings documenting prospective, longitudinal associations, powerful and increasingly causal understandings of mechanism and mediation, and new levels of observation made possible by dramatic technological advances. Among the discrete, foundational discoveries that have become the products of this science are the following:

1. Epidemiologic and population-based studies have soundly documented the propensity for morbidities and difficulties of all kinds—biomedical diseases, psychiatric disorders, injuries, and academic, professional, and personal underachievement—to aggregate by population, space, and time, thereby disproportionately affecting small subgroups of individuals, during constrained periods of historical or developmental time. Thus, especially during periods of strife, war, or economic decline, those people whose health and well-being are most harshly and persistently vulnerable are likely to issue from impoverished, alienated, or otherwise marginalized groups. Misfortune is neither stochastically nor evenly distributed within human populations, and the inequalities that ensue from maldistribution are serious, ethical, and public health challenges to society's commitments to justice and health equity. Our societal aspirations to create a more "empathic civilization" (Rifkin 2009) will demand a more human practice of medicine (Halpern 2001), a broader allegiance to unbiased opportunity (Robert Wood Johnson Foundation Commission to Build a Healthier America 2009), and a deeper commitment to the rich pluripotentiality of young lives (Shonkoff and Phillips 2000).
2. Studies examining the developmental biology of social adversity have positioned this new

science on the cusp of deep mechanistic explanations for the important, earlier insights of Waddington (Waddington 1959, 2012), Gottlieb (Gottlieb 1991), and others (Gilbert 2002; Karmiloff-Smith 2007; Meaney 2010)—insight that organismic development is guided by the *combined, interactive influences of genes and experiences*. We now know that development includes not only gene expression regulation through experiential modification of chromatin structure but also by real GxE interactions and the joint, interactive effects of allelic variation and chromatin modification together (see, e.g., Lam et al. 2012; Pezawas et al. 2005; Rutter 2012). As asserted here and elsewhere, the simple partitioning of developmental variance into genetic and environmentally determined components now falls far short of a truly interactive view of the operation of nature and nurture (Meaney 2010). Coming now steadily into view are the actual molecular mechanisms by which constitution and context conjointly determine differences in health and development, both in childhood and over the lifespan.

3. The origins, dimensions, and consequences of *individual differences in phenotype* are emerging as essential components in a full understanding of the biology of social adversity. Biology is replete with both between- and within-species variation that bears convincing witness to the evolutionary uses of diversity, and elegant ethological and epigenetic work, such as that by Meaney (Meaney 2010), Szyf (McGowan and Szyf 2010), and Suomi (Suomi 2006), reveals the adaptive benefits of phenotypic diversification. There is the nearly tautological reality that the operation of natural selection demands the genetic diversity achieved through spontaneous mutation, but beyond such self-evident principles, there are clear examples of how species diversification enhances survival and fitness. Thus, maternally and epigenetically regulated differentiation of rat pups' adrenocortical responsivity produces a range of low to high reactivity phenotypes, each of which may maximize survival and fitness within particular, early and later life environments (Weaver et al. 2004). Similarly, neither the aggressively uninhibited nor the shy, neophobic phenotypes of young rhesus macaques can be warranted as "normal" or optimal; rather, each has adaptive value within specific social and physical contexts (Cirulli et al. 2009; Stevens et al. 2009). What is salient and important about phenotypic variants is their capacity for enhancing fitness within the diversity of species-typical environments encountered. One illustrative variant are those children and young nonhuman primates that evince an exceptional neurobiological susceptibility to aspects of social settings, a phenotype likely representing a conditional adaptation to early environmental signals (Barr et al. 2004; Belsky 2005; Boyce and Ellis 2005; Ellis et al. 2011a). Such individuals show a heightened risk of morbidity under conditions of stress and adversity but exceptionally good health and positive development in settings characterized by support, nurturance, and stability.
4. Increasingly visible within the emerging literature on the neurobiological consequences of early life adversity is a new collection of studies and papers examining the *social brain* (Adolphs 2009; Blakemore 2010, 2012; Lesch 2007; Norman et al. 2012; Robinson et al. 2005, 2008). The brain has evolved to acquire specific organizational circuits, cortical regions, and subcortical structures dedicated to the detection of survival threats, and social experiences of loneliness, abandonment, or neglect may chronically activate such circuitry, creating long-term perceptual and affective biases and fundamentally altering a child's view of the social world (Eisenberger and Cole 2012). Such circuitry is also represented in the periphery, with both animal (Insel 2010) and human (Norman et al. 2012) studies documenting effects on social affiliative processes mediated in part by hormonal events such as the expression of oxytocin and vasopressin.
5. As also discussed, a remarkable diversity of early, *social environmental dimensions* has been linked to important differences in mental

and physical health, trajectories of development, and individual differences in behavior. Such dimensions include, but are not limited to, acute and chronic stressors, poverty and subjective social marginalization, and the absence of positive contextual factors, such as good parenting or a child-supportive community. Of apparently particular importance to social epidemiologic perspectives on early development are studies describing and documenting the effects of social hierarchies, structural subordination, bullying, discrimination, and victimization. The hierarchical and networked social structures found across phylogeny—literally from fruit flies (fish and primates) to human kindergartners (see Boyce et al. 2012a; Fernald and Maruska 2012; Schneider et al. 2012)—suggest an evolved predisposition with implications for survival, reproduction, and safety. Although such hierarchies may be a heritable legacy from our evolutionary past, promising new work addresses approaches to minimizing the health effects of subordinate social positions at the levels of societies, communities, and schools. Such work also attests to the individual and societal benefits of fostering the development of empathy, altruism, and sociality.

6. The central role of *time*—evolutionary, historical, developmental, neurogenomic, and neurophysiological—in determining phenotypic variation is another recurrent if often implicit theme in emerging developmental science. Much of the biological embedding of current social contexts reflects response predispositions established, selectively and epigenetically, through adaptations to the temporally distant environments of early hominids (Dubos 1965; Nesse and Young 2000). Social disparities in health—products, in part, of the social, economic, and health policies of contemporary societies—wax and wane within historical time according to the era's dominant sociopolitical philosophies (Beckfield and Krieger 2009; Krieger 2001). Further, developmental time is strikingly uneven in its potency, intensity of change, and accessibility to environmental influence. Thus, at quite different levels of temporal resolution, time and timing appear to play crucial, but not yet fully explored, roles in guiding societal, organismic, and neurobiological responses to the conditions of early life.

Taken together, these points of emerging empirical evidence form a constellation of discoveries defining a new and lively research field and the social and developmental biology of early adversity and its influences on life course development and health. Although substantial recent progress has been made within a broad assortment of disciplines, much new research, conceptual integration, and thought remains to be accomplished. The promise of this new field, however, lies in a stunning prospect that understanding the social determinants of morbidities in childhood might unlock new approaches to the prevention and treatment of disorders over the entire life course. A final agenda for future research now outlines a set of proposals for new, promising, and possibly heuristic directions of investigation.

7 An Agenda for Future Research

1. As the fields reporting various forms of interplay between genes and environments exponentially grow, what is now needed are programs of research examining the questions of how and by what mechanisms genes and early social contexts co-determine trajectories of behavioral and biological development. With respect to differences in complex behavior and its disorders, a focus on proximal, neurobiological processes must come strongly to the foreground. Although pursuing the epigenetic pathogenesis of early psychiatric and other disorders is a powerful first step (Docherty and Mill 2008; Robison and Nestler 2011), it must be followed by studies examining the brain structures and neural processes that mediate GxE associations with mental and physical health (Ladd-Acosta et al. 2007; Turecki et al. 2012). As new knowledge of the

interactive genetic and environmental influences on social brain development becomes available, a major challenge will be the integration of mechanistic observations across levels of analysis and scale (Norman et al. 2012).

2. A systematic and useful biology of social adversity will necessarily involve not only a search for the mechanisms (i.e., mediators) underpinning associations among stress, development, and morbidity but also the effects of modifiers (i.e., moderators) that reveal when, at what ages, or in what subgroups such associations hold (Baron and Kenny 1986; Kraemer et al. 2001, 2008). Understanding the mechanistic processes by which an environmental exposure is linked to disordered development can be a powerful aid to elucidating pathogenesis (e.g., the role of high-density lipoprotein transport of cholesterol as a mediator of the association between dietary fat and coronary heart disease (Lloyd et al. 2012)) and imagining novel interventions (e.g., changing mother-infant relationships as a means of altering the association between poverty and child development (Olds et al. 2010)). On the other hand, grasping mediational linkages may be a necessary but insufficient condition for understanding causation, and the parsing of populations into subgroups of varying exposure susceptibility, through the discovery of moderator variables, can also advance comprehension and the tractability of a given association (e.g., changes in the potency of stress-illness associations by differences in individual sensitivity to social contextual effects (Belsky and Pluess 2009; Boyce and Ellis 2005; Ellis et al. 2011a)).
3. As attention to epigenetic development grows, the capacity to place a finer, more exacting point on the specific kinds of environments that interact with particular allelic and epigenetic variants will be important and likely illuminating. Evolutionary perspectives on social adversity will also be essential to understand how difficult "environments of evolutionary adaptedness" shaped human and infra-human biology (e.g., Boyce and Ellis 2005; Sapolsky 2003), how contextual stressors might have generated species diversity (Wolf et al. 2005), and how adversity may have contributed to the emergence of social cooperation (Andras et al. 2007). We need far finer and more precise renditions of the social-environmental dimensions that interact with genes and produce negative and positive outcomes salient to population and public health. An important subtext to such work is the extraordinary value of cross-species, animal-human, comparative studies, which together not only inform the evolutionary biology of social environments and its consequences but also enable experimental studies capable of bolstering the causal inferences disallowed by human research.
4. Successfully pursuing a new developmental science of childhood adversity will surely also involve the perspective of complex adaptive systems. Social causation is nonlinear, rather than Newtonian, in character. Traditional epidemiologic strategies for understanding the health effects of social-environmental factors involve the ascertainment of such factors' "independent" influences on a health endpoint through the use of multiple hierarchical regression models (Diez Roux 2007). Although such an approach allows estimation of the isolated effects of single independent variables, it belies the reality that most human disorders are etiologically complex, with multiple interacting "causes." Even detecting GxE interactions almost certainly underserves the true complexity of pathogenic processes, because allelic variation in a single gene likely interacts with polymorphisms in many other genes, and multiple dimensions of the environment may also interactively influence outcomes. In such circumstances—circumstances that may eventually prove to predominate in disease causation—the use of more sophisticated models and analytic tools may be required to understand the multiply interactive networks of risk factors involved in the ontogeny of disordered development and health (Kauffman 1993; Koopman and Lynch 1999). If so, one such approach with increasingly demonstrable efficacy is the use of complex

systems analysis, involving descriptive inventories of system components, nonlinear mathematical modeling, and the construction of agent-based models of causal networks (Diez Roux 2007; Galea et al. 2010).

5. Finally, as highlighted by Garner, Shonkoff, and others (Garner et al. 2012; Shonkoff 2012), prevention science is powerfully in need of new ideas for and approaches to the design of interventions based on the emerging science of early development. The Nurse-Family Partnership program conceived and elegantly studied by David Olds and colleagues (see http://www.nursefamilypartnership.org), for example, departed dramatically from prior, outmoded early childhood enrichment programs by envisioning the mother-infant dyad as the unit of intervention and by using nurses as home visitors to effectively place the intervention within a medical frame of reference. Nonetheless, even more radical departures are needed from the conventions of traditional early development programs, including careful consideration of how complex dynamic systems thinking might be wed to novel, preventive interventions. Attending closely to discoveries emanating from the disciplines and sciences surveyed here could potentially prompt approaches to targeting and conceiving imaginative interventions with far greater efficacy and whole population effects. However complex and challenging that task might be, all such efforts could be potentially rewarded with a level of health and well-being for our children and grandchildren that is more enduring, robust, and enabling.

The new developmental biology of early life effects on health development over the life course is a now flourishing science, nearing readiness to transform conventional understandings of disease ontogeny, to foster clearer and more vivid perspectives on the temporally distant effects of childhood events, and to broaden and transform approaches to ensuring the health of our children and the developmental sturdiness of their futures. Although much careful and innovative thought will be a prerequisite for such a demanding journey, the road ahead looks promising, indeed.

References

Abbott, D. H., Keverne, E. B., Bercovitch, F. B., Shively, C. A., Mendoza, S. P., Saltzman, W., et al. (2003). Are subordinates always stressed? A comparative analysis of rank differences in cortisol levels among primates. *Hormones and Behavior, 43*(1), 67–82.

Adler, N. E., Boyce, W. T., Chesney, M. A., Folkman, S., & Syme, S. L. (1993). Socioeconomic inequalities in health: No easy solution. *JAMA, 269*(24), 3140–3145.

Adler, N. E., Boyce, W. T., Chesney, M. A., Cohen, S., Folkman, S., Kahn, R. L., & Syme, S. L. (1994). Socioeconomic status and health: The challenge of the gradient. *The American Psychologist, 49*(1), 15–24.

Adler, N. E., Epel, E. S., Castellazzo, G., & Ickovics, J. R. (2000). Relationship of subjective and objective social status with psychological and physiological functioning: Preliminary data in healthy, White women. *Health Psychology, 19*(6), 586–592.

Adolphs, R. (2009). The social brain: Neural basis of social knowledge. *Annual Review of Psychology, 60*, 693–716. doi:10.1146/annurev.psych.60.110707.163514.

Alexander, N., Klucken, T., Koppe, G., Osinsky, R., Walter, B., Vaitl, D., et al. (2012). Interaction of the serotonin transporter-linked polymorphic region and environmental adversity: Increased amygdala-hypothalamus connectivity as a potential mechanism linking neural and endocrine hyperreactivity. *Biological Psychiatry, 72*(1), 49–56. doi:10.1016/j.biopsych.2012.01.030.

Alkon, A., Lippert, S., Vujan, N., Rodriquez, M. E., Boyce, W. T., & Eskenazi, B. (2006). The ontogeny of autonomic measures in 6- and 12-month-old infants. *Developmental Psychobiology, 48*(3), 197–208. doi:10.1002/dev.20129.

Andras, P., Lazarus, J., & Roberts, G. (2007). Environmental adversity and uncertainty favour cooperation. *BMC Evolutionary Biology, 7*, 240. doi:10.1186/1471-2148-7-240.

Ariès, P. (1962). *Centuries of childhood: A social history of family life*. New York: Alfred A. Knopf.

Aron, E. N., Aron, A., & Jagiellowicz, J. (2012). Sensory processing sensitivity: A review in the light of the evolution of biological responsivity. *Personality and Social Psychology Review, 16*(3), 262–282. doi:10.1177/1088868311434213.

Arseneault, L., Walsh, E., Trzesniewski, K., Newcombe, R., Caspi, A., & Moffitt, T. E. (2006). Bullying victimization uniquely contributes to adjustment problems in young children: A nationally representative cohort study. *Pediatrics, 118*(1), 130–138. doi:10.1542/peds.2005-2388.

Bagot, R. C., & Meaney, M. J. (2010). Epigenetics and the biological basis of gene x environment interactions. *Journal of the American Academy of Child and Adolescent Psychiatry, 49*(8), 752–771. doi:10.1016/j.jaac.2010.06.001.

Bakermans-Kranenburg, M. J., & Van Ijzendoorn, M. H. (2015). The hidden efficacy of interventions: Genexenvironment experiments from a differential susceptibility perspective. *Annual*

Review of Psychology, 66, 381–409. doi 10.1146/annurev-psych-010814-015407.

Bakermans-Kranenburg, M. J., Van Ijzendoorn, M. H., Mesman, J., Alink, L. R., & Juffer, F. (2008a). Effects of an attachment-based intervention on daily cortisol moderated by dopamine receptor D4: A randomized control trial on 1- to 3-year-olds screened for externalizing behavior. *Development and Psychopathology, 20*(3), 805–820. doi:10.1017/S0954579408000382.

Bakermans-Kranenburg, M. J., Van Ijzendoorn, M. H., Pijlman, F. T., Mesman, J., & Juffer, F. (2008b). Experimental evidence for differential susceptibility: Dopamine D4 receptor polymorphism (DRD4 VNTR) moderates intervention effects on toddlers' externalizing behavior in a randomized controlled trial. *Developmental Psychology, 44*(1), 293–300. doi:10.1037/0012-1649.44.1.293.

Barker, D. J. (1990). The fetal and infant origins of adult disease. *BMJ, 301*(6761), 1111.

Barker, D. J., & Bagby, S. P. (2005). Developmental antecedents of cardiovascular disease: A historical perspective. *Journal of the American Society of Nephrology, 16*(9), 2537–2544. doi:10.1681/ASN.2005020160.

Baron, R., & Kenny, D. (1986). The moderator-mediator variable distinction in social psychological research: Conceptual, strategic, and statistical considerations. *Journal of Personality and Social Psychology, 51*(6), 1173–1182.

Barr, R. G., Konner, M., Bakeman, R., & Adamson, L. (1991). Crying in !Kung San infants: A test of the cultural specificity hypothesis. *Developmental Medicine and Child Neurology, 33*(7), 601–610.

Barr, C. S., Newman, T. K., Lindell, S., Shannon, C., Champoux, M., Lesch, K. P., et al. (2004). Interaction between serotonin transporter gene variation and rearing condition in alcohol preference and consumption in female primates. *Archives of General Psychiatry, 61*(11), 1146–1152.

Bateson, P., & Gluckman, P. (2011). *Plasticity, robustness, development and evolution*. Cambridge CB2 8RU, UK: Cambridge University Press, The Edinburgh Building.

Bavelier, D., Levi, D. M., Li, R. W., Dan, Y., & Hensch, T. K. (2010). Removing brakes on adult brain plasticity: From molecular to behavioral interventions. *The Journal of Neuroscience, 30*(45), 14964–14971.

Beckfield, J., & Krieger, N. (2009). Epi + demos – cracy: Linking political systems and priorities to the magnitude of health inequities--evidence, gaps, and a research agenda. *Epidemiologic Reviews, 31*, 152–177. doi:10.1093/epirev/mxp002.

Belsky, J. (2005). Differential susceptibility to rearing influence: An evolutionary hypothesis and some evidence. In B. J. Ellis & D. F. Bjorklund (Eds.), *Origins of the social mind: Evolutionary psychology and child development* (pp. 139–163). New York: Guilford.

Belsky, J., & Pluess, M. (2009). Beyond diathesis stress: Differential susceptibility to environmental influences. *Psychological Bulletin, 135*(6), 885–908. doi:10.1037/a0017376.

Belsky, J., Bakermans Kranenburg, M. J., & Van IJzendoorn, M. H. (2007). For better and for worse: Differential susceptibility to environmental influences. *Current Directions in Psychological Science, 16*(6), 300–304.

Blakemore, S. J. (2010). The developing social brain: Implications for education. *Neuron, 65*(6), 744–747. doi:10.1016/j.neuron.2010.03.004.

Blakemore, S. J. (2012). Development of the social brain in adolescence. *Journal of the Royal Society of Medicine, 105*(3), 111–116. doi:10.1258/jrsm.2011.110221.

Blumenshine, P., Egerter, S., Barclay, C. J., Cubbin, C., & Braveman, P. A. (2010). Socioeconomic disparities in adverse birth outcomes: A systematic review. *American Journal of Preventive Medicine, 39*(3), 263–272. doi:10.1016/j.amepre.2010.05.012.

Bock, G. R., & Whelan, J. (Eds.). (1991). *The childhood environment and adult disease*. West Sussez: Ciba Foundation.

Boivin, M., & Hertzman, C. (2012). *Early childhood development: Adverse experiences and developmental health*. Ottawa: Royal Society of Canada.

Borghol, N., Suderman, M., McArdle, W., Racine, A., Hallett, M., Pembrey, M., et al. (2012). Associations with early life socio-economic position in adult DNA methylation. *International Journal of Epidemiology, 41*(1), 62–74.

Bowlby, J. (1969). *Attachment and loss*. London: Hogarth.

Boyce, W. T. (1985). Stress and child health: An overview. *Pediatric Annals, 14*(8), 539–542.

Boyce, W. T. (2016). Differential susceptibility of the developing brain to contextual adversity and stress. *Neuropsychopharmacology Reviews, 41*(1), 142–162.

Boyce, W. T., & Ellis, B. J. (2005). Biological sensitivity to context: I. An evolutionary-developmental theory of the origins and functions of stress reactivity *Development and Psychopathology, 17*(2), 271–301.

Boyce, W. T., & Kobor, M. S. (2015). Development and the epigenome: The 'synapse' of gene-environment interplay. *Developmental Science, 18*(1), 1–23. doi:10.1111/desc.12282.

Boyce, W. T., Chesney, M., Alkon-Leonard, A., Tschann, J., Adams, S., Chesterman, B., et al. (1995). Psychobiologic reactivity to stress and childhood respiratory illnesses: Results of two prospective studies. *Psychosomatic Medicine, 57*, 411–422.

Boyce, W. T., O'Neill-Wagner, P., Price, C. S., Haines, M., & Suomi, S. J. (1998). Crowding stress and violent injuriesamong behaviorally inhibited rhesus macaques. *Health Psychology, 17*(3), 285–289.

Boyce, W. T., Den Besten, P. K., Stamperdahl, J., Zhan, L., Jiang, Y., Adler, N. E., & Featherstone, J. D. (2010). Social inequalities in childhood dental caries: The convergent roles of stress, bacteria and disadvantage. *Social Science & Medicine, 71*(9), 1644–1652. doi:10.1016/j.socscimed.2010.07.045.

Boyce, W. T., Obradović, J., Bush, N., Stamperdahl, J., Kim, Y. S., & Adler, N. (2012a). Social stratification, classroom 'climate' and the behavioral adaptation of kindergarten children. *Proceedings of the National Academy of Sciences, 109*(Suppl 2), 17168–17173.

Boyce, W. T., Sokolowski, M. B., & Robinson, G. E. (2012b). Toward a new biology of social adversity. *Proceedings of the National Academy of Sciences of the United States of America, 109*(Suppl 2), 17143–17148. doi:10.1073/pnas.1121264109.

Brim, O. G., & Kagan, J. (Eds.). (1980). *Constancy and change in human development.* Cambridge, MA: Harvard University Press.

Bronfenbrenner, U., & Morris, P. A. (2006). The bioecological model of human development. In R. M. Lerner & W. Damon (Eds.), *Handbook of child psychology: Vol. 1. Theoretical models of human development* (6th ed., pp. 793–828). Hoboken: John Wiley & Sons, Inc.

Brown, R. L. (2010). Epidemiology of injury and the impact of health disparities. *Current Opinion in Pediatrics, 22*(3), 321–325. doi:10.1097/MOP.0b013e3283395f13.

Brown, D. W., Anda, R. F., Tiemeier, H., Felitti, V. J., Edwards, V. J., Croft, J. B., & Giles, W. H. (2009). Adverse childhood experiences and the risk of premature mortality. *American Journal of Preventive Medicine, 37*(5), 389–396. doi:10.1016/j.amepre.2009.06.021.

Carpiano, R. M., Lloyd, J. E., & Hertzman, C. (2009). Concentrated affluence, concentrated disadvantage, and children's readiness for school: A population-based, multi-level investigation. *Social Science & Medicine, 69*(3), 420–432. doi:10.1016/j.socscimed.2009.05.028.

Caspi, A., McClay, J., Moffitt, T. E., Mill, J., Martin, J., Craig, I. W., et al. (2002). Role of genotype in the cycle of violence in maltreated children. *Science, 297*(5582), 851–854.

Caspi, A., Sugden, K., Moffitt, T. E., Taylor, A., Craig, I. W., Harrington, H., et al. (2003). Influence of life stress on depression: Moderation by a polymorphism in the 5-HTT gene. *Science, 301*(5631), 386–389.

Champagne, F. A., Weaver, I. C., Diorio, J., Dymov, S., Szyf, M., & Meaney, M. J. (2006). Maternal care associated with methylation of the estrogen receptor-alpha1b promoter and estrogen receptor-alpha expression in the medial preoptic area of female offspring. *Endocrinology, 147*(6), 2909–2915. doi:10.1210/en.2005-1119.

Chedgzoy, K., Greenhalgh, S., & Shaughnessy, R. (2007). *Shakespeare and childhood.* Cambridge, UK: Cambridge University Press.

Chen, E., Miller, G. E., Kobor, M. S., & Cole, S. W. (2011). Maternal warmth buffers the effects of low early-life socioeconomic status on pro-inflammatory signaling in adulthood. *Molecular Psychiatry, 16*(7), 729–737. doi:10.1038/mp.2010.53.

Cirulli, F., Francia, N., Berry, A., Aloe, L., Alleva, E., & Suomi, S. J. (2009). Early life stress as a risk factor for mental health: Role of neurotrophins from rodents to non-human primates. *Neuroscience and Biobehavioral Reviews, 33*(4), 573–585. doi:10.1016/j.neubiorev.2008.09.001.

Cohen, S., Line, S., Manuck, S. B., Rabin, B. S., Heise, E. R., & Kaplan, J. R. (1997). Chronic social stress, social status, and susceptibility to upper respiratory infections in nonhuman primates [see comments]. *Psychosomatic Medicine, 59*(3), 213–221.

Cohen, S., Janicki-Deverts, D., Chen, E., & Matthews, K. A. (2010). Childhood socioeconomic status and adult health. *Annals of the New York Academy of Sciences, 1186*, 37–55. doi:10.1111/j.1749-6632.2009.05334.x.

Cole, S. W. (2009). Social regulation of human gene expression. *Current Directions in Psychological Science, 18*(3), 132–137. doi:10.1111/j.1467-8721.2009.01623.x.

Cole, S. W., Hawkley, L. C., Arevalo, J. M., Sung, C. Y., Rose, R. M., & Cacioppo, J. T. (2007). Social regulation of gene expression in human leukocytes. *Genome Biology, 8*(9), R189. doi:10.1186/gb-2007-8-9-r189.

Committee on a Framework for Development a New Taxonomy of Disease. (2011). *Toward precision medicine: Building a knowledge network for biomedical research and a new taxonomy of disease*. Washington, DC: National Academies Press.

Cummings, E. M., El-Sheikh, M., Kouros, C. D., & Keller, P. S. (2007). Children's skin conductance reactivity as a mechanism of risk in the context of parental depressive symptoms. *Journal of Child Psychology and Psychiatry, 48*(5), 436–445. doi:10.1111/j.1469-7610.2006.01713.x.

Cupello, A., Albano, C., Gatta, E., Scarrone, S., Villa, E., & Zona, G. (2009). Binding of paroxetine to the serotonin transporter in membranes from different cells, subcellular fractions and species. *Neurochemical Research, 34*(2), 255–259. doi:10.1007/s11064-008-9764-z.

Curley, J. P., Jensen, C. L., Mashoodh, R., & Champagne, F. A. (2011). Social influences on neurobiology and behavior: Epigenetic effects during development. *Psychoneuroendocrinology, 36*(3), 352–371. doi:10.1016/j.psyneuen.2010.06.005.

Cushing, B. S., & Kramer, K. M. (2005). Mechanisms underlying epigenetic effects of early social experience: The role of neuropeptides and steroids. *Neuroscience and Biobehavioral Reviews, 29*(7), 1089–1105. doi:10.1016/j.neubiorev.2005.04.001.

Dancause, K. N., Laplante, D. P., Fraser, S., Brunet, A., Ciampi, A., Schmitz, N., & King, S. (2012). Prenatal exposure to a natural disaster increases risk for obesity in 5(1/2)-year-old children. *Pediatric Research, 71*(1), 126–131. doi:10.1038/pr.2011.18.

Danese, A., Moffitt, T. E., Pariante, C. M., Ambler, A., Poulton, R., & Caspi, A. (2008). Elevated inflammation levels in depressed adults with a history of childhood maltreatment. *Archives of General Psychiatry, 65*(4), 409–416.

de Quervain, D. J., Kolassa, I. T., Ackermann, S., Aerni, A., Boesiger, P., Demougin, P., et al. (2012). PKCalpha is genetically linked to memory capacity in healthy subjects and to risk for posttraumatic stress disorder in genocide survivors. *Proceedings of the National Academy of Sciences of the United States of America, 109*(22), 8746–8751. doi:10.1073/pnas.1200857109.

Diamond, J. (2012). *The world until yesterday: What can we learn from traditional societies*. New York: Penguin Group.

Diaz, C., Starfield, B., Holtzman, N., Mellits, E. D., Hankin, J., Smalky, K., & Benson, P. (1986). Ill health and use of medical care: Community-based assessment of morbidity in children. *Medical Care, 24*(9), 848–856.

Diez Roux, A. V. (2007). Integrating social and biologic factors in health research: A systems view. *Annals of Epidemiology, 17*(7), 569–574. doi:10.1016/j.annepidem.2007.03.001.

Docherty, S., & Mill, J. (2008). Epigenetic mechanisms as mediators of environmental risks for psychiatric disorders. *Psychiatry, 7*(12), 500–506.

Dowd, J. B., Zajacova, A., & Aiello, A. (2009). Early origins of health disparities: Burden of infection, health, and socioeconomic status in U.S. children. *Social Science & Medicine, 68*(4), 699–707. doi:10.1016/j.socscimed.2008.12.010.

Dubos, R. J. (1965). *Man adapting*. New Haven: Yale University Press.

Dubos, R., Savage, D., & Schaedler, R. (1966). Biological freudianism. Lasting effects of early environmental influences. *Pediatrics, 38*(5), 789–800.

Dunn, E. C., Uddin, M., Subramanian, S. V., Smoller, J. W., Galea, S., & Koenen, K. C. (2011). Research review: Gene-environment interaction research in youth depression – a systematic review with recommendations for future research. *Journal of Child Psychology and Psychiatry, 52*(12), 1223–1238. doi:10.1111/j.1469-7610.2011.02466.x.

Egan, S. K., & Perry, D. G. (1998). Does low self-regard invite victimization? *Developmental Psychology, 34*(2), 299–309.

Egan, M. F., Goldberg, T. E., Kolachana, B. S., Callicott, J. H., Mazzanti, C. M., Straub, R. E., et al. (2001). Effect of COMT Val108/158 Met genotype on frontal lobe function and risk for schizophrenia. *Proceedings of the National Academy of Sciences of the United States of America, 98*(12), 6917–6922. doi:10.1073/pnas.111134598.

Eisenberger, N. I., & Cole, S. W. (2012). Social neuroscience and health: Neurophysiological mechanisms linking social ties with physical health. *Nature Neuroscience, 15*(5), 669–674. doi:10.1038/nn.3086.

Ellis, B. J., McFadyen-Ketchum, S., Dodge, K. A., Pettit, G. S., & Bates, J. E. (1999). Quality of early family relationships and individual differences in the timing of pubertal maturation in girls: A longitudinal test of an evolutionary model. *Journal of Personality and Social Psychology, 77*(2), 387–401.

Ellis, B. J., Jackson, J. J., & Boyce, W. T. (2006). The stress response systems: Universality and adaptive individual differences. *Developmental Review, 26*(2), 175–212.

Ellis, B. J., Boyce, W. T., Belsky, J., Bakermans-Kranenburg, M. J., & van Ijzendoorn, M. H. (2011a). Differential susceptibility to the environment: An evolutionary--neurodevelopmental theory. *Development and Psychopathology, 23*(1), 7–28. doi:10.1017/S0954579410000611.

Ellis, B. J., Shirtcliff, E. A., Boyce, W. T., Deardorff, J., & Essex, M. J. (2011b). Quality of early family relationships and the timing and tempo of puberty: Effects depend on biological sensitivity to context. *Development and Psychopathology, 23*(1), 85–99. doi:10.1017/S0954579410000660.

El-Sheikh, M. (2005). Stability of respiratory sinus arrhythmia in children and young adolescents: A longitudinal examination. *Developmental Psychobiology, 46*(1), 66–74. doi:10.1002/dev.20036.

El-Sheikh, M., Keller, P. S., & Erath, S. A. (2007). Marital conflict and risk for child maladjustment over time: Skin conductance level reactivity as a vulnerability factor. *Journal of Abnormal Child Psychology, 35*(5), 715–727. doi:10.1007/s10802-007-9127-2.

Essex, M. J., Thomas Boyce, W., Hertzman, C., Lam, L. L., Armstrong, J. M., Neumann, S. M., & Kobor, M. S. (2013). Epigenetic vestiges of early developmental adversity: Childhood stress exposure and DNA methylation in adolescence. *Child Development, 84*(1), 58–75. doi:10.1111/j.1467-8624.2011.01641.x.

Evans, G. W. (2004). The environment of childhood poverty. *The American Psychologist, 59*(2), 77–92.

Evans, G. W., & Kim, P. (2007). Childhood poverty and health: Cumulative risk exposure and stress dysregulation. *Psychological Science, 18*(11), 953–957. doi:10.1111/j.1467-9280.2007.02008.x.

Evans, G. W., Gonnella, C., Marcynyszyn, L. A., Gentile, L., & Salpekar, N. (2005). The role of chaos in poverty and children's socioemotional adjustment. *Psychological Science, 16*(7), 560–565.

Evans, G. W., Chen, E., Miller, G., & Seeman, T. (2012). How poverty gets under the skin: A life-course perspective. In V. Maholmes & R. B. King (Eds.), *The Oxford handbook of poverty and child development* (pp. 13–36). Oxford: Oxford University Press.

Falconi, A. M., Catalano, R., & Boyce, W. T. (2017). Early life predictors of late life health. In W. Satariano & M. Maus (Eds.), *Aging, Place, and Health: A Global Perspective*. Burlington: Jones & Bartlett Learning.

Fehr, E., Bernhard, H., & Rockenbach, B. (2008). Egalitarianism in young children. *Nature, 454*(7208), 1079–1083. doi:10.1038/nature07155.

Fernald, R. D., & Maruska, K. P. (2012). How does social information change the brain? PNAS.

Fraga, M. F., Ballestar, E., Paz, M. F., Ropero, S., Setien, F., Ballestar, M. L., et al. (2005). Epigenetic differences arise during the lifetime of monozygotic twins. *Proceedings of the National Academy of Sciences of the United States of America, 102*(30), 10604–10609.

Freud, S. (1940). An outline of psychoanalysis. In J. Strachey (Ed.), *The standard edition of the complete psychological works of Sigmund Freud* (Vol. 23). London: Hogarth Press.

Galea, S., Riddle, M., & Kaplan, G. A. (2010). Causal thinking and complex system approaches in epidemiology. *International Journal of Epidemiology, 39*(1), 97–106.

Galobardes, B., Lynch, J. W., & Davey Smith, G. (2004). Childhood socioeconomic circumstances and cause-specific mortality in adulthood: Systematic review and interpretation. *Epidemiologic Reviews, 26*, 7–21.

Garner, A. S., Shonkoff, J. P., Siegel, B. S., Dobbins, M. I., Earls, M. F., Garner, A. S., et al. (2012). Early childhood adversity, toxic stress, and the role of the pediatrician: Translating developmental science into lifelong health. *Pediatrics, 129*(1), e224–e231. doi:10.1542/peds.2011-2662.

Gianaros, P. J., & Manuck, S. B. (2010). Neurobiological pathways linking socioeconomic position and health. *Psychosomatic Medicine, 72*(5), 450–461. doi:10.1097/PSY.0b013e3181e1a23c.

Gilbert, S. F. (2002). The genome in its ecological context: Philosophical perspectives on interspecies epigenesis. *Annals of the New York Academy of Sciences, 981*, 202–218.

Gilbert, S. F., & Epel, D. (2009). *Ecological developmental biology: Integrating epigenetics, medicine, and evolution*. Sunderland: Sinauer Associates.

Gini, G., & Pozzoli, T. (2009). Association between bullying and psychosomatic problems: A meta-analysis. *Pediatrics, 123*(3), 1059–1065. doi:10.1542/peds.2008-1215.

Glew, G. M., Fan, M. Y., Katon, W., Rivara, F. P., & Kernic, M. A. (2005). Bullying, psychosocial adjustment, and academic performance in elementary school. *Archives of Pediatrics & Adolescent Medicine, 159*(11), 1026–1031. doi:10.1001/archpedi.159.11.1026.

Gluckman, P. D., Hanson, M. A., & Pinal, C. (2005). The developmental origins of adult disease. *Maternal & Child Nutrition, 1*(3), 130–141.

Gluckman, P. D., Hanson, M. A., & Beedle, A. S. (2007). Non-genomic transgenerational inheritance of disease risk. *BioEssays, 29*(2), 145–154.

Gluckman, P. D., Hanson, M. A., Bateson, P., Beedle, A. S., Law, C. M., Bhutta, Z. A., et al. (2009). Towards a new developmental synthesis: Adaptive developmental plasticity and human disease. *Lancet, 373*(9675), 1654–1657. doi:10.1016/S0140-6736(09)60234-8.

Goodman, E., Adler, N. E., Daniels, S. R., Morrison, J. A., Slap, G. B., & Dolan, L. M. (2003). Impact of objective and subjective social status on obesity in a biracial cohort of adolescents. *Obesity Research, 11*(8), 1018–1026.

Gottlieb, G. (1991). Experiential canalization of behavioral development: Theory. *Developmental Psychology, 27*(1), 4–13.

Greenfield, E. A. (2010). Child abuse as a life-course social determinant of adult health. *Maturitas, 66*(1), 51–55. doi:10.1016/j.maturitas.2010.02.002.

Gump, B. B., Reihman, J., Stewart, P., Lonky, E., Darvill, T., & Matthews, K. A. (2007). Blood lead (Pb) levels: A potential environmental mechanism explaining the relation between socioeconomic status and cardiovascular reactivity in children. *Health Psychology, 26*(3), 296–304. doi:10.1037/0278-6133.26.3.296.

Hackman, D. A., & Farah, M. J. (2009). Socioeconomic status and the developing brain. *Trends in Cognitive Sciences, 13*(2), 65–73. doi:10.1016/j.tics.2008.11.003.

Hackman, D. A., Farah, M. J., & Meaney, M. J. (2010). Socioeconomic status and the brain: Mechanistic insights from human and animal research. *Nature Reviews Neuroscience, 11*(9), 651–659. doi:10.1038/nrn2897.

Halpern, J. (2001). *From detached concern to empathy: Humanizing medical practice*. New York: Oxford University Press.

Hane, A. A., & Fox, N. A. (2006). Ordinary variations in maternal caregiving influence human infants' stress reactivity. *Psychological Science, 17*(6), 550–556. doi:10.1111/j.1467-9280.2006.01742.x.

Hariri, A. R., & Weinberger, D. R. (2003). Imaging genomics. *British Medical Bulletin, 65*, 259–270.

Hariri, A. R., Drabant, E. M., Munoz, K. E., Kolachana, B. S., Mattay, V. S., Egan, M. F., & Weinberger, D. R. (2005). A susceptibility gene for affective disorders and the response of the human amygdala. *Archives of General Psychiatry, 62*(2), 146–152.

Harlow, H. F., Harlow, M. K., & Suomi, S. J. (1971). From thought to therapy: Lessons from a primate laboratory. *American Scientist, 59*(5), 538–549.

Hart, T., & Risley, T. R. (1995). *Meaningful differences in the everyday experience of young American children*. Baltimore, MD: Paul H. Brookes.

Hawley, P. H. (1999). The ontogenesis of social dominance: A strategy-based evolutionary perspective. *Developmental Review, 19*, 97–132.

Hazani, E., & Shasha, S. M. (2008). Effects of the Holocaust on the physical health of the offspring of survivors. *The Israel Medical Association Journal, 10*(4), 251–255.

Heijmans, B. T., Tobi, E. W., Stein, A. D., Putter, H., Blauw, G. J., Susser, E. S., et al. (2008). Persistent epigenetic differences associated with prenatal exposure to famine in humans. *Proceedings of the National Academy of Sciences of the United States of America, 105*(44), 17046–17049. doi:10.1073/pnas.0806560105.

Hensch, T. K. (2005). Critical period plasticity in local cortical circuits. *Nature Reviews. Neuroscience, 6*(11), 877–888. doi:10.1038/nrn1787.

Hertzman, C. (2010). Social geography of developmental health in the early years. *Healthcare Quarterly, 14*(1), 32–40.

Hertzman, C., & Boyce, W. T. (2010). How experience gets under the skin to create gradients in developmental health. *Annual Review of Public Health, 31*, 329–347. 323p following 347. doi:10.1146/annurev.publhealth.012809.103538.

Hillis, S. D., Anda, R. F., Dube, S. R., Felitti, V. J., Marchbanks, P. A., & Marks, J. S. (2004). The association between adverse childhood experiences and adolescent pregnancy, long-term psychosocial consequences, and fetal death. *Pediatrics, 113*(2), 320–327.

Houweling, T. A., & Kunst, A. E. (2010). Socio-economic inequalities in childhood mortality in low- and middle-income countries: A review of the international evidence. *British Medical Bulletin, 93*, 7–26. doi:10.1093/bmb/ldp048.

Hrdy, S. B. (1999). *Mother nature: Maternal instincts and how they shape the human species*. New York: Ballantine Books.

Insel, T. R. (2010). The challenge of translation in social neuroscience: A review of oxytocin, vasopressin, and affiliative behavior. *Neuron, 65*(6), 768–779. doi:10.1016/j.neuron.2010.03.005.

Isles, A. R., & Wilkinson, L. S. (2008). Epigenetics: What is it and why is it important to mental disease? *British Medical Bulletin, 85*, 35–45. doi:10.1093/bmb/ldn004.

Janus, M., & Offord, D. (2000). Reporting on readiness to learn at school in Canada. *Canadian Journal of Policy Research, 1*, 71–75.

Javidi, H., & Yadollahie, M. (2012). Post-traumatic stress disorder. *Journal of Occupational and Environmental Medicine, 3*(1), 2–9.

Jirtle, R. L., & Skinner, M. K. (2007). Environmental epigenomics and disease susceptibility. *Nature Reviews. Genetics, 8*(4), 253–262. doi:10.1038/nrg2045.

Kaplan, J. R., Manuck, S. B., Clarkson, T. B., Lusso, F. M., & Taub, D. M. (1982). Social status, environment, and athersclerosis in cynomolgus monkeys. *Arteriosclerosis, 2*, 359–368.

Karmiloff-Smith, A. (2007). Atypical epigenesis. *Developmental Science, 10*(1), 84–88. doi:10.1111/j.1467-7687.2007.00568.x.

Kauffman, S. A. (1993). *The origins of order: Self-organization and selection in evolution*. New York: Oxford University Press.

Kawachi, I., Adler, N. E., & Dow, W. H. (2010). Money, schooling, and health: Mechanisms and causal evidence. *Annals of the New York Academy of Sciences, 1186*, 56–68. doi:10.1111/j.1749-6632.2009.05340.x.

Keating, D. P., & Hertzman, C. (1999). *Developmental health and the wealth of nations: Social, biological, and educational dynamics*. New York: The Guilford Press.

Keltner, D., Gruenfeld, D., & Anderson, C. (2003). Power, approach, and inhibition. *Psychological Review, 110*(2), 265–284.

Kershaw, P., Forer, B., Lloyd, J. E. V., Hertzman, C., Boyce, W. T., Zumbo, B. D., et al. (2009). The use of population-level data to advance interdisciplinary methodology: A cell-through-society sampling framework for child development research. *International Journal of Social Research Methodology, 12*(5), 387–403.

Kessler, R. C., Duncan, G. J., Gennetian, L. A., Katz, L. F., Kling, J. R., Sampson, N. A., et al. (2014). Associations of housing mobility interventions for children in high-poverty neighborhoods with subsequent mental disorders during adolescence. *JAMA, 311*(9), 937–948. doi:10.1001/jama.2014.607.

Keverne, E. B., Martensz, N. D., & Tuite, B. (1989). Beta-endorphin concentrations in cerebrospinal fluid of monkeys are influenced by grooming relationships. *Psychoneuroendocrinology, 14*(1–2), 155–161.

Khan, Y., & Bhutta, Z. A. (2010). Nutritional deficiencies in the developing world: Current status and opportunities for intervention. *Pediatric Clinics of North America, 57*(6), 1409–1441. doi:10.1016/j.pcl.2010.09.016.

Kim, Y. S., Koh, Y. J., & Leventhal, B. L. (2004). Prevalence of school bullying in Korean middle school students. *Archives of Pediatrics & Adolescent Medicine, 158*(8), 737–741.

Kim, Y. S., Leventhal, B. L., Koh, Y. J., & Boyce, W. T. (2009). Bullying increased suicide risk: Prospective study of Korean adolescents. *Archives of Suicide Research, 13*(1), 15–30. doi:10.1080/13811110802572098.

King, M. L. (2007). Concepts of childhood: What we know and where we might go. *Renaissance Quarterly, 60*(2), 371–407.

Kinnally, E. L., Capitanio, J. P., Leibel, R., Deng, L., LeDuc, C., Haghighi, F., & Mann, J. J. (2010a). Epigenetic regulation of serotonin transporter expression and behavior in infant rhesus macaques. *Genes, Brain, and Behavior, 9*(6), 575–582. doi:10.1111/j.1601-183X.2010.00588.x.

Kinnally, E. L., Karere, G. M., Lyons, L. A., Mendoza, S. P., Mason, W. A., & Capitanio, J. P. (2010b). Serotonin pathway gene-gene and gene-environment interactions influence behavioral stress response in infant rhesus macaques. *Development and Psychopathology, 22*(1), 35–44. doi:10.1017/S0954579409990241.

Kinnally, E. L., Feinberg, C., Kim, D., Ferguson, K., Leibel, R., Coplan, J. D., & John Mann, J. (2011). DNA methylation as a risk factor in the effects of early life stress. *Brain Behavior and Immunity*. doi:10.1016/j.bbi.2011.05.001.

Kittleson, M. M., Meoni, L. A., Wang, N. Y., Chu, A. Y., Ford, D. E., & Klag, M. J. (2006). Association of childhood socioeconomic status with subsequent coronary heart disease in physicians. *Archives of Internal Medicine, 166*(21), 2356–2361.

Knafo, A., Israel, S., & Ebstein, R. P. (2011). Heritability of children's prosocial behavior and differential susceptibility to parenting by variation in the dopamine receptor D4 gene. *Development and Psychopathology, 23*(1), 53–67. doi:10.1017/S0954579410000647.

Koopman, J. S., & Lynch, J. W. (1999). Individual causal models and population system models in epidemiology. *American Journal of Public Health, 89*(8), 1170–1174.

Kraemer, H. C., Stice, E., Kazdin, A., Offord, D., & Kupfer, D. (2001). How do risk factors work together? Mediators, moderators, independent, overlapping and proxy-risk factors. *The American Journal of Psychiatry, 158*, 848–856.

Kraemer, H. C., Kiernan, M., Essex, M., & Kupfer, D. J. (2008). How and why criteria defining moderators and mediators differ between the Baron & Kenny and MacArthur approaches. *Health Psychology, 27*(2 Suppl), S101–S108. doi:10.1037/0278-6133.27.2(Suppl.).S101.

Krieger, N. (2001). Theories for social epidemiology in the 21st century: An ecosocial perspective. *International Journal of Epidemiology, 30*, 668–677.

Kuh, D., & Ben-Shlomo, Y. (2004). *A life course approach to chronic disease epidemiology* (2nd ed.). Oxford: Oxford University Press.

Kuzawa, C. W., & Thayer, Z. M. (2011). Timescales of human adaptation: The role of epigenetic processes. *Epigenomics, 3*(2), 221–234. doi:10.2217/epi.11.11.

Ladd-Acosta, C., Pevsner, J., Sabunciyan, S., Yolken, R. H., Webster, M. J., Dinkins, T., et al. (2007). DNA methylation signatures within the human brain.

American Journal of Human Genetics, 81(6), 1304–1315. doi:10.1086/524110.

Lam, L. L., Emberly, E., Fraser, H. B., Neumann, S. M., Chen, E., Miller, G. E., & Kobor, M. S. (2012). Biological and environmental predictors of variable DNA methylation in a human community cohort. *PNAS.*

Lawlor, D. A., Sterne, J. A., Tynelius, P., Davey Smith, G., & Rasmussen, F. (2006). Association of childhood socioeconomic position with cause-specific mortality in a prospective record linkage study of 1,839,384 individuals. *American Journal of Epidemiology, 164*(9), 907–915. doi:10.1093/aje/kwj319.

Lesch, K. P. (2007). Linking emotion to the social brain. The role of the serotonin transporter in human social behaviour. *EMBO Reports, 8*, S24–S29. doi:10.1038/sj.embor.7401008.

Liew, C. C., Ma, J., Tang, H. C., Zheng, R., & Dempsey, A. A. (2006). The peripheral blood transcriptome dynamically reflects system wide biology: A potential diagnostic tool. *The Journal of Laboratory and Clinical Medicine, 147*(3), 126–132. doi:10.1016/j.lab.2005.10.005.

Liu, L., Li, Y., & Tollefsbol, T. O. (2008). Gene-environment interactions and epigenetic basis of human diseases. *Current Issues in Molecular Biology, 10*(1–2), 25–36.

Liu, L., Johnson, H. L., Cousens, S., Perin, J., Scott, S., Lawn, J. E., et al. (2012). Global, regional, and national causes of child mortality: An updated systematic analysis for 2010 with time trends since 2000. *Lancet, 379*(9832), 2151–2161. doi:10.1016/S0140-6736(12)60560-1.

Lloyd, L. J., Langley-Evans, S. C., & McMullen, S. (2012). Childhood obesity and risk of the adult metabolic syndrome: A systematic review. *International Journal of Obesity, 36*(1), 1–11. doi:10.1038/ijo.2011.186.

Lumey, L. H., Stein, A. D., & Susser, E. (2011). Prenatal famine and adult health. *Annual Review of Public Health, 32*, 237–262. doi:10.1146/annurev-publhealth-031210-101230.

Lupien, S. J., King, S., Meaney, M. J., & McEwen, B. S. (2001). Can poverty get under your skin? Basal cortisol levels and cognitive function in children from low and high socioeconomic status. *Development and Psychopathology, 13*, 653–676.

MacDonald, J. L., & Roskams, A. J. (2009). Epigenetic regulation of nervous system development by DNA methylation and histone deacetylation. *Progress in Neurobiology, 88*(3), 170–183.

Manuck, S. B., Craig, A. E., Flory, J. D., Halder, I., & Ferrell, R. E. (2011). Reported early family environment covaries with menarcheal age as a function of polymorphic variation in estrogen receptor-alpha. *Development and Psychopathology, 23*(1), 69–83. doi:10.1017/S0954579410000659.

Marmot, M. (2010). *Fair society, healthy lives*. Firenze: L.S. Olschki.

Mazumdar, S., King, M., Liu, K. Y., Zerubavel, N., & Bearman, P. (2010). The spatial structure of autism in California, 1993-2001. *Health & Place, 16*(3), 539–546. doi:10.1016/j.healthplace.2009.12.014.

McDade, T. (2012). Early environments and the ecologics of inflammation. *Proceedings of the National Academy of Sciences of the United States of America, 109*(Suppl 2), 17281–17288.

McEwen, B. S., & Gianaros, P. J. (2010). Central role of the brain in stress and adaptation: Links to socioeconomic status, health, and disease. *Annals of the New York Academy of Sciences, 1186*, 190–222. doi:10.1111/j.1749-6632.2009.05331.x.

McGowan, P. O., & Szyf, M. (2010). The epigenetics of social adversity in early life: Implications for mental health outcomes. *Neurobiology of Disease, 39*(1), 66–72. doi:10.1016/j.nbd.2009.12.026.

McGowan, P. O., Sasaki, A., Huang, T. C., Unterberger, A., Suderman, M., Ernst, C., et al. (2008). Promoter-wide hypermethylation of the ribosomal RNA gene promoter in the suicide brain. *PloS One, 3*(5), e2085.

McGowan, P. O., Sasaki, A., D'Alessio, A. C., Dymov, S., Labonte, B., Szyf, M., et al. (2009). Epigenetic regulation of the glucocorticoid receptor in human brain associates with childhood abuse. *Nature Neuroscience, 12*(3), 342–348. doi:10.1038/nn.2270.

Meaney, M. J. (2010). Epigenetics and the biological definition of gene x environment interactions. *Child Development, 81*(1), 41–79. doi:10.1111/j.1467-8624.2009.01381.x.

Meaney, M. J., & Ferguson-Smith, A. C. (2010). Epigenetic regulation of the neural transcriptome: The meaning of the marks. *Nature Neuroscience, 13*(11), 1313–1318. doi:10.1038/nn1110-1313.

Mehler, M. F. (2008). Epigenetic principles and mechanisms underlying nervous system functions in health and disease. *Progress in Neurobiology, 86*(4), 305–341.

Miller, G. E., Chen, E., Fok, A. K., Walker, H., Lim, A., Nicholls, E. F., et al. (2009a). Low early-life social class leaves a biological residue manifested by decreased glucocorticoid and increased proinflammatory signaling. *Proceedings of the National Academy of Sciences of the United States of America, 106*(34), 14716–14721. doi:10.1073/pnas.0902971106.

Miller, A. H., Maletic, V., & Raison, C. L. (2009b). Inflammation and its discontents: The role of cytokines in the pathophysiology of major depression. *Biological Psychiatry, 65*(9), 732–741. doi:10.1016/j.biopsych.2008.11.029.

Moffitt, T. E., Caspi, A., & Rutter, M. (2005). Strategy for investigating interactions between measured genes and measured environments. *Archives of General Psychiatry, 62*(5), 473–481.

Mohr, S., & Liew, C. C. (2007). The peripheral-blood transcriptome: New insights into disease and risk assessment. *Trends in Molecular Medicine, 13*(10), 422–432. doi:10.1016/j.molmed.2007.08.003.

Morita, K., Saito, T., Ohta, M., Ohmori, T., Kawai, K., Teshima-Kondo, S., & Rokutan, K. (2005). Expression analysis of psychological stress-associated genes in peripheral blood leukocytes. *Neuroscience Letters, 381*(1–2), 57–62.

Msall, M. E., Bier, J. A., LaGasse, L., Tremont, M., & Lester, B. (1998). The vulnerable preschool child: The impact of biomedical and social risks on neurodevelopmental function. *Seminars in Pediatric Neurology, 5*(1), 52–61.

Nesse, R. M., & Young, E. A. (2000). Evolutionary origins and functions of the stress response. In G. Fink (Ed.), *Encyclopedia of stress* (Vol. 2, pp. 79–84). San Diego: Academic Press.

Norman, G. J., Hawkley, L. C., Cole, S. W., Berntson, G. G., & Cacioppo, J. T. (2012). Social neuroscience: The social brain, oxytocin, and health. *Social Neuroscience, 7*(1), 18–29. doi:10.1080/17470919.2011.568702.

Oberg, C. (2008). Children of genocide: A legacy of lost dreams. *Pediatrics, 121*(3), 611–615. doi:10.1542/peds.2007-2208.

Oberlander, T. F., Weinberg, J., Papsdorf, M., Grunau, R., Misri, S., & Devlin, A. M. (2008). Prenatal exposure to maternal depression, neonatal methylation of human glucocorticoid receptor gene (NR3C1) and infant cortisol stress response. *Epigenetics, 3*(2), 97–106.

Obradovic, J., Bush, N. R., Stamperdahl, J., Adler, N. E., & Boyce, W. T. (2010). Biological sensitivity to context: The interactive effects of stress reactivity and family adversity on socio-emotional behavior and school readiness. *Child Development, 81*(1), 270–289.

Offord, D. R. (1995). Child psychiatric epidemiology: Current status and future prospects. *Canadian Journal of Psychiatry. Revue Canadienne de Psychiatrie, 40*(6), 284–288.

Olds, D. L., Kitzman, H. J., Cole, R. E., Hanks, C. A., Arcoleo, K. J., Anson, E. A., et al. (2010). Enduring effects of prenatal and infancy home visiting by nurses on maternal life course and government spending: Follow-up of a randomized trial among children at age 12 years. *Archives of Pediatrics and Adolescent Medicine, 164*(5), 419–424. doi:10.1001/archpediatrics.2010.49.

Ollikainen, M., Smith, K. R., Joo, E. J., Ng, H. K., Andronikos, R., Novakovic, B., et al. (2010). DNA methylation analysis of multiple tissues from newborn twins reveals both genetic and intrauterine components to variation in the human neonatal epigenome. *Human Molecular Genetics, 19*(21), 4176–4188. doi:10.1093/hmg/ddq336.

Ostrove, J. M., Adler, N. E., Kuppermann, M., & Washington, A. E. (2000). Objective and subjective assessments of socioeconomic status and their relationship to self-rated health in an ethnically diverse sample of pregnant women. *Health Psychology, 19*(6), 613–618.

Overton, W. F., & Lerner, R. M. (2014). Fundamental concepts and methods in developmental science: A relational perspective. *Research in Human Development, 11*, 63–73.

Painter, R. C., Roseboom, T. J., & Bleker, O. P. (2005). Prenatal exposure to the Dutch famine and disease in later life: An overview. *Reproductive Toxicology, 20*(3), 345–352.

Painter, R., Osmond, C., Gluckman, P., Hanson, M., Phillips, D., & Roseboom, T. (2008). Transgenerational effects of prenatal exposure to the Dutch famine on neonatal adiposity and health in later life. *BJOG: An International Journal of Obstetrics & Gynaecology, 115*(10), 1243–1249.

Panter-Brick, C., Lende, D., & Kohrt, B. (2012). Children in global adversity: Physical health, mental health, behavioral health, and symbolic health. In V. Maholmes & R. B. King (Eds.), *The Oxford handbook of poverty and child development* (pp. 603–621). Oxford: Oxford University Press.

Pellegrini, A. D., Roseth, C. J., Mliner, S., Bohn, C. M., Van Ryzin, M., Vance, N., et al. (2007). Social dominance in preschool classrooms. *Journal of Comparative Psychology, 121*(1), 54–64. doi:10.1037/0735-7036.121.1.54.

Pellegrini, A. D., Van Ryzin, M. J., Roseth, C., Bohn-Gettler, C., Dupuis, D., Hickey, M., & Peshkam, A. (2010). Behavioral and social cognitive processes in preschool children's social dominance. *Aggressive Behavior, 37*(3), 248–257. doi:10.1002/ab.20385.

Pezawas, L., Meyer-Lindenberg, A., Drabant, E. M., Verchinski, B. A., Munoz, K. E., Kolachana, B. S., et al. (2005). 5-HTTLPR polymorphism impacts human cingulate-amygdala interactions: A genetic susceptibility mechanism for depression. *Nature Neuroscience, 8*(6), 828–834.

Pluess, M., & Belsky, J. (2013). Vantage sensitivity: Individual differences in response to positive experiences. *Psychological Bulletin, 139*(4), 901–916. doi:10.1037/a0030196.

Quas, J. A., Bauer, A., & Boyce, W. T. (2004). Physiological reactivity, social support, and memory in early childhood. *Child Development, 75*(3), 797–814.

Rifkin, J. (2009). *The empathic civilization: The race to global consciousness in a world in crisis*. New York: Jeremy P. Tarcher/Penguin.

Robert Wood Johnson Foundation Commission to Build a Healthier America. (2009). Beyond Health Care: New Directions to a Healthier America. Retrieved from Princeton, NJ:

Robinson, G. E., Grozinger, C. M., & Whitfield, C. W. (2005). Sociogenomics: Social life in molecular terms. *Nature Reviews Genetics, 6*, 257–270.

Robinson, G. E., Fernald, R. D., & Clayton, D. F. (2008). Genes and social behavior. *Science, 322*(5903), 896–900. doi:10.1126/science.1159277.

Robison, A. J., & Nestler, E. J. (2011). Transcriptional and epigenetic mechanisms of addiction. *Nature Reviews. Neuroscience, 12*(11), 623–637. doi:10.1038/nrn3111.

Roseboom, T. J., van der Meulen, J. H., Osmond, C., Barker, D. J., Ravelli, A. C., Schroeder-Tanka, J. M., et al. (2000). Coronary heart disease after prenatal exposure to the Dutch famine, 1944-45. *Heart, 84*(6), 595–598.

Roth, T. L., Lubin, F. D., Funk, A. J., & Sweatt, J. D. (2009). Lasting epigenetic influence of early-life adversity on the BDNF gene. *Biological Psychiatry, 65*(9), 760–769. doi:10.1016/j.biopsych.2008.11.028.

Russo, V. E. A., Cove, D. J., Edgar, L. G., Jaenisch, R., & Salamini, F. (Eds.). (1999). *Development: Genetics, epigenetics and environmental regulation*. Berlin: Springer-Verlag.

Rutter, M. (2006). *Genes and behaviour: Nature/nurture interplay explained*. Oxford, UK: Blackwell Publishing.

Rutter, M. (2012). Achievements and challenges in the biology of environmental effects. *PNAS*.

Sapolsky, R. M. (2003). Stress and plasticity in the limbic system. *Neurochemical Research, 28*(11), 1735–1742.

Sapolsky, R. M. (2005). The influence of social hierarchy on primate health. *Science, 308*(5722), 648–652.

Schneider, J., Dickinson, M., & Levine, J. (2012). Social structures depend on innate determinants and chemosensory processing in Drosophila. *PNAS*.

Sentenac, M., Arnaud, C., Gavin, A., Molcho, M., Gabhainn, S. N., & Godeau, E. (2012). Peer victimization among school-aged children with chronic conditions. *Epidemiologic Reviews, 34*(1), 120–128. doi:10.1093/epirev/mxr024.

Shannon, K. E., Beauchaine, T. P., Brenner, S. L., Neuhaus, E., & Gatzke-Kopp, L. (2007). Familial and temperamental predictors of resilience in children at risk for conduct disorder and depression. *Development and Psychopathology, 19*(3), 701–727. doi:10.1017/S0954579407000351.

Shonkoff, J. (2012). Leveraging the biology of adversity and resilience to address the roots of disparities in health and development. *Proceedings of the National Academy of Sciences of the United States of America,109*(Suppl 2), 17302–17307.

Shonkoff, J. P., & Garner, A. S. (2012). The lifelong effects of early childhood adversity and toxic stress. *Pediatrics, 129*(1), e232–e246. doi:10.1542/peds.2011-2663.

Shonkoff, J. P., & Phillips, D. A. (Eds.). (2000). *From neurons to neighborhoods: The science of early child development*. Washington, DC: National Academy Press.

Shorter, E. (1975). *The making of the modern family*. New York: Basic Books.

Slavich, G. M., & Cole, S. W. (2013). The emerging field of human social genomics. *Clinical Psychological Science: A Journal of the Association for Psychological Science, 1*(3), 331–348.

Sourander, A., Jensen, P., Ronning, J. A., Elonheimo, H., Niemela, S., Helenius, H., et al. (2007). Childhood bullies and victims and their risk of criminality in late adolescence: The Finnish From a Boy to a Man study. *Archives of Pediatrics & Adolescent Medicine, 161*(6), 546–552. doi:10.1001/archpedi.161.6.546.

Stearns, P. N. (2011). *Childhood in world history* (2nd ed.). New York, NY: Routledge.

Steptoe, A., Feldman, P. J., Kunz, S., Owen, N., Willemsen, G., & Marmot, M. (2002). Stress responsivity and socioeconomic status: A mechanism for increased cardiovascular disease risk? *European Heart Journal, 23*, 1757–1763.

Stevens, H. E., Leckman, J. F., Coplan, J. D., & Suomi, S. J. (2009). Risk and resilience: Early manipulation of macaque social experience and persistent behavioral and neurophysiological outcomes. *Journal of the American Academy of Child and Adolescent Psychiatry, 48*(2), 114–127. doi:10.1097/CHI.0b013e318193064c.

Suomi, S. J. (2006). Risk, resilience, and gene x environment interactions in rhesus monkeys. *Annals of the New York Academy of Sciences, 1094*, 52–62. doi:10.1196/annals.1376.006.

Syme, S. L. (2008). Reducing racial and social-class inequalities in health: The need for a new approach. *Health Affairs (Millwood), 27*(2), 456–459. doi:10.1377/hlthaff.27.2.456.

Szyf, M., McGowan, P., & Meaney, M. J. (2008). The social environment and the epigenome. *Environmental and Molecular Mutagenesis, 49*(1), 46–60. doi:10.1002/em.20357.

Thompson, P. M., Martin, N. G., & Wright, M. J. (2010). Imaging genomics. *Current Opinion in Neurology, 23*(4), 368–373. doi:10.1097/WCO.0b013e32833b764c.

Tsankova, N., Renthal, W., Kumar, A., & Nestler, E. J. (2007). Epigenetic regulation in psychiatric disorders. *Nature Reviews. Neuroscience, 8*(5), 355–367. doi:10.1038/nrn2132.

Turecki, G., Ernst, C., Jollant, F., Labonte, B., & Mechawar, N. (2012). The neurodevelopmental origins of suicidal behavior. *Trends in Neurosciences, 35*(1), 14–23. doi:10.1016/j.tins.2011.11.008.

Turner, J. D., Pelascini, L. P., Macedo, J. A., & Muller, C. P. (2008). Highly individual methylation patterns of alternative glucocorticoid receptor promoters suggest individualized epigenetic regulatory mechanisms. *Nucleic Acids Research, 36*(22), 7207–7218. doi:10.1093/nar/gkn897.

Turner, H. A., Finkelhor, D., Shattuck, A., & Hamby, S. (2012). Recent victimization exposure and suicidal ideation in adolescents. *Archives of Pediatrics & Adolescent Medicine*, 1–6. doi:10.1001/archpediatrics.2012.1549.

U.S. Department of Health and Human Services. (2011). *CDC Health Disparities and Inequalities Report—United States, 2011*. Atlanta: U.S. Department of Health and Human Services, Centers for Disease Control and Prevention.

Uebelhack, R., Franke, L., Herold, N., Plotkin, M., Amthauer, H., & Felix, R. (2006). Brain and platelet serotonin transporter in humans-correlation between [123I]-ADAM SPECT and serotonergic measurements in platelets. *Neuroscience Letters, 406*(3), 153–158. doi:10.1016/j.neulet.2006.06.004.

van IJzendoorn, M. H., Caspers, K., Bakermans-Kranenburg, M. J., Beach, S. R., & Philibert, R. (2010). Methylation matters: Interaction between methylation density and serotonin transporter genotype predicts unresolved loss or trauma. *Biological Psychiatry, 68*(5), 405–407. doi:10.1016/j.biopsych.2010.05.008.

Vogel, E. F., & Bell, N. W. (1961). The emotionally disturbed child as the family scapegoat. In N. W. Bell & E. F. Vogel (Eds.), *A Modern introduction to the family*. London: Routledge & Kegan Paul.

Waddington, C. H. (1959). Canalization of development and genetic assimilation of acquired characters. *Nature, 183*(4676), 1654–1655.

Waddington, C. H. (2012). The epigenotype. 1942. *International Journal of Epidemiology, 41*(1), 10–13. doi:10.1093/ije/dyr184.

Wadsworth, M. E., Raviv, T., Reinhard, C., Wolff, B., Santiago, C. D. C., & Einhorn, L. (2008). An indirect effects model of the association between poverty and child functioning: The role of children. *Journal of Loss and Trauma, 30*.

Weaver, I. C. (2009). Epigenetic effects of glucocorticoids. *Seminars in Fetal and Neonatal Medicine, 14*(3), 143–150. doi:10.1016/j.siny.2008.12.002.

Weaver, I. C., Cervoni, N., Champagne, F. A., D'Alessio, A. C., Sharma, S., Seckl, J. R., et al. (2004). Epigenetic programming by maternal behavior. *Nature Neuroscience, 7*(8), 847–854.

Weikum, W. M., Oberlander, T. F., Hensch, T. K., & Werker, J. F. (2012). Prenatal exposure to antidepressants and depressed maternal mood alter trajectory of infant speech perception. *Proceedings of the National Academy of Sciences, 109*(2), 17221–17227. doi:10.1073/pnas.1121263109.

West-Eberhard, M. J. (2003). *Developmental plasticity and evolution*. New York: Oxford University Press.

Whittle, S., Yap, M. B., Sheeber, L., Dudgeon, P., Yucel, M., Pantelis, C., et al. (2010). Hippocampal volume and sensitivity to maternal aggressive behavior: A prospective study of adolescent depressive symptoms. *Development and Psychopathology, 23*(1), 115–129. doi:10.1017/S0954579410000684.

Wolf, D. M., Vazirani, V. V., & Arkin, A. P. (2005). Diversity in times of adversity: Probabilistic strategies in microbial survival games. *Journal of Theoretical Biology, 234*(2), 227–253. doi:10.1016/j.jtbi.2004.11.020.

Wright, R. O., & Christiani, D. (2010). Gene-environment interaction and children's health and development. *Current Opinion in Pediatrics, 22*(2), 197–201. doi:10.1097/MOP.0b013e328336ebf9.

Wu, H., & Sun, Y. E. (2006). Epigenetic regulation of stem cell differentiation. *Pediatric Research, 59*(4 Pt 2), 21R–25R. doi:10.1203/01.pdr.0000203565.76028.2a.

Yang, E.-J., Lin, E. W., & Hensch, T. K. (2012). A critical period for acoustic preference in mice. *Proceedings of the National Academy of Sciences, 109*(Suppl 2), 17213–17220.

Zhang, T. Y., & Meaney, M. J. (2010). Epigenetics and the environmental regulation of the genome and its function. *Annual Review of Psychology, 61*, 439–466, C431–433.. doi:10.1146/annurev.psych.60.110707.163625.

2

Middle Childhood: An Evolutionary-Developmental Synthesis

Marco DelGiudice

Middle childhood—conventionally going from about 6–11 years of age—is a crucial yet under-appreciated phase of human development. On the surface, middle childhood may appear like a slow-motion interlude between the spectacular transformations of infancy and early childhood and those of adolescence. In reality, this life stage is anything but static: the transition from early to middle childhood heralds a global shift in cognition, motivation, and social behavior, with profound and wide-ranging implications for the development of personality, sex differences, and even psychopathology (Table 1).

In the last two decades, converging theories and findings from anthropology, primatology, evolutionary psychology, endocrinology, and behavior genetics have revolutionized our understanding of middle childhood. In this chapter, I show how these diverse contributions can be synthesized into an integrated evolutionary-developmental model of middle childhood. I begin by reviewing the main evolved functions of middle childhood and the cognitive, behavioral, and hormonal processes that characterize this life stage. Then, I introduce the idea that the transition to middle childhood works as a switch point in the development of life history strategies (Del Giudice et al. 2009, 2012; Del Giudice and Belsky 2011) and discuss three insights in the nature of middle childhood that arise from an integrated approach. This chapter was originally published as a short paper in the journal *Child Development Perspectives* (Del Giudice 2014a). It is reprinted here with updated references and a new section on the model's implications for health development in a life course perspective (LCHD).

1 What Is Middle Childhood?

Middle childhood is one of the main stages of human development, marked by the eruption of the first permanent molars around age 6 and the onset of androgen secretion by the adrenal glands at about 6–8 years (Bogin 1997). In middle childhood, body growth slows considerably, usually following a small mid-growth spurt. At the same time, muscularity increases and the body starts accumulating fat (the *adiposity rebound*; Hochberg 2008), while sex differences in body composition become more pronounced (Del Giudice et al. 2009; Wells

This chapter contains a modified version of a previously published review and analysis of existing research, written by Marco Del Giudice, that appeared in *Child Development Perspectives*.
Reprinted with permission from:
Del Giudice, M. (2014), Middle Childhood: An Evolutionary-Developmental Synthesis. Child Dev Perspect, 8: 193–200. doi:10.1111/cdep.12084.

M. DelGiudice (✉)
Department of Psychology, University of New Mexico, Logan Hall, 2001 Redondo Dr. NE, Albuquerque, NM 87131, USA
e-mail: marcodg@unm.edu

Table 1 Development in middle childhood

Body growth	Eruption of permanent molars
	Mid-growth spurt, followed by decelerating skeletal growth
	Increased muscle mass
	Increased adiposity and BMI (adiposity rebound)
	Initial development of axillary hair and body odor
	Increased sex differences in adiposity (F > M), bone strength, and muscularity (M > F)
	Emergence of sex differences in vocal characteristics
Brain growth	Approaching peak of overall brain volume
	Peak of gray matter volume
	Continuing increase in white matter volume/integrity
Motor and perceptual skills	Increased gross motor skills (e.g., walking)
	Increased fine motor skills
	Local-global shift in visual processing preferences
Cognitive skills	Increased reasoning and problem-solving skills (e.g., concrete operations)
	Increased self-regulation and executive functions (inhibition, attention, planning, etc.)
	Increased mentalizing skills (multiple perspectives, conflicting goals)
	Increased navigational skills (working memory, ability to understand maps)
Motivation and social behavior	Acquisition of cultural norms (e.g., prosociality)
	Complex moral reasoning (conflicting points of view)
	Increased pragmatic abilities (gossiping, storytelling, verbal competition, etc.)
	Consolidation of status/dominance hierarchies
	Changes in aggression levels (individual trajectories)
	Development of disgust
	Changes in food preferences (e.g., spicy foods)
	Onset of sexual/romantic attraction
	Increased frequency of sexual play
	Increased sense of gender identity
	Peak of sex segregation
	Peak of sex differences in social play (including play fighting vs. play parenting)
	Increased sex differences in physical aggression (M > F)
	Emergence of sex differences in attachment styles
Psychopathology	Early peak of psychopathology onset (externalizing, anxiety, phobias, ADHD)
	Peak onset of fetishistic attractions
	Emergence of sex differences in conduct disorders (M > F)
Social context	Active involvement in caretaking, foraging, domestic tasks, helping
	Expectations of responsible behavior
	Attribution of individuality and personhood ("getting noticed")
Behavior genetics	Increased heritability of general intelligence and language skills
	New genetic influences on general intelligence, language, aggression, and prosociality

See the main text for supporting references
BMI body mass index, *M* male, *F* female, *ADHD* attention deficit hyperactivity disorder

2007). Figure 1 places middle childhood in the broader context of human growth from conception to adolescence.

In biological terms, middle childhood corresponds to human *juvenility*—a stage in which the individual is still sexually immature, but no longer dependent on parents for survival. In social mammals and primates, juvenility is a phase of intense learning—often accomplished through play—in which youngsters practice adult behavioral patterns and acquire essential social and foraging skills. Indeed, the duration of juvenility in

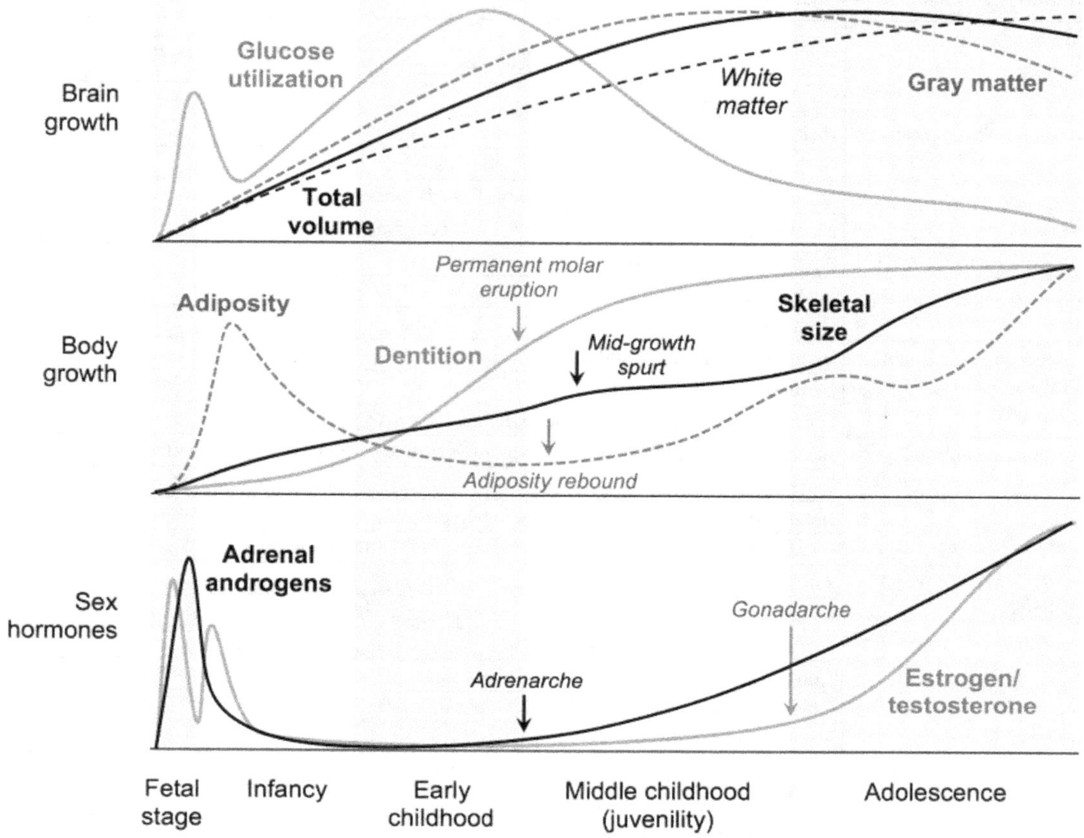

Fig. 1 Developmental trajectories of human growth and sex hormones production, from conception to adolescence. Arrows show the landmark events that characterize middle childhood (Reproduced from Del Giudice 2014a)

primates correlates strongly with the size and complexity of social groups, as well as with cortical brain volume (Joffe 1997). Social learning in juvenility can be understood as investment in *embodied capital*—skills and knowledge that cost time and effort to acquire but increase an individual's performance and reproductive success (Kaplan et al. 2000).

Human children are no exception to this pattern. Social learning is universally recognized as a key evolved function of middle childhood and is enabled by a global reorganization of cognitive functioning known as the *five-to-seven shift* (Weisner 1996). By age 6, the brain has almost reached its maximum size and receives a decreasing share of the body's glucose after the consumption peak of early childhood (Fig. 1; Giedd and Rapoport 2010; Kuzawa et al. 2014). However, brain development proceeds at a sustained pace, with intensive synaptogenesis in cortical areas (gray matter) and rapid maturation of axonal connections (white matter; Lebel et al. 2008). The transition to middle childhood is marked by a simultaneous increase in perceptual abilities (including a transition from local to global visual processing), motor control (including the emergence of adult-like walking), and complex reasoning skills (Bjorklund 2011; Poirel et al. 2011; Weisner 1996). The most dramatic changes probably occur in the domain of self-regulation and executive functions: children become much more capable of inhibiting unwanted behavior, maintaining sustained attention, making and following plans, and so forth (Best et al. 2009; Weisner 1996; see also McClelland et al. 2017). Parallel improvements take place in mentalizing (the ability to understand and represent mental states) and moral reasoning, as children become able to consider multiple perspectives and conflicting goals (Jambon and Smetana 2014; Lagattuta et al. 2009).

In traditional societies, older relatives—especially parents and grandparents—are the main sources of knowledge for juveniles, supplemented by peers and—where available—professional teachers. Storytelling—both fictional and based in real events—is a powerful technology for transmitting knowledge about foraging and social skills, avoidance of dangers, topography, wayfinding, and social roles and norms (Scalise Sugiyama 2011). Storytelling mimics the format of episodic memories, providing the child with a rich source of indirect experience (Scalise Sugiyama 2011). Intriguingly, episodic memory shows dramatic and sustained improvements across middle childhood (Ghetti and Bunge 2012).

However, children at this age are not just learning and playing. Cross-culturally, middle childhood is the time when children are expected to start helping with domestic tasks—such as caring for younger siblings, collecting food and water, tending animals, and helping adults prepare food (Bogin 1997; Lancy and Grove 2011; Scalise Sugiyama 2011; Weisner 1996). In favorable ecologies, juveniles can contribute substantially to family subsistence (Kramer 2011). Thanks to marked increases in spatial cognition—reflected in the emerging ability to understand maps—and navigational skills, children become able to memorize complex routes and find their way without adult supervision (Bjorklund 2011; Piccardi et al. 2014). The important role of juveniles in collecting and preparing food may explain why the emotion of disgust does not fully develop until middle childhood (Rozin 1990a).

The transition to middle childhood is typically associated with a strong separation in gender roles, even in societies where tasks are not rigidly assigned by sex. Spontaneous sex segregation of boys and girls peaks during these years, as does the frequency of sexually differentiated play (Del Giudice et al. 2009). On a broader social level, cross-cultural evidence shows that juveniles start "getting noticed" by adults—that is, they begin to be viewed fully as people with their own individuality, personality, and social responsibility (Lancy and Grove 2011).

In summary, the life stage of juvenility/middle childhood has two major interlocking functions: *social learning* and *social integration* in a system of roles, norms, activities, and shared knowledge. While children are still receiving sustained investment from parents and other relatives—in the form of food, protection, knowledge, and so forth—they also start to actively contribute to their family economy. By providing resources and sharing the burden of child care, juveniles can boost their parents' reproductive potential. The dual nature of juveniles as both *receivers* and *providers* explains many psychological features of middle childhood and has likely played a major role in the evolution of human life history (Kramer 2011).

1.1 Adrenarche

The transition to middle childhood is coordinated by a remarkable endocrinological event: the awakening of the adrenal glands, or *adrenarche* (Auchus and Rainey 2004; Hochberg 2008). Starting at about 6–8 years—with much individual variation and only minor differences between males and females—adrenal glands begin to secrete increasing amounts of androgens (see Fig. 1), mainly dehydroepiandrosterone (DHEA) and its sulfate (DHEAS). Adrenal androgens have only minor effects on physical development, but they have powerful effects on brain functioning. DHEA and DHEAS promote neurogenesis and modulate gamma-aminobutyric acid (GABA) and glutamate receptors; moreover, DHEA can act directly on androgen and estrogen receptors. Even more important, adrenal androgens can be converted to estrogen or testosterone in the brain (Campbell 2006; Del Giudice et al. 2009). As sex hormones, adrenal androgens play a twofold role: They activate sexually differentiated brain pathways that had been previously organized by the hormonal surges of prenatal development and infancy (Fig. 1), and they further organize brain development along sexually differentiated trajectories (Del Giudice et al. 2009).

Adrenal androgens likely provide a major impulse for many of the psychological changes of middle childhood (Campbell 2006, 2011; Del Giudice et al. 2009), including the emergence and intensification of sex differences across domains (see Table 1). Since the age of adrenarche correlates strongly with that of *gonadarche* (the awakening of the testes/ovaries that marks the beginning of puberty; Hochberg 2008), human development shows a peculiar pattern in which sexually differentiated brain pathways are activated several years *before* the development of secondary sexual characteristics. This developmental pattern (shared by chimpanzees and, to a lesser extent, gorillas; Bernstein et al. 2012) results in a temporary decoupling between physical and behavioral development, consistent with the idea of middle childhood as a sexually differentiated phase of social learning and experimentation (Geary 2010). Moreover, adrenal androgens promote extended brain plasticity through synaptogenesis and may play an important role in shifting the allocation of the body's energetic resources away from brain development and toward the accumulation of muscle and fat in preparation for puberty (Campbell 2006, 2011; see also Kuzawa et al. 2014).

2 The Transition to Middle Childhood as a Developmental Switch Point

The evolutionary model of middle childhood sketched in the previous section can be enriched and extended by considering the role of adrenarche as a *developmental switch* (Del Giudice et al. 2009). The concept of a developmental switch was introduced by West-Eberhard (2003); a switch is a regulatory mechanism that activates at a specific point in development, collects input from the external environment or the state of the organism, and shifts the individual along alternative pathways—ultimately resulting in the development of alternative phenotypes (morphological, physiological, or behavioral traits of an organism). For example, a switch may regulate the development of aggressive behavior so that safe conditions entrain the development of low levels of aggression, whereas threatening environments trigger high levels of aggression. Developmental switches enable *adaptive plasticity*—the ability of an organism to adjust its phenotype to match the local environment in a way that promotes biological fitness (West-Eberhard 2003). In other words, plastic organisms track the state of the environment—usually through indirect cues—and use this information to develop alternative phenotypes that tend to promote survival or reproduction under different conditions.

Developmental switches work in a *modular* fashion (see Fig. 2). Activation of a switch leads to the coordinated expression of different genes—both those involved in the regulatory mechanism itself and those involved in the production of the new phenotype. Moreover, alternative phenotypes (A and B in Fig. 2) involve the expression of modular packages of genes specific to each phenotype. Another key aspect of developmental switches is that they integrate variation in the environment with individual differences in the genes that regulate the switch. For example, different individuals may have genetically different thresholds for switching between aggressive and nonaggressive phenotypes. Finally, the embodied effects of past experiences and conditions (e.g., an individual's previous exposure to stress or nutritional conditions early in life) may also modulate how the switch functions, allowing the organism to integrate information over time and across different life stages (Del Giudice 2014b; Ellis 2013). In many instances, the effects of past experience on developmental switches may be mediated by epigenetic mechanisms (see Meaney 2010).

The concept of a developmental switch point resembles that of a *sensitive period*, in that the organism is maximally responsive to some environmental input. The crucial difference is that, because genetic and environmental inputs converge in the regulatory mechanism, a developmental switch amplifies both environmental *and*

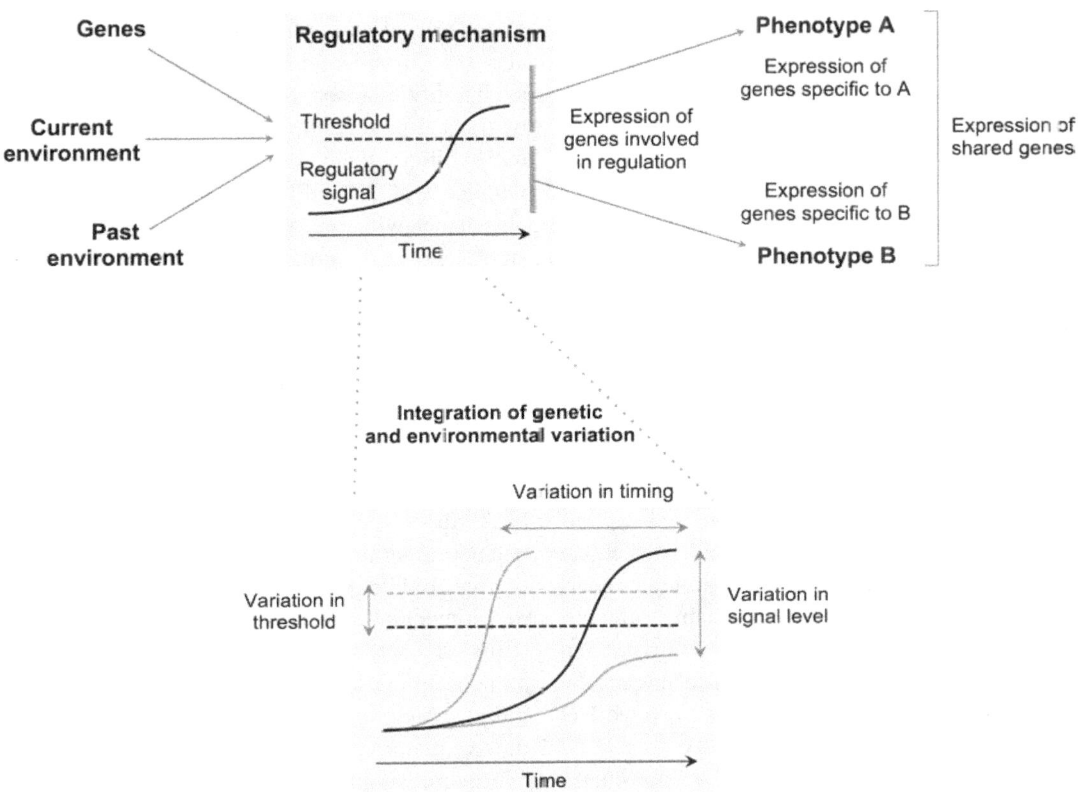

Fig. 2 The concept of a developmental switch. A regulatory mechanism, which may operate through hormonal signals, integrates current and past information from the environment with the individual's genotype. As a result, the individual's developmental trajectory is shifted along alternative pathways—here, A and B—depending on whether a threshold is reached within the mechanism. The location of the threshold, the intensity of the signal, and the timing of the switch point all depend on the joint action of the current state of the environment, the embodied effect of past environmental conditions, and individual variation in the genes involved in the regulatory mechanism. Each alternative pathway involves the modular expression of a set of specific genes, in addition to the shared genes expressed in the new developmental stage. A developmental switch may integrate many sources of input from the environment or produce graded phenotypes rather than discrete alternatives such as A and B

genetic effects on the phenotype (West-Eberhard 2003). Indeed, the activation of a developmental switch exposes many new potential sources of genetic variation, including the genes involved in the regulatory mechanism and in the expression of the new phenotypes (Fig. 2).

2.1 A Switch Point in Life History Development

The role of adrenarche as a developmental switch is not limited to a single trait; in fact, the transition to middle childhood (or *juvenile transition*; Del Giudice et al. 2009) encompasses all the major domains of behavior—from learning and self-regulation to attachment and sexuality (see Table 1). My colleagues and I (Del Giudice and Belsky 2011; Del Giudice et al. 2009, 2012) have argued that the transition to middle childhood is a switch point in the development of *life history strategies*, which are coordinate suites of morphological, physiological, and behavioral traits that determine how organisms allocate their resources to key biological activities such as growth, reproduction, mating, and parenting (for a non-technical overview of life history theory, see Del Giudice et al. 2015). At the level of behavior, individual differences in life history strategy are reflected in patterns of self-regulation, aggression, cooperation and prosociality, attachment, sexuality, and so forth (Del Giudice and Belsky 2011; Del Giudice et al. 2009, 2011; Ellis et al. 2009). Although life history strategies are partly heritable, they also show a degree of plasticity in response to the quality of the environment, including the level of danger and unpredictability –embodied in the experience of early stress—and the availability of adequate nutritional resources. In a nutshell, dangerous and unpredictable environments tend to favor *fast* strategies characterized by early reproduction, sexual promiscuity, unstable relationships, impulsivity, risk taking, aggression, and exploitative tendencies, whereas safe and predictable environments tend to entrain *slow* strategies characterized by late reproduction, stable relationships, high self-control, aversion to risk, and prosociality. Slow strategies are also favored by nutritional scarcity when danger is low (see Del Giudice et al. 2016; Ellis et al. 2009).

Our argument is that adrenarche coordinates the expression of individual differences in life history strategy by integrating individual genetic variation with information about the child's social and physical environment collected throughout infancy and early childhood (Belsky et al. 1991). The stress response system plays a major role in gathering and storing information about environmental safety, predictability, and availability of resources; adrenarche contributes by translating that information into adaptive, sexually differentiated patterns of behavior (Del Giudice et al. 2011; Ellis and Del Giudice 2014). Consistent with this view, both early relational stress and early nutrition have been found to modulate the timing of adrenarche (Ellis and Essex 2007; Hochberg 2008). It is no coincidence that the first sexual and romantic attractions typically develop in middle childhood, in tandem with the intensification of sexual play (Bancroft 2003; Herdt and McClintock 2000). By interacting with peers and adults, juveniles receive feedback about the effectiveness of their nascent behavioral strategies. The information collected during middle childhood feeds into the next developmental switch point, that of gonadarche (Ellis 2013); the transition to adolescence offers an opportunity for youth to adjust or revise their initial strategy before attaining sexual and reproductive maturity (Del Giudice and Belsky 2011).

The role of adrenarche as a switch point in life history development adds another level of complexity to the biological profile of juvenility. Figure 3 outlines an integrated evolutionary-developmental model that brings together the various strands of theory and evidence reviewed in this chapter.

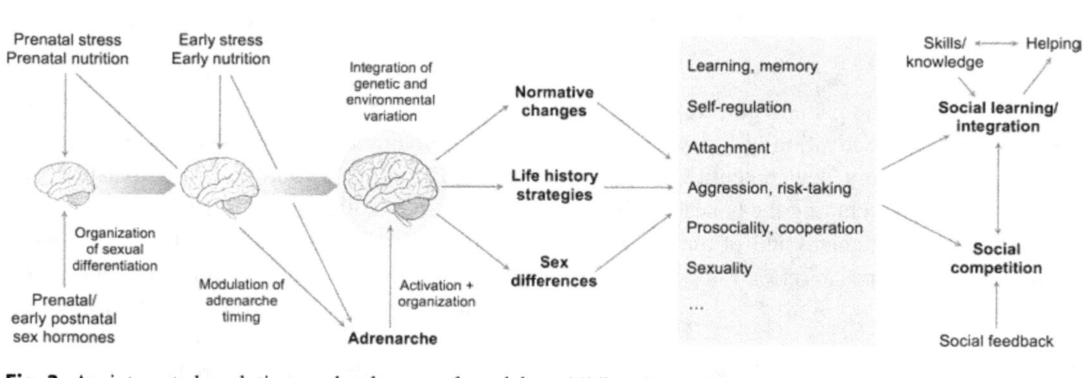

Fig. 3 An integrated evolutionary-developmental model of middle childhood. Adrenarche is shown as a switch in the development of life history strategies, as well as a key mechanism underlying the normative changes of middle childhood and the emergence and intensification of sex differences. At a broader level, development in middle childhood serves two complementary functions, social integration and social competition

3 Three Insights in the Nature of Middle Childhood

3.1 Insight 1: Social Integration and Social Competition Are Complementary Functions of Middle Childhood

Evolutionary accounts of middle childhood typically focus on learning, helping, and other forms of social integration. A life history approach emphasizes the need to consider social competition as a crucial, complementary function of human juvenility. In the peer group, children compete for vital social resources—status, reputation, allies, and friends. While learning and play are relatively risk-free, they are not without consequences. The social position achieved in middle childhood is a springboard for adolescence and adulthood; popularity and centrality within the peer network put a child at a considerable advantage, with potentially long-term effects on mating and reproductive success (Del Giudice et al. 2009).

Physical and relational aggression are obvious tactics for gaining influence, but social competition also occurs through prosocial behaviors such as forming alliances, doing favors, and displaying valuable skills. Indeed, managing the balance between prosocial and coercive tactics is an important part of developing social skills (Hawley 2014). More broadly, competition shapes many aspects of cognitive and behavioral development in middle childhood; for example, increased pragmatic abilities allow children to gossip, joke, tease, and engage in verbal duels—all forms of social competition mediated by language (Locke and Bogin 2006). Intensifying social competition also contributes to explain the early peak of psychopathology onset observed in middle childhood, characterized by increasing rates of externalizing disorders (e.g., conduct disorder), anxiety disorders (including social phobia), and attention deficit hyperactivity disorder (ADHD; Del Giudice et al. 2009).

3.2 Insight 2: Sexual Selection Contributes to the Emergence and Intensification of Sex Differences in Middle Childhood

By determining children's initial place in social networks and hierarchies, competition in middle childhood indirectly affects their ability to attract sexual and romantic partners later. In other words, middle childhood is a likely target for *sexual selection*—that is, natural selection arising from the processes of choosing mates (*mate choice*) and competing for mates (mating *competition*). My colleagues and I (Del Giudice et al. 2009) argued that sexual selection is one reason why sex differences emerge and intensify in middle childhood. In particular, sex differences in physical aggression increase markedly, in tandem with sex differences in muscularity and play fighting. At the same time, attachment styles begin to diverge between males and females, with insecurely attached boys becoming more avoidant and insecure girls becoming more preoccupied/ambivalent (Del Giudice 2009; Del Giudice and Belsky 2010). Different attachment styles are conducive to different social strategies and may be adaptive in regulating children's nascent relationships with peers. There is initial evidence that attachment styles in middle childhood reflect the effects of prenatal sex hormones, which according to our model are activated by adrenal androgens (Del Giudice and Angeleri 2016). Sexual selection also has indirect implications for the development of psychopathology; for example, marked sex differences in the prevalence of conduct disorders become apparent at the beginning of middle childhood, likely reflecting the stronger role of aggression in boys' social competition (see Del Giudice et al. 2009; Martel 2013).

3.3 Insight 3: In Middle Childhood, Heightened Sensitivity to the Environment Goes Hand in Hand with the Expression of New Genetic Factors

When an organism goes through a developmental switch point, inputs from the environment combine with the individual's genotype to determine the resulting phenotype. For example, when adrenal androgens begin to increase during the transition to middle childhood, they activate many hormone-sensitive brain pathways that have been dormant since infancy. In doing so, they release previously hidden genetic variation (Del Giudice et al. 2009). Thus, middle childhood should be characterized by a mixture of heightened sensitivity to the environment—possibly mediated by newly activated epigenetic mechanisms (Meaney 2010) and expression of new genetic factors.

Evidence of increased sensitivity to the environment in middle childhood is not hard to find. Two intriguing and little-known examples concern the development of food preferences and erotic fetishes. In cultures where chili pepper is an essential part of the diet, children tend to dislike spicy food until middle childhood and then increase rapidly their preference for the flavor of chili as a result of social learning (Rozin 1990b). Fetishistic attractions also tend to form in middle childhood, with the onset of pleasurable sensations toward the object of the fetish (e.g., rubber, shoes) that later become fully eroticized (Lawrence 2009). The onset of fetishistic attractions is part of a generalized awakening of sexuality in middle childhood (Table 1) and illustrates the potential for rapid plasticity with long-lasting outcomes. Enhanced sensitivity to the environment extends beyond individual learning to acquiring social norms: for example, cross-cultural differences in prosocial behavior are absent in young children but emerge clearly during middle childhood (House et al. 2013).

On the genetic side of the equation, general intelligence and language skills increase markedly in heritability from early to middle childhood. In both cases, new genetic factors come into play around age 7 (Davis et al. 2009; Hayiou-Thomas et al. 2012). Studies of prosociality and aggression find the same pattern, with new genetic influences on behavior emerging during the transition to middle childhood (Knafo and Plomin 2006; van Beijsterveldt et al. 2003). These genetic findings dovetail with converging evidence that individual changes in levels of aggression are especially frequent during the transition to juvenility (Del Giudice et al. 2009).

4 Implications for Health Development

The main focus of this chapter has been on psychological development, but the implications of the evolutionary-developmental synthesis extend to both mental and physical health. The transition to middle childhood seems to be a switch point for a number of growth and metabolic processes that have long-term impact on health, including the risk for obesity and type 2 diabetes (Hochberg 2008, 2010). These processes become apparent in middle childhood (e.g., anticipated onset of the adiposity rebound, rapid weight gain, onset of insulin resistance), but respond to the accumulated effects of early nutrition and other sources of stress, starting from prenatal life (e.g., intrauterine growth restriction; see Salsberry et al. 2017). From the standpoint of the model presented here, one can predict that metabolic changes in middle childhood will reflect both the "programming" effects of the early environment (Gluckman et al. 2005) and the activation of new genetic factors. Consistent with this view, a recent study has documented significant genetic correlations between puberty timing, insulin levels, type 2 diabetes, and cardiovascular disease (Day et al. 2015). Moreover, some of those factors are likely to be expressed in sexually differentiated ways, and the different patterns of health risk associated with early adrenarche and puberty in boys and girls may be usefully interpreted in light of different constraints on life history trade-offs in the two sexes (see Hochberg 2010). These predictions are consistent with the nonlinear and multilevel nature of developmental processes—one of the guiding principles of LCHD emphasized in this volume.

Another intriguing implication of this perspective is that the juvenile transition may be a promising—and still virtually unexplored—developmental window for intervention. While intervening to change early life conditions may be desirable in view of their long-term effects, this approach is not always possible or realistic. In addition, prenatal factors such as fetal nutrition and gestational stress may be especially difficult to target, as they do not simply mirror the mother's conditions but reflect a complex—and partially conflictual—interplay between fetal and maternal factors (e.g., Del Giudice 2012; Gangestad et al. 2012; Haig 1993). However, the logic of developmental switches (Fig. 2) suggests that the activation of the mechanisms that initiate the switch (e.g., adrenarche) may correspond to a transient phase of instability and openness in the system. If so, it should be possible to exploit that phase to maximize the efficacy of focused interventions—including pharmacological ones. Of course, this would require a better understanding of how different hormonal and neurobiological systems interact during the transition to middle childhood; the existing evidence points to a central role of the hypothalamic-pituitary-adrenal (HPA) axis, the hypothalamic-pituitary-adrenal-thyroid (HPT) axis, and the insulin/insulin-like growth factor 1 (IGF-1) signaling systems as mediators of life history allocations, not just in humans but in other vertebrates as well (see Del Giudice et al. 2015; Ellis and Del Giudice 2014). Those systems might be used as direct targets for intervention, but also as "endophenotypes" or early indicators of the efficacy of interventions. Importantly, neurobiological systems such as the HPA axis regulate both metabolism and behavior—as components of coordinated life history allocations—so that many of the same processes may be relevant to both physical and mental health. The idea that intervening *during* a biological transition may afford more leverage to alter developmental trajectories resonates with two key principles of LCHD, that is, the nonlinearity of developmental processes and their time sensitivity.

Probably the most important take-home point of an evolutionary-developmental approach is that researchers should be more cautious in assuming that undesirable developmental outcomes reflect dysregulation of a biological system (e.g., see Kim et al. 2017) and more open to the possibility that those outcomes may be part of adaptive—or formerly adaptive—strategies for survival and reproduction. As I have argued in detail elsewhere (Del Giudice 2014b, c), a life history framework is especially useful in teasing out the logic of potentially adaptive combinations of traits, highlighting critical factors in the environment, and bridging behavioral development with physical growth trajectories. As an example, consider the association between intrauterine growth restriction and early maturation in children (Hochberg 2008, 2010). This can be interpreted as a manifestation of physiological dysregulation due to prenatal adversity or as an adaptive programming effect on children's metabolic processes and life history trajectories. This alternative interpretation is supported by the association between low birth weight, anticipated puberty, and early childbearing in women (e.g., Nettle et al. 2013). A third possibility is that low birth weight partly reflects reduced energetic and metabolic investment by the mother during pregnancy, which may be adaptive as a component of a fast life history strategy. If so, the association between reduced fetal growth and earlier sexual maturation may not be fully causal, but rather result—at least in part—from shared genetic, or epigenetic, factors that influence life history strategy in both the mother and the offspring. Clearly, the implications for intervention are going to be quite different depending on which of these scenarios apply.

Another recent example is the finding that early adrenarche is associated with reduced white matter volume in the frontal lobe of children (Klauser et al. 2015). Again, the standard interpretation is that early DHEA exposure has a disruptive effect on neurodevelopmental processes; however, it is also possible that different trajectories of brain development—and even associated "symptoms" such as anxiety and aggressive behaviors—may instead reflect alternative strategies on a fast-slow continuum of life history variation. Ellis et al. (2012) present an extended analysis of adolescent risk-taking from this perspective and discuss several implications for the design of interventions. The LCHD principle that evolution both enables and constrains plasticity is especially relevant in this regard; evolutionary scenarios are not just interesting explanatory "stories," but can illuminate limits as well as opportunities for intervention. For example, when considering mother-fetus interactions, the existence of partial conflicts of interest on nutrition, cortisol production, and so on suggests that interventions designed to favor the fetus may sometimes have detrimental side effects for the mother and vice versa (see Del Giudice 2014b; Haig 1993).

In considering potential adaptive explanations for apparently pathological outcomes, it is important to remember that biologically adaptive traits may carry substantial costs. Fitness is ultimately about reproductive success; natural selection does not necessarily promote psychological well-being or physical health and may sacrifice survival in exchange for enhanced reproduction. Moreover, even adaptive developmental processes may result in genuinely maladaptive outcomes for some individuals (Frankenhuis and Del Giudice 2012). It follows that the existence of substantial psychological, social, or health costs does not automatically qualify a trait or behavior as biologically maladaptive (see Del Giudice 2014b; Ellis et al. 2012; Ellis and Del Giudice 2014).

5 Conclusions

We cannot make sense of human development without understanding middle childhood and its many apparent paradoxes. An evolutionary-developmental approach illuminates the complexity of this life stage and shows how different levels of analysis—from genes to society—can be tied together in a coherent synthesis. This emerging view of middle childhood can help developmental scientists appreciate its centrality in the human life history and stimulate ideas for research and intervention. The study of middle childhood may finally be ready to come of age, opening up promising avenues for a better understanding of health development across the life course.

References

Auchus, R. J., & Rainey, W. E. (2004). Adrenarche–physiology, biochemistry and human disease. *Clinical Endocrinology, 60*, 288–296.

Bancroft, J. (Ed.). (2003). *Sexual development in childhood*. Bloomington: Indiana University Press.

Belsky, J., Steinberg, L., & Draper, P. (1991). Childhood experience, interpersonal development, and reproductive strategy: An evolutionary theory of socialization. *Child Development, 62*, 647–670.

Bernstein, R. M., Sterner, K. N., & Wildman, D. E. (2012). Adrenal androgen production in catarrhine primates and the evolution of adrenarche. *American Journal of Physical Anthropology, 147*, 389–400.

Best, J. R., Miller, P. H., & Jones, L. L. (2009). Executive functions after age 5: Changes and correlates. *Developmental Review, 29*, 180–200.

Bjorklund, D. F. (2011). *Children's thinking: Cognitive development and individual differences* (5th ed.). Belmont: Wadsworth.

Bogin, B. (1997). Evolutionary hypotheses for human childhood. *Yearbook of Physical Anthropology, 40*, 63–89.

Campbell, B. C. (2006). Adrenarche and the evolution of human life history. *American Journal of Human Biology, 18*, 569–589.

Campbell, B. C. (2011). Adrenarche and middle childhood. *Human Nature, 22*, 327–349.

Davis, O. S. P., Haworth, C. M. A., & Plomin, R. (2009). Dramatic increase in heritability of cognitive development from early to middle childhood: An 8-year longitudinal study of 8,700 pairs of twins. *Psychological Science, 20*, 1301–1308.

Day, F. R., Bulik-Sullivan, B., Hinds, D. A., Finucane, H. K., Murabito, J. M., Tung, J. Y., et al. (2015). Genetic determinants of puberty timing in men and women: Shared genetic aetiology between sexes and with health-related outcomes. *Nature Communications, 6*, 8842.

Del Giudice, M. (2009). Sex, attachment, and the development of reproductive strategies. *Behavioral and Brain Sciences, 32*, 1–21.

Del Giudice, M. (2012). Fetal programming by maternal stress: Insights from a conflict perspective. *Psychoneuroendocrinology, 37*, 1614–1629.

Del Giudice, M. (2014a). Middle childhood: An evolutionary-developmental synthesis. *Child Development Perspectives, 8*, 193–200.

Del Giudice, M. (2014b). Early stress and human behavioral development: Emerging evolutionary perspectives. *Journal of Developmental Origins of Health and Disease, 5*, 270–280.

Del Giudice, M. (2014c). An evolutionary life history framework for psychopathology. *Psychological Inquiry, 25*, 261–300.

Del Giudice, M., & Angeleri, R. (2016). Digit ratio (2D:4D) and attachment styles in middle childhood: Indirect evidence for an organizational effect of sex hormones. *Adaptive Human Behavior and Physiology, 2*, 1–10.

Del Giudice, M., & Belsky, J. (2010). Sex differences in attachment emerge in middle childhood: An evolutionary hypothesis. *Child Development Perspectives, 4*, 97–105.

Del Giudice, M., & Belsky, J. (2011). The development of life history strategies: Toward a multi-stage theory. In D. M. Buss & P. H. Hawley (Eds.), *The evolution of personality and individual differences*, (pp. 154–176). New York: Oxford University Press.

Del Giudice, M., Angeleri, R., & Manera, V. (2009). The juvenile transition: A developmental switch point in human life history. *Developmental Review, 29*, 1–31.

Del Giudice, M., Ellis, B. J., & Shirtcliff, E. A. (2011). The adaptive calibration model of stress responsivity. *Neuroscience & Biobehavioral Reviews, 35*, 1562–1592.

Del Giudice, M., Angeleri, R., & Manera, V. (2012). Juvenility and the juvenile transition. In R. J. R. Levesque (Ed.), *Encyclopedia of adolescence*, (pp. 1534–1537). New York: Springer.

Del Giudice, M., Gangestad, S. W., & Kaplan, H. S. (2015). Life history theory and evolutionary psychology. In D. M. Buss (Ed.), *The handbook of evolutionary psychology – Vol 1: Foundations* (2nd ed., pp. 88–114). New York: Wiley.

Del Giudice, M., & Angeleri, R. (2016). Digit ratio (2D:4D) and attachment styles in middle childhood: Indirect evidence for an organizational effect of sex hormones. *Adaptive Human Behavior and Physiology, 2*, 1–10.

Ellis, B. J. (2013). The hypothalamic-pituitary-gonadal axis: A switch-controlled, condition-sensitive system in the regulation of life history strategies. *Hormones and Behavior, 64*, 215–225.

Ellis, B. J., & Del Giudice, M. (2014). Beyond allostatic load: Rethinking the role of stress in regulating human development. *Development and Psychopathology, 26*, 1–20.

Ellis, B. J., & Essex, M. J. (2007). Family environments, adrenarche and sexual maturation: A longitudinal test of a life history model. *Child Development, 78*, 1799–1817.

Ellis, B. J., Figueredo, A. J., Brumbach, B. H., & Schlomer, G. L. (2009). The impact of harsh versus unpredictable environments on the evolution and development of life history strategies. *Human Nature, 20*, 204–268.

Ellis, B. J., Del Giudice, M., Dishion, T. J., Figueredo, A. J., Gray, P., Griskevicius, V., et al. (2012). The evolutionary basis of risky adolescent behavior: Implications for science, policy, and practice. *Developmental Psychology, 48*, 598–623.

Frankenhuis, W. E., & Del Giudice, M. (2012). When do adaptive developmental mechanisms yield maladaptive outcomes? *Developmental Psychology, 48*, 628–642.

Gangestad, S. W., Caldwell Hooper, A. E., & Eaton, M. A. (2012). On the function of placental corticotropin-releasing hormone: A role in maternal-fetal conflicts over blood glucose concentrations. *Biological Reviews, 87*, 856–873.

Geary, D. C. (2010). *Male, female: The evolution of human sex differences*. Washington, DC: American Psychological Association.

Ghetti, S., & Bunge, S. A. (2012). Neural changes underlying the development of episodic memory during middle childhood. *Developmental Cognitive Neuroscience, 2*, 381–395.

Giedd, J. N., & Rapoport, J. L. (2010). Structural MRI of pediatric brain development: What have we learned and where are we going? *Neuron, 67*, 728–734.

Gluckman, P. D., Hanson, M. A., & Spencer, H. G. (2005). Predictive adaptive responses and human evolution. *Trends in Ecology & Evolution, 20*, 527–533.

Haig, D. (1993). Genetic conflicts in human pregnancy. *QUARTERLY REVIEW OF BIOLOGY, 68*, 495–532.

Hawley, P. H. (2014). Ontogeny and social dominance: A developmental view of human power patterns. *Evolutionary Psychology, 12*, 318–342.

Hayiou-Thomas, M. E., Dale, P. S., & Plomin, R. (2012). The etiology of variation in language skills changes with development: A longitudinal twin study of language from 2 to 12 years. *Developmental Science, 15*, 233–249.

Herdt, G., & McClintock, M. (2000). The magical age of 10. *Archives of Sexual Behavior, 29*, 587–606.

Hochberg, Z. (2008). Juvenility in the context of life history theory. *Archives of Disease in Childhood, 93*, 534–539.

Hochberg, Z. (2010). Evo-devo of child growth III: Premature juvenility as an evolutionary trade-off. *Hormone Research in Pædiatrics, 73*, 430–437.

House, B. R., Silk, J. B., Henrich, J., Barrett, H. C., Scelza, B. A., Boyette, A. H., et al. (2013). Ontogeny of prosocial behavior across diverse societies. *Proceedings of the National Academy of Sciences USA, 110*, 14586–14591.

Jambon, M., & Smetana, J. G. (2014). Moral complexity in middle childhood: Children's evaluations of necessary harm. *Developmental Psychology, 50*, 22–33.

Joffe, T. H. (1997). Social pressures have selected for an extended juvenile period in primates. *Journal of Human Evolution, 32*, 593–605.

Kaplan, H., Hill, K., Lancaster, J., & Hurtado, A. M. (2000). A theory of human life history evolution: Diet, intelligence, and longevity. *Evolutionary Anthropology, 9*, 156–185.

Kim, P., Evans, G. W., Chen, E., Miller, G., & Seeman, T. (2017). How socioeconomic disadvantages get under the skin and into the brain to influence health development across the lifespan. In N. Halfon, C. B. Forrest, R. M. Lerner, & E. Faustman (Eds.), *Handbook of life course health-development science*. Cham: Springer.

Klauser, P., Whittle, S., Simmons, J. G., Byrne, M. L., Mundy, L. K., Patton, G. C., et al. (2015). Reduced frontal white matter volume in children with early onset of adrenarche. *Psychoneuroendocrinology, 52*, 111–118.

Knafo, A., & Plomin, R. (2006). Prosocial behavior from early to middle childhood: Genetic and environmental influences on stability and change. *Developmental Psychology, 42*, 771–786.

Kramer, K. L. (2011). The evolution of human parental care and recruitment of juvenile help. *Trends in Ecology and Evolution, 26*, 533–540.

Kuzawa, C. W., Chugani, H. T., Grossman, L. I., Lipovich, L., Muzik, O., Hof, P. R., et al. (2014). Metabolic costs and evolutionary implications of human brain development. *Proceedings of the National Academy of Sciences of the United States of America, 111*, 13010–13015.

Lagattuta, K. H., Sayfan, L., & Blattman, A. J. (2009). Forgetting common ground: Six- to seven-year-olds have an overinterpretive theory of mind. *Developmental Psychology, 46*, 1417–1432.

Lancy, D. F., & Grove, M. A. (2011). Getting noticed: Middle childhood in cross-cultural perspective. *Human Nature, 22*, 281–302.

Lawrence, A. A. (2009). Erotic target location errors: An underappreciated paraphilic dimension. *Journal of Sex Research, 46*, 194–215.

Lebel, C., Walker, L., Leemans, A., Phillips, L., & Beaulieu, C. (2008). Microstructural maturation of the human brain from childhood to adulthood. *NeuroImage, 40*, 1044–1055.

Locke, J. L., & Bogin, B. (2006). Language and life history: A new perspective on the development and evolution of human language. *Behavioral and Brain Sciences, 29*, 259–280.

Martel, M. M. (2013). Sexual selection and sex differences in the prevalence of childhood externalizing and adolescent internalizing disorders. *Psychological Bulletin, 139*, 1221–1259.

McClelland, M., Morrison, F., Gestsdóttir, S., Cameron, C., Bowers, E. D., Duckworth, A., Little, T., & Grammer. J. (2017). Self-regulation. In N. Halfon, C. B. Forrest, R. M. Lerner, & E. Faustman (Eds.), *Handbook of life course health-development science*. Cham: Springer.

Meaney, M. J. (2010). Epigenetics and the biological definition of gene x environment interactions. *Child Development, 81*, 41–79.

Nettle, D., Dickins, T. E., Coall, D. A., & de Mornay Davies, P. (2013). Patterns of physical and psychological development in future teenage mothers. *Evolution, Medicine, and Public Health, 2013*, 187–196.

Piccardi, L., Leonzi, M., D'Amico, S., Marano, A., & Guariglia, C. (2014). Development of navigational working memory: Evidence from 6- to 10-year-old children. *British Journal of Developmental Psychology, 32*, 205–217.

Poirel, N., Simon, G., Cassotti, M., Leroux, G., Perchey, G., Lanoë, C., Lubin, A., Turbelin, M. R., Rossi, S., Pineau, A., & Houdé, O. (2011). The shift from local to global visual processing in 6-year-old children is associated with grey matter loss. *PloS One, 6*, e20879.

Rozin, P. (1990a). Development in the food domain. *Developmental Psychology, 26*, 555–562.

Rozin, P. (1990b). Getting to like the burn of chili pepper: Biological, psychological, and cultural perspectives. In B. G. Green, J. R. Mason, & M. R. Kare (Eds.), *Chemical senses – Volume 2: Irritation*. New York: Dekker.

Salsberry, P., Tanda, R., Anderson, S. E., & Kamboj, M. K. (2017). Pediatric type 2 diabetes: Prevention and treatment through a life course health development framework. In N. Halfon, C. B. Forrest, R. M. Lerner, & E. Faustman (Eds.), *Handbook of life course health-development science*. Cham: Springer.

Scalise Sugiyama, M. (2011). The forager oral tradition and the evolution of prolonged juvenility. *Frontiers in Psychology, 2*, 133.

van Beijsterveldt, T. C. E. M., Bartels, M., Hudziak, J. J., & Boomsma, D. I. (2003). Causes of stability of aggression from early childhood to adolescence: A longitudinal genetic analysis in Dutch twins. *Behavior Genetics, 33*, 591–605.

Weisner, T. S. (1996). The 5–7 transition as an eco-cultural project. In A. Sameroff & M. Haith (Eds.), *The five to seven year shift: The age of reason and responsibility* (pp. 295–326). Chicago: University of Chicago Press.

Wells, J. C. K. (2007). Sexual dimorphism of body composition. *Best Practice & Research Clinical Endocrinology & Metabolism, 21*, 415–430.

West-Eberhard, M. J. (2003). *Developmental plasticity and evolution*. New York: Oxford University Press.

3

Adolescent Health Development: A Relational Developmental Systems Perspective

Richard M. Lerner, Claire D. Brindis, Milena Batanova, and Robert Wm. Blum

Consistent with the United Nations Conventions, adolescence encompasses the second decade of life (Lerner and Steinberg 2009). Since the emergence of the study of this portion of the life course (Hall 1904), adolescence has been regarded as a period characterized by purportedly troublesome transformations (e.g., in bodily attributes associated with puberty; Susman and Dorn 2009, 2013) and allegedly problematic transitions (e.g., in regard to socioemotional functions linked to self-definition or identity, Erikson 1959, or to changes in the focus of social relationships, from parents to peers, Freud 1969). When viewed from this "deficit" model, adolescents were seen by both scholars and the general public as both dangerous to themselves and to society (Anthony 1969). They were regarded as "problems to be managed" (Roth and Brooks-Gunn 2003a, b).

Certainly, it may be argued that adolescence is the most profound period of change within the life span. As in infancy and early to middle childhood, the individual's physiological, psychological, behavioral, and social relationship characteristics undergo both quantitative and qualitative changes, that is, transitions and transformations. For instance, changes in the prefrontal cortex, increases in the interconnectivity among brain regions, and increases in dopamine levels provide both vulnerabilities to risk and opportunities for growth in cognitive control (Steinberg 2010). At the same time, most youth in Western societies are experiencing great contextual changes, such as changing schools (e.g., Eccles 2004) and the increased relevance of peer influences on behavior (e.g., Gardner and Steinberg 2005). Moreover, in adolescence, the individual has the cognitive, behavioral, and social relational skills to contribute actively and often effectively to his or her own developmental changes (Lerner 1982; Lerner and Busch-Rossnagel 1981; Lerner and Walls 1999; Ricco and Overton 2011). In contrast to earlier developmental periods, adolescents have a burgeoning capacity

---

The writing of this chapter was supported in part by grants from the John Templeton Foundation. We are grateful to Elizabeth Goodman for her comments

R.M. Lerner, PhD (✉)
Tufts University, Medford, MA, USA
e-mail: Richard.lerner@tufts.edu

M. Batanova, PhD
Institute for Applied Research in Youth Development, Tufts University, Medford, MA, USA

C.D. Brindis, DrPH
University of California-San Francisco (UCSF), Philip R. Lee Institute for Health Policy Studies and the Adolescent and Young Adult Health National Resource Center, San Francisco, CA, USA

R.Wm. Blum, MD, MPH, PhD
Johns Hopkins Bloomberg School of Public Health, Baltimore, MD, USA

for self-governance, for formulating and taking actions that exert at least some control over their own development. That is, there is uniquely marked development of intentional agency in adolescence. Agency involves self-regulatory skills that include, for instance, the *selection* of goals or the formulation of purposes that are of importance to adolescents' developing senses of self and growing attempts to find a means to "matter" in their world (Eccles 2004; Freund and Baltes 2002; Mascolo and Fischer 2015). There is also growth in the use of executive functioning, strategic thinking, and behavioral skills in recruiting goal-related resources that enable actions *optimizing* the chances of fulfilling their purposes. Furthermore, there is also development of the ability to *compensate* effectively when goals are blocked and/or to select new goals when initial optimization attempts fail and the chances of attaining an initial goal are lost (Gestsdottir and Lerner 2008; McClelland et al. 2015).

In general, scholars who study the adolescent period acknowledge that multiple dimensions of change involving the individual and his or her context characterize this portion of the life span (Lerner et al. 2015; Lerner and Steinberg 2009). However, substantial variation has emerged in scholars' approach to this individual-context relationship. Analogous to interpreting only main effects of statistical analyses framed by the General Linear Model, some scholars have focused on one domain of change (e.g., adolescent identity development) and have not emphasized other levels of organization within the ecology of human development (e.g., see Marcia 1980). Other scholars have taken a reductionist orientation to the phenomena of adolescence and have sought to use biogenic ideas (e.g., genetic or evolutionary biological ideas; see Bjorkland and Ellis, 2005) to interpret all psychological and social relationship phenomena of the period (see Elder 1980, 1998; Elder et al. 2015, for critiques of the main effect or reductionist approaches).

In turn, however, in 2003, Roth and Brooks-Gunn (2003a, b) reviewed the literature on youth development programs aimed at enhancing health and thriving among adolescents. They concluded that adolescents should be regarded not as problems to be managed but, instead, as resources to be developed. Their insight built on at least three sources. First, Larson (2000) provided a compelling vision for research aimed at emphasizing the strengths of adolescence (e.g., involving their burgeoning capacities for intentional self-regulation) and for using these strengths to promote positive youth development (PYD). Instead of health or positive development being conceptualized as the diminution or the absence of disease or of problem behaviors, respectively, the PYD perspective suggested that there were facets of thriving that, when promoted, resulted in healthy and positive development. Second, Eccles and Gootman (2002) edited a field-defining report issued by the National Academy of Sciences about the ways in which community programs for youth development could promote several attributes of psychological and behavioral functioning believed to be indicative of such development. The report included a summary of the attributes of positive development as involving constructs that could be summarized by "Five Cs:" competence, confidence, character, connection, and caring (see too, Lerner et al. 2005). Third, Hamilton (1999) explained that the idea of PYD was being used in the developmental science literature in three ways: (a) as a label for a model of the processes through which health and thriving developed in adolescence, (b) as a philosophy for or an approach to designing community-based programs aimed at promoting thriving, and (c) as instances of such programs.

The emphasis on strengths as compared to deficits and on links between the positive development of youth and their engagement with contextual resources or ecological "developmental assets" (Benson et al. 2006), represented by community-based youth development programs, reflected the spirit of the times (the *zeitgeist*) of developmental science during the latter years of the twentieth century and the first decade of the twenty-first century (Lerner 2012; Lerner et al. 2015). Conceptions of human development, which in earlier periods stressed genetic or maturational determinants of development or approaches to development that reduced human behavior to stimulus-response relations, were being replaced by ideas emphasizing that development involved mutually influential relations among a person's biological and psychological characteristics, social relationships, and influences from families, schools, community institutions, out-of-school-time (OST) programs, and both the designed and natural environment.

Developmental scientists argued that all of these influences, although always present across life, change in their significance across both life and across historical periods (e.g., Bronfenbrenner and Morris 2006; Lerner 2012; Overton 2013, 2015). Indeed, we explain below that, today, these ideas have a new manifestation quite compatible with the PYD perspective: They are found in the seven principles of life course health development (see Halfon and Forrest 2017) that address the conceptualization of the nature and bases of health and positive behavior development across the life span.

Therefore, in the contemporary study of adolescent development, the main effect and reductionist approaches of the past are regarded as anachronistic ideas incapable of producing models that adequately account for the integration of multiple levels of organization within the ecology of human development (Lerner 2015; Lerner and Benson 2013a, b; Lerner et al. 2015). In particular, such traditional approaches overlook the burgeoning information indicating that this integration reflects systemic relations, that is, mutually influential patterns of covariation within and across these levels (e.g., see von Bertalanffy 1933, 1968). At this writing, then, models of adolescent development that are associated with what Overton has explained as a relational developmental systems (RDS) metatheory define the cutting edge of theory-predicated scholarship about adolescent development. This metatheory is derived from a process-relational paradigm (Overton 2015), and the concepts associated with RDS thinking are being used to describe, explain, and optimize the course of development in the second decade of life and, as such, to frame applied research aimed at promoting health and positive development among diverse adolescents (Lerner et al. 2015).

It is not coincidental that concepts associated with the RDS metatheory are entirely consistent with the seven life course health development principles proposed by Halfon and Forrest (2017). This congruence of ideas is based on a few common scholarly roots of these two sets of ideas for understanding human development. For example, the life course conceptions of Elder (1998; Elder et al. 2015), the life span developmental ideas of Baltes (e.g., 1997; Baltes et al. 2006), and the constructs associated with Bronfenbrenner's (1979, 2005; Bronfenbrenner and Morris 2006) bioecological model of human development have shaped both RDS thinking and the life course health development principles. It will be useful, then, to discuss the features of the RDS metatheory and, in this context, point to the compatibility between RDS concepts and the life course health development principles. This discussion will enable us to illustrate how the ideas associated with both approaches to adolescent development can innovatively integrate and extend scholarship about transitions and transformations characterizing the adolescent period. In addition, because of the emphasis in both sets of ideas on the concept of relative *plasticity* in human development—that is, on the potential for systematic changes in the structure and function of health assets across the life course—we will discuss how these two approaches afford optimism that relational changes linked to positive change in the health developmental system can be identified and used to promote thriving in adolescence.

1 Viewing Adolescent Development Through the Lens of the Relational Developmental Systems Metatheory

The study of human development, in general, and adolescent development, more specifically, has evolved from a field dominated by split, reductionist (psychogenic or biogenic) approaches to a multidisciplinary scholarly field (Lerner and Steinberg 2009), one that seeks to integrate variables from biological through cultural and historical levels of organization across the life span into a synthetic, coactional system (e.g., Elder 1998; Ford and Lerner 1992; Gottlieb 1997, 1998; Lerner 2012). Reductionist accounts of development that adhere to a Cartesian dualism pull apart (split) facets of the integrated developmental system (Overton 2015). For instance, reductionist views typically elevate the importance of such split formulations as nature versus nurture, continuity versus discontinuity, stability versus instability, or basic versus applied science (Lerner 2002, 2006).

Split approaches are rejected by proponents of theories derived from an RDS metatheory (e.g., Mistry and Wu 2010; Overton 2013; Overton and Lerner 2014), which in turn are derived from a process-relational paradigm (Overton 2015). Across the past four plus decades, several scholars have provided ideas contributing to the evolution of this paradigm (e.g., Baltes 1997; Baltes, et al., 2006; Brandtstädter 1998; Bronfenbrenner 1979, 2005; Bronfenbrenner and Morris 2006; Elder 1998; Elder et al. 2015; Ford and Lerner 1992; Nesselroade 1988; Overton 1973; Overton and Reese 1981; Riegel 1975, 1976; and, even earlier, see von Bertalanffy 1933).

Overton (e.g., 2013, 2015) has integrated and extended this scholarship. Overton explains that, compared to a Cartesian worldview, the process-relational paradigm focuses on process (systematic changes in the developmental system), becoming (moving from potential to actuality; a developmental process as having a past, present, and future; Whitehead 1929/1978), holism (the meanings of entities and events derive from the context in which they are embedded), relational analysis (assessment of the mutually influential relations within the developmental system), and the use of multiple perspectives and explanatory forms (employment of ideas from multiple theory-based models of change within and of the developmental system) in understanding human development. Within the process-relational paradigm, the organism is seen as inherently active, self-creating (autopoietic), self-organizing, self-regulating (agentic), nonlinear/complex, and adaptive (Overton 2015; see too Sokol et al. 2015). Similarly, these ideas are echoed in the life course health development principles (specifically, Nos. 1 and 3) that health development emerges as a consequence of complex, nonlinear process that results from person⇔environment coactions that are multidimensional, multidirectional, and multilevel.

Accordingly, both within the RDS approach to theory and the life course health development principles, split conceptions are eschewed in favor of a metatheory that emphasizes the study and integration of different levels of organization, ranging from biology/physiology to culture and history, as a means to understand life span human development (Lerner 2006; Overton 2013, 2015), the production of health, and the development of disease. Accordingly, conceptual emphasis is placed on mutually influential relations between individuals and contexts, represented as individual ⇔ context relations.

This representation of the coactions between person and setting within RDS-based models is not meant to convey a person-context interaction—which is typically represented in the developmental literature as person X context. An interaction connotes that the entities involved in the relation are separate and independent (as in a statistical interaction) and that, as such, their association involves a linear combination of discrete and separate variables. Both before and after the interaction, these entities (variables) are independent and unchanged by each other. The bidirectional arrow used in the RDS illustration of person ⇔ context relations is intended to emphasize that the coaction of individual and context involves the entire developmental system. As such, the relations among levels of the autopoietic system, and not independent linear combinatorial attributes, are the focus in such a model. Indeed, the fusion of individual and context within the developmental system means that across ontogeny (across the life span), any portion of the system is inextricably embedded with—or embodied by, in Overton's (2013, 2015) conceptualization—all other portions of the developmental system. Embodiment refers to the way individuals behave, experience, and live in the world by being active agents with particular kinds of bodies; the body is integratively understood as a form (a biological referent), as lived experience (a psychological referent), and as an entity in active engagement with the world (a sociocultural referent) (Overton 2015).

Similarly, within the life course health development perspective, health development is also embodied: It is an emergent property of living systems (Principle 1), and it develops continuously across the life span (Principle 2).

Within the context of such a bidirectional relational system, the embeddedness within history (temporality) is of fundamental significance (Elder 1998; Elder et al. 2015). We may note that the developmental system is embedded in history (temporality). This embeddedness means that change is constant in the developmental system and that, as such, there may be either stochastic or systematic changes in person⇔context relations *across time and place* (Elder 1998; Elder et al. 2015; Misteli 2013). Sensitivity of change to time and place is also a key idea within the life course health development Principle 4, which states that health development is highly sensitive to the timing and social structure of environmental exposures. The presence of such temporality in individual ⇔ context relations within the developmental system means that there always exists some potential for systematic change and, thus, for (relative) plasticity in human development. In short, potential plasticity in individual ⇔ context relations derives from the "arrow of time" (Lerner 1984; Lerner and Benson 2013a, b; Overton 2013) running through the integrated (relational) developmental system.

2 Three Moments of Analysis in an RDS Approach to Adolescent Health Development

To elucidate the role of time and place in contributing to the bidirectional relations of focal concern within RDS metatheory, developmental scientists may focus on either the role of the individual or the context, in particular instantiations of individual⇔context exchanges. This focus may seem contradictory to the fusion among levels of organization emphasized in this approach. However, as we noted earlier, Overton (2015) embeds the RDS metatheory in the process-relational paradigm (see, as well, Sokol et al. 2015). Overton uses this paradigm to explain the possibility of this changing focus in developmental analysis. He notes that the process-relational paradigm involves different moments within a research program.

One moment involves the idea of the identity of opposites, a second moment involves the opposites of identity, and a third (relationally integrative) moment involves the synthesis of wholes. In discussing these three moments of scientific analysis within RDS approaches to developmental science, we point to the predominant trait model of individuality, the Five-Factor Theory (FFT, involving the purported Big Five "personality traits" of conscientiousness, agreeableness, neuroticism, openness to experience, and extraversion; Costa and McCrae 1980, 2006; McCrae et al. 2000). The FFT example is a means to explain these RDS-based moments and to contrast their use with thinking associated with Cartesian, split, reductionist approaches to the study of the individual development.

The first moment recognizes that both individual and context define— and are mutually constituted by—each other in one moment, or point, in a program of developmental inquiry. Overton (2010, p. 14) notes that:

> The principle of the identity of opposites establishes the identity among parts of a whole by casting them not as exclusive contradictions as in the split epistemology, but as differentiated polarities (i.e., coequals) of a unified (i.e., indissociable) inclusive matrix—as a relation. As differentiations, each pole defines and is defined by its opposite.

The identity of opposites, therefore, emphasizes the fused person ⇔ context relationship as the primary unit of analysis for understanding development. As such, in this moment of research, developmental scientists would reject the idea that there are any aspects of human *behavioral* development— for instance, entities such as traits—that "are more or less immune to environmental influences" (McCrae et al. 2000, pp. 175); the idea that such entities are indicators of split notions reflecting "nature over nurture" (McCrae et al. 2000, p. 173) would also be rejected by developmental scientists working within this first moment of analysis.

The second moment that Overton (2010, 2013, 2015; Overton and Müller 2013) discusses is the opposites of identity. This moment allows one, in effect, to hold the other parts of the integrated system in abeyance and focus on one part of the system; however, the ultimate aim is one of reintegrating the part into the whole at a subsequent moment. Overton (2013, pp. 47–48) explains that:

> The limitation of the identity moment of analysis is that, in establishing a flow of categories of one into the other, a stable base for inquiry that was provided by bedrock material atoms of the split metatheory is eliminated...Reestablishing a stable base—not an absolute fixity, nor an absolute relativity, but a relative relativity (Latour 1993)—within relational metatheory requires moving to a second moment of analysis. In this moment of opposition, the law of contradiction is reasserted and categories again exclude each other. As a consequence of this exclusion, parts exhibit unique identities that differentiate each from the other.

Therefore, when functioning within this second moment of analysis, developmental scientists could focus solely on attributes of individuals, for instance, the purported traits of conscientiousness, agreeableness, neuroticism, openness to experience, and extraversion that comprise the Big Five components of the FFT (Costa and McCrae 1980, 2006; McCrae et al. 2000) and, for instance, study the psychometric properties of these constructs to provide "objective," or quantitative, indices of these attributes. Indeed, such psychometric work has often been a part of research programs framed by RDS models (e.g., Damon 2008; Lerner et al. 2015). Thus, working within this second moment of analysis, developmental scientists following an RDS-based model, and social or personality researchers using a Cartesian split model, would be engaging in commensurate work. However, the difference between these two groups of scholars is brought to the fore when the third moment of analysis discussed by Overton (2015) is considered.

The third moment, the synthesis of wholes, occurs when the first two moments are embedded in a multi-perspective process-relational paradigm and are recognized as mutually necessary in a systematic, integrative program of research, wherein one needs both of the first two moments. That is, "A complete relational program requires principles according to which the individual identity of each concept of a formerly dichotomous pair is maintained while simultaneously it is affirmed that each concept constitutes, and is constituted by the other" (Overton and Müller 2013, p. 35).

Accordingly, the developmental scientist working within an RDS model would use an "objective" measure studied within the second moment of analysis within an integrated, relational empirical approach that focused on the individual⇔context relation. Clearly, the trait theorist would not take such a step, given that the work of such scholars is framed by the ideas, noted above, that context is irrelevant to the understanding (i.e., successful prediction) of the life course of the manifestation of traits. Indeed, in their belief "that personality traits are more or less immune to environmental influences" (McCrae et al. 2000, pp. 175), trait theorists maintain that contextual conditions, whether similar or not, are irrelevant to prediction; given the purported biological base of traits, only nature variables have predictive efficacy.

However, there is abundant evidence that purported traits are in fact not "trait-like" at all, that is, these attributes reflect relations between individuals and contexts, as they occur at particular times and places (Ardelt 2000; Block 1995, 2010; Elder 1998; Elder et al. 2015; Roberts et al. 2006). Indeed, methodological work framed by RDS concepts (e.g., Molenaar and Nesselroade 2014, 2015; Nesselroade 1988; Nesselroade and Molenaar 2010) indicates that the purported life span stability of traits, as well as the purported immunity to contextual influences, is empirically counterfactual. Moreover, underscoring the importance of this third moment of analysis discussed by Overton (2015), these methodological innovations demonstrate the ability to index with psychometric precision integrative individual ⇔ context (including individual ⇔ individual) units of analysis (e.g., Molenaar 2014; Molenaar et al. 2014; Molenaar and Nesselroade 2015). This innovation in developmental methodology is important for understanding key features of the individual⇔context relational process propelling developmental change in adolescence.

3 Developmental Regulations, Adaptive Developmental Regulations, and Human Agency in RDS Metatheory

Given the analytic moment of the identity of opposites—that each component of the developmental system constitutes, and is constituted by, the other components of the system—RDS metatheory focuses on the "rules" or processes which govern, or regulate, exchanges between individuals and their contexts. Such processes are the function of the developmental system. An RDS program of research might seek to understand the nature of relations between individuals and their contexts, including the dynamics of those relations across the life course. For instance, RDS-based research might ask how specific features of the individual and specific features of the context coalesce to influence the substantive course of individual⇔individual relations.

Brandtstädter (1998) termed these bidirectional relations "developmental regulations" and noted that, when developmental regulations involve mutually beneficial individual⇔context relations, then these developmental regulations are adaptive. Developmental regulations are the fundamental feature of human life, that is, all human life exists in a context and involves bidirectional exchanges with it (Darwin 1859; Forrest 2014; Tobach and Schneirla 1968). These exchanges involve physiological systems and functions (e.g., respiration, circulation, digestion, reproduction) and behaviors (e.g., social affiliation and cooperation, or aggression and competition, as might be involved in protection, hunting, and scavenging; Johanson and Edey 1981) and involve both organismic self-regulation (e.g., hypothalamic functioning, circadian rhythms) and intentional self-regulation (e.g., goal selection, resource recruitment, and executive functioning; Gestsdóttir and Lerner 2008).

Gestsdóttir et al. (2014) note that self-regulation is a multidimensional construct, involving a range of behaviors, from basic physiological functions to complex intentional cognitive processes (e.g., Bandura 2001; Brandtstädter 1998; McClelland et al. 2015). As such, self-regulation pertains to all aspects of adaption, as people alter their thoughts, attention, emotions, and behaviors to react to contextual events and, as well, to influence selected features of their contexts. Here, culture plays a key moderating role. Trommsdorff (2012) notes that self-regulation "is assumed to develop by organizing inner mental processes and behavior in line with cultural values, social expectations, internalized standards, and one's self-construal" (p. 19).

The developmental course of self-regulation is, in effect, the developmental course of human agency in the context of individual desires, purposes, needs, goals and identity, perceptions of and coactions with other people, the physical ecology, and culture (e.g., Damon 2008; Geldhof et al. 2010; Gestsdóttir and Lerner 2008; Lerner et al. 2001). Agency is a defining feature of the active, self-creating (autopoietic, enactive), and nonlinear adaptive living system (Overton and Lerner 2014; Narvaez 2008; Witherington 2014). Such agency is the individual's contribution to adaptive developmental regulations (Brandtstädter 1998, 1999).

The development of agency begins in early life, primarily with organismic self-regulation processes. However, as we have noted, by the time of adolescence, self-regulation is increasingly intentional and purposeful (Damon 2008) and involves the self-system and the phenomena associated with identity development (Gestsdóttir and Lerner 2008; Lerner et al. 2001). The adolescent instantiation of agency reflects ideas associated with the work of comparative psychologists Tobach and Schneirla (1968), who distinguished between the biosocial functioning of insects (e.g., ants) and the psychosocial functioning of organisms with higher psychological levels, levels that are marked by greater plasticity, rather than stereotypy, in their eventual highest levels of ontogenetic change. Such higher levels provide the physiological base for symbolic functioning.

In turn, reflecting the life course health development principles that evolution enables as well as constrains health development pathways and plasticity (Principle No. 5) and that optimal health development promotes survival, enhances thriving, and protects against disease (Principle No. 6), evolutionary biologists Jablonka and Lamb (2005) note that both psychological processes and cultural processes are integrated with the genetic and epigenetic processes of evolution to make human adaptiveness and contributions qualitatively different than corresponding instances of adaptiveness of social contributions among other organisms. Together, these comparative psychology and evolutionary biology literatures suggest that, among humans, adaptiveness and positive contributions reflect integrated cognitive, emotional, and behavioral processes that involve abstract, symbolic constructs, such as language or moral reasoning, or character virtues (e.g., Lerner and Callina 2014).

4 Implications for Research About Adolescent Health Development

Empirically, indexing such facets of adolescent health development, in general, or the complex dimensions of evolutionary change linked to adolescent health development more specifically (e.g., Gissis and Jablonka 2011; Lerner et al. 2015; Slavich and Cole 2013) may involve both point-in-time (cross-sectional) assessments and historical (longitudinal) assessments (Lerner 2004). Scientists must conduct such assessments within the context of recognizing that contexts are complex (e.g., they exist at multiple levels of organization; Bronfenbrenner 1979). Individuals cannot necessarily act in ways that benefit all levels and all components of the context at all times and places (Elder 1998). Thus, adaption is not treated as a categorical concept (as something that either exists or not) but, instead, as a multivariate concept comprised of ordinal or interval dimensions. Researchers studying adaptation would not ask, then, whether it exists or not; rather, the question would be how beneficial is the developmental regulation (the individual⇔context relation) for specific people or specific social institutions of the context, at specific times and in specific places (e.g., see Bornstein 2006, 2017).

Consistent both with the seventh principle of life course health development, that is, that the cadence of human health development results from the synchronized timing of variables from all levels of the developmental systems—that is, molecular, physiological, behavioral, cultural, and evolutionary processes (e.g., Cole 2014; Meaney 2014; Slavich and Cole 2013)—and with the Bornstein (2017) "specificity principle," we suggest, therefore, that addressing a multipart "what" question is the key to conducting programmatic research about the function, structure, and content of health development in adolescence. In other words, to test RDS-based ideas about the ontogenetically changing structure of adolescent development in general and health development more specifically, researchers need to ascertain answers to the following multipart "what" questions:

1. What specific structure-content relations emerge; at
2. What specific levels of organization within the relational developmental system that are linked to;
3. What specific antecedent and consequent adaptive developmental regulations (to what trajectory of individual⇔context relations); at
4. What specific points in adolescent development; for
5. What specific groups of youth; living in
6. What specific contexts; at
7. What specific points in time (history)?

Such work may have several benefits. Questions about coherence and reliability or consistency of indicators of health development with respect to variation in context may be especially useful for understanding the developmental course of multidimensional, latent variable conceptions of health among diverse adolescents. For instance, are specific indicators of, say, cardiovascular, respiratory, nutritional, or mental health manifested consistently across time and place? To what extent and for whom and under which conditions can biologic propensities to such health developmental challenges be moderated?

Consider nutrition more closely. How do adolescents' diets influence their cardio-metabolic risk as adolescents and adults? Do adolescents maintain a healthy diet across different settings involving peers and family members? Is there age-associated variation in answers to this question, for instance, variation associated with pubertal development or pubertal status/stage (e.g., early, on time, or late)? Do answers to these questions vary in relation to gender? As well, do they vary in relation to normative social transitions (e.g., moving from elementary school to middle school)? How do peer social networks influence these behaviors or family mealtime behaviors? Are answers moderated or changed by the socioeconomic, cultural, religious, or national contexts of youth? In turn, do answers here vary in relation to media exposure about eating and about desirable body types that may be prevalent for youth living in particular settings at particular times in history? Given the synchronization issues raised by the seventh life course health development principle, how are all these answers moderated or changed by what may be nonnormative life or historical events in the lives of adolescents (Baltes et al. 2006)? Examples here may be the death of a parent or deployment in the military (Cozza and Lerner 2013), family disruption due to divorce or separation, or family challenges in the face of environmental tragedies such as weather-related calamities or living in settings beset by violence.

The life course health development principles remind us that health development is highly sensitive to the timing and social structure of environmental events (Principle 4), and these examples of questions reflecting the specificity of health-related individual⇔context relations that may impinge on the thriving of adolescents underscore the subtle and nuanced nature of the developmental system within which adolescent health development is embodied.

The idea of embodiment and of adolescent health development being an emergent property of the living system (Principle 1) underscores that it is insufficient to take a "main effect" approach to the study of even a facet of health development as complex as the effects of nutrition. Scientists and practitioners framing their research and applications, respectively, within RDS-based models and/or life course health development principles must also ask how do answers to all the questions we have posed regarding nutrition covary with comparable questions pertaining to adolescent lifestyle changes (e.g., involving sleep, exercise, or sexual debut), healthy status of bodily systems, and the presence of chronic and acute health challenges, of both more biological (e.g., hormonal changes) and more social origins (e.g., school bullying).

5 Conclusions

The interrelated "what" questions we have presented, illustrated by the example of nutrition's effects on health development, will, then, help developmental and medical science collaborate to understand the assuredly complex questions that need to be addressed in a scholarly agenda that comprehensively describes, explains, and optimizes the course of individual health development across the adolescent period. Developmental scientists know that in some senses each adolescent is like every other adolescent (e.g., there are nomothetic principles that apply to functioning of the physiological and psychological changes prototypic of the period), that each adolescent is like only some other adolescent (e.g., group differential variation exists as, for instance, when both the presence of good health status and healthy disparities vary across gender, race, socioeconomic level, culture, and nation of residence), and that each adolescent is like no other adolescent (e.g., there are idiographic characteristics pertinent to every young person, for instance, resulting from the relations among his/her timing of molecular, physiological, behavioral, cultural, and evolutionary processes brought into high relief by life course health development Principle 7). Therefore, the scholarly agenda brought to the fore by RDS metatheory and by the principles of life course health development will require scholars seeking to understand and to promote adolescent health to accept that their work will be exceedingly more complex than work predicated on main effect or reductionist approaches.

However, the relative plasticity in the development of human health and positive development that is found in studies that have been derived from or associated with RDS-based or life course health development-related scholarship, respectively (e.g., Lerner et al. 2015), is a basis for *optimism* that embracing such complexity is not only the intellectually correct path to take. It is also a feasible approach to adopt. The advances in relational developmental systems-predicated methods that we have discussed (e.g., Molenaar et al. 2014; Molenaar and Nesselroade 2014, 2015; Nesselroade and Molenaar 2010) provide powerful research and data analytic tools enabling such complexity to be integratively assessed.

The adolescent decade is "privileged" because of the generally disease-free status of individuals within it, as compared to subsequent decades of life (e.g., Susman and Dorn 2009; Paus 2009). Nevertheless, application of methods linked to the ideas of RDS metatheory and the principles of life course health development hold the promise of narrowing the disparities that exist across time and place in adolescent health development. In addition, therefore, these conceptions have one other vital asset; their use in research and application will enhance the probability that all youth will transition from adolescence into the adult years in manners that will enable their life course trajectories to more prominently be marked by health and thriving. Such a contribution by these conceptual frameworks will make quite vivid the insight of Lewin (1954) that there is nothing more practical than a good theory.

Acknowledgement Supported (in full or in part) by Grant # U45MC27709 from the Department of Health and Human Services, Health Resources and Services Administration, Maternal and Child Health Bureau (Title V, Social Security Act), Division of Child, Adolescent and Family Health, Adolescent Health Branch.

References

Anthony, E. J. (1969). The reactions of adults to adolescents and their behavior. In G. Caplan & S. Lebovici (Eds.), *Adolescence: Psychosocial perspectives* (p. 77). New York: Basic Books.

Ardelt, M. (2000). Still stable after all these years? Personality stability theory revisited. *Social Psychology Quarterly, 63*(4), 392–405.

Baltes, P. B. (1997). On the incomplete architecture of human ontogeny: Selection, optimization, and compensation as foundations of developmental theory. *American Psychologist, 52*, 366–380.

Baltes, P. B., Lindenberger, U., & Staudinger, U. M. (2006). Lifespan theory in developmental psychology. In W. Damon & R. M. Lerner (Eds.), *Theoretical models of human development. Vol. 1: Handbook of child psychology* (6th ed., pp. 569–664). Hoboken: Wiley.

Bandura, A. (2001). Social cognitive theory: An agentic perspective. *Annual Review of Psychology, 52* 1–26. Palo Alto: Annual Reviews, Inc.

Benson, P. L., Scales, P. C., Hamilton, S. F., & Semsa, A., Jr. (2006). Positive youth development: Theory, research, and applications. In R. M. Lerner (Ed.), *Theoretical models of human development, Volume 1 of handbook of child psychology* (6th ed., pp. 894–941). Editors-in-chief: W. Damon & R. M. Lerner. Hoboken: Wiley.

Bjorklund, D. F., & Ellis, B. J. (2005). Evolutionary psychology and child development: An emerging synthesis. In B. J. Ellis & D. F. Bjorklund (Eds.), *Origins of the social mind: Evolutionary psychology and child development* (pp. 3–18). New York: Guilford.

Block, J. (1995). A contrarian view of the five-factor approach to personality description. *Psychological Bulletin, 117*, 187–215.

Block, J. (2010). The five-factor framing of personality and beyond: Some ruminations. *Psychological Inquiry, 21*(1), 2–25.

Bornstein, M. H. (2006). Parenting science and practice. In K. A. Renninger, & I. E. Sigel (Vol. Eds.), *Handbook of child psychology,* Vol. 4*: Child psychology in practice* (6th ed., pp. 893–949). Editors-in-Chief: W. Damon, & R. M. Lerner. Hoboken: Wiley.

Bornstein, M. H. (2017). The specificity principle in acculturation science. *Perspectives on Psychological Science, 12*(1), 3–45.

Brandtstädter, J. (1998). Action perspectives on human development. In R. M. Lerner (Ed.), *Handbook of child psychology, Vol. 1* (5th ed., pp. 807–866). New York: Wiley.

Brandtstädter, J. (1999). The self in action and development: Cultural, biosocial, and ontogenetic bases of intentional self-development. In J. Brandtstädter & R. M. Lerner (Eds.), *Action and self-development: Theory and research through the life-span* (pp. 37–65). Thousand Oaks: Sage.

Bronfenbrenner, U. (1979). *The ecology of human development*. Cambridge, MA: Harvard University Press.

Bronfenbrenner, U. (2005). *Making human beings human*. Thousand Oaks: Sage Publications.

Bronfenbrenner, U., & Morris, P. A. (2006). The bioecological model of human development. In R. M. Lerner (Ed.), *Theoretical models of human development.* Volume 1 of *Handbook of child psychology* (6th ed., pp. 795–828). Editors-in-chief: W. Damon & R. M. Lerner. Hoboken: Wiley.

Cole, S. W. (2014). Human social genomics. *PLoS Genetics, 10*(8), 1–7.

Costa, P. T., Jr., & McCrae, R. R. (1980). Still stable after all these years: Personality as a key to some issues in adulthood and old age. In P. B. Baltes & O. G. Brim Jr. (Eds.), *Life span development and behavior* (Vol. 3, pp. 65–102). New York: Academic Press.

Costa, P. T., Jr., & McCrae, R. R. (2006). Age changes in personality and their origins: Comment on Roberts,

Walton, and Viechtbauer (2006). *Psychological Bulletin, 132*, 28–30.

Cozza, S. J., & Lerner, R. M. (Eds.). (2013). Military children and families. *The Future of Children, 23*(2), 3–11.

Damon, W. (2008). *The path to purpose: Helping our children find their calling in life*. New York: Simon and Schuster.

Darwin, C. (1859). *The origin of species by means of natural selection or the preservation of favoured races in the struggle for life*. London: J. Murray.

Eccles, J. S. (2004). Schools, academic motivation, and stage-environment fit. In R. M. Lerner & L. Steinberg (Eds.), *Handbook of adolescent psychology* (2nd ed., pp. 125–153). Hoboken: Wiley.

Eccles, J. S., & Gootman, J. A. (Eds.). (2002). *Community programs to promote youth development/committee on community-level programs for youth*. Washington, DC: National Academy Press.

Elder, G. H., Jr. (1980). Adolescence in historical perspective. In J. Adelson (Ed.), *Handbook of adolescent psychology* (pp. 3–46). New York: Wiley.

Elder, G. H., Jr. (1998). The life course and human development. In R. M. Lerner (Ed.), *Handbook of child psychology, Volume 1: Theoretical models of human development* (5th ed., pp. 939–991). Editor-in-chief: W. Damon. New York: Wiley.

Elder, G. H., Jr., Shanahan, M. J., & Jennings, J. A. (2015). Human development in time and place. In M. H. Bornstein and T. Leventhal (Eds.), *Handbook of child psychology and developmental science*, Volume 4: *Ecological settings and processes in developmental systems* (7th ed., pp. 6–54). Editor-in-chief: R. M. Lerner. Hoboken: Wiley.

Ford, D. L., & Lerner, R. M. (1992). *Developmental systems theory: An integrative approach*. Newbury Park: Sage.

Forrest, C. B. (2014). A living systems perspective on health. *Medical Hypotheses, 82*, 209–2143.

Freud, A. (1969). Adolescence as a developmental disturbance. In G. Caplan & S. Lebovici (Eds.), *Adolescence* (pp. 5–10). New York: Basic Books.

Freund, A. M., & Baltes, P. B. (2002). Life-management strategies of selection, optimization and compensation: Measurement by self-report and construct validity. *Journal of Personality and Social Psychology, 82*(4), 642–662.

Gardner, M., & Steinberg, L. (2005). Peer influence on risk taking, risk preference, and risky decision making in adolescence and adulthood: An experimental study. *Developmental Psychology, 41*, 625–635.

Geldhof, G. J., Little, T. D., & Colombo, J. (2010). Self-regulation across the lifespan. In M. E. Lamb & A. M. Freund (Vol. Eds.), *Social and emotional development*. Volume 2 of the *Handbook of lifespan development*. Editor-in-Chief: R. M. Lerner. Hoboken: Wiley.

Gestsdóttir, G., & Lerner, R. M. (2008). Positive development in adolescence: The development and role of intentional self regulation. *Human Development, 51*, 202–224.

Gestsdottir, S., Geldhof, G. J., Paus, T., Freund, A. M., Aðalbjarnardóttir, S., Lerner, J. V., & Lerner, R. M. (2014). Self-regulation among youth in four Western cultures: Is there an adolescence-specific structure of the Selection-Optimization-Compensation (SOC) model? *International Journal of Behavioral Development, 39*(4), 346–358.

Gissis, S. B., & Jablonka, E. (Eds.). (2011). *Transformations of Lamarchism: From subtle fluids to molecular biology*. Cambridge, MA: The MIT Press.

Gottlieb, G. (1997). *Synthesizing nature-nurture: Prenatal roots of instinctive behavior*. Mahwah: Erlbaum.

Gottlieb, G. (1998). Normally occurring environmental and behavioral influences on gene activity: From central dogma to probabilistic epigenesis. *Psychological Review, 105*(4), 792–802.

Halfon, N., & Forrest, C. B. (2017). The emerging theoretical framework of life course health development. In N. Halfon, C. B. Forrest, R. M. Lerner, & E. Faustman (Eds.), *Handbook of life course health-development science*. Cham: Springer.

Hall, G. S. (1904). *Adolescence: Its psychology and its relations to psychology. anthropology, sociology, sex, crime, religion, and education*. New York: Appleton

Hamilton, S. F. (1999). *A three-part definition of youth development*. Unpublished manuscript. Ithaca: Cornell University College of Human Ecology.

Jablonka, E., & Lamb, M. J. (2005). *Evolution in four dimensions: Genetic, epigenetic, behavioral, and symbolic variation in the history of life*. Cambridge, MA: MIT Press.

Johanson, D. C., & Edey, M. A. (1981). *Lucy: The beginnings of humankind*. New York: Simon & Schuster.

Larson, R. W. (2000). Toward a psychology of positive youth development. *American Psychologist, 55*(1), 170–183.

Latour, B. (1993). *We have never been modern* (trans. Catherine Porter), Cambridge, MA: Harvard University Press.

Lerner, R. M., & Busch-Rossnagel, N. A. (Eds.). (1981). *Individuals as producers of their development: A life-span perspective*. New York: Academic Press.

Lerner, R. M. (1982). Children and adolescents as producers of their own development. *Developmental Review, 2*, 342–370.

Lerner, R. M. (1984). *On the nature of human plasticity*. New York: Cambridge University Press.

Lerner, R. M., & Walls, T. (1999). Revisiting individuals as producers of their development: From dynamic interactionism to developmental systems. In J. Brandtstädter & R. M. Lerner (Eds.), *Action and self-development: Theory and research through the life-span* (pp. 3–36). Thousand Oaks: Sage.

Lerner, R. M. (2002). *Concepts and theories of human development* (3rd ed.). Mahwah: Lawrence Erlbaum Associates.

Lerner, R. M. (2004). *Liberty: Thriving and civic engagement among America's youth*. Thousand Oaks: Sage Publications.

Lerner, R. M., Lerner, J. V., Almerigi, J. B., Theokas, C., Phelps, E., Gestsdottir, S., et al. (2005). Positive Youth Development, Participation in community youth development programs, and community contributions of fifthgrade adolescents: Findings from the first wave of the 4-H study of Positive Youth Development. *Journal of Early Adolescence, 25*(1), 17–71.

Lerner, R. M. (Ed.). (2006). *Theoretical models of human development.* Volume 1 of *Handbook of child psychology* (6th ed.). Editors-in-chief: W. Damon & R. M. Lerner. Hoboken: Wiley.

Lerner, R. M. (2012). Essay review: Developmental science: Past, present, and future. *International Journal of Developmental Science, 6*(1–2), 29–36.

Lerner, R. M., & Callina, K. S. (2014). The study of character development: Towards tests of a relational developmental systems model. *Human Development, 57*(6), 322–346.

Lerner, R. M. (Editor-in-Chief). (2015). *Handbook of child psychology and developmental science* (7th ed.). Hoboken: Wiley.

Lerner, R. M., & Benson, J. B. (Eds.). (2013a). *Embodiment and epigenesis: Theoretical and methodological issues in understanding the role of biology within the relational developmental system. Volume 1: Philosophical, theoretical, and biological dimensions. advances in child development and behavior* (Vol. 44). London: Elsevier.

Lerner, R. M., & Benson, J. B. (Eds.). (2013b). *Embodiment and epigenesis: Theoretical and methodological issues in understanding the role of biology within the relational developmental system. Volume 2: Ontogenetic dimensions. Advances in child development and behavior* (Vol. 45). London: Elsevier.

Lerner, R. M., & Callina, K. S. (2015). The study of character development: Towards tests of a relational developmental systems model. *Human Development, 57*(6), 322–346.

Lerner, R. M., & Steinberg, L. (2009). The scientific study of adolescent development. In R. M. Lerner & L. Steinberg (Eds.), *Handbook of adolescent psychology* (3rd ed., pp. 3–14). Hoboken: Wiley.

Lerner, R. M., Freund, A. M., De Stefanis, I., & Habermas, T. (2001). Understanding developmental regulation in adolescence: The use of the selection, optimization, and compensation model. *Human Development, 44*, 29–50.

Lerner, R. M., Lerner, J. V., Bowers, E., & Geldhof, G. J. (2015). Positive youth development: A relational developmental systems model. In W. F. Overton & P. C. Molenaar (Eds.), *Theory and method.* Volume 1 of the *Handbook of child psychology and developmental science* (7th ed., pp. 607–651). Editor-in-chief: R. M. Lerner. Hoboken: Wiley.

Lewin, K. (1954). Behavior and development as a function of the total situation. In L. Carmichael (Ed.), *Manual of child psychology* (2nd ed.). New York: Wiley.

Marcia, J. E. (1980). Identity in adolescence. In J. Adelson (Ed.), *Handbook of adolescent psychology* (pp. 159–187). New York: Wiley.

Mascalo, M. F., & Fischer, K. W. (2015). The dynamic development of thinking, feeling, and acting: Infancy through adulthood In W. F. Overton & P. C. M. Molenaar (Eds.), *Handbook of child psychology and developmental science* (7th ed.), Volume 1*: Theory and method.* Editor-in-chief: R. M. Lerner. Hoboken: Wiley.

McClelland, M. M., Geldhof, G. J., Cameron, C. E., & Wanless, S. B. (2015). Development and self-regulation. In W. F. Overton & P. C. Molenaar (Eds.), *Theory and method.* Volume 1 of the *Handbook of child psychology and developmental science* (7th ed.). Editor-in-chief: R. M. Lerner. Hoboken: Wiley.

McCrae, R. R., Costa, P. T., Hrebickova, M., Ostendord, F., Angleitner, A., & Avia, M. D. (2000). Nature over nurture: Temperament, personality, and life span development. *Journal of Personality and Social Psychology, 78*(1), 173–186.

Meaney, M. (2014, October 10). *Epigenetics offer hope for disadvantaged children.* [Children and family: Blog]. Retrieved from http://childandfamilyblog.com/epigenetics-offer-hope-disadvantaged-children/

Misteli, T. (2013). The cell biology of genomes: Bringing the double helix to life. *Cell, 152*(6), 1209–1212.

Mistry, J., & Wu, J. (2010). Navigating cultural worlds and negotiating identities: A conceptual model. *Human Development, 53*(1), 5–25.

Molenaar, P. C. (2014). Dynamic models of biological pattern formation have surprising implications for understanding the epigenetics of development. *Research in Human Development, 11*(1), 50–62.

Molenaar, P. C., & Nesselroade, J. R. (2014). New trends in the inductive use of relation developmental systems theory: Ergodicity, nonstationarity, and heterogeneity. In P. C. Molenaar, R. M. Lerner, & K. M. Newell (Eds.), *Handbook of developmental systems and methodology* (pp. 442–462). New York: Guilford Press.

Molenaar, P. C. M., & Nesselroade, J. R. (2015). Systems methods for developmental research. In W. F. Overton & P. C. M. Molenaar (Eds.), *Handbook of child psychology and developmental science* (7th ed.), Volume 1*: Theory and method.* Editor-in-chief: R. M. Lerner. Hoboken: Wiley.

Molenaar, P. C., Lerner, R. M., & Newell, K. M. (2014). Developmental systems theory and methodology: A review of the issues. In P. C. Molenaar, R. M. Lerner, & K. M. Newell (Eds.), *Handbook of developmental systems and methodology* (pp. 3–18). New York: Guilford Press.

Narvaez, D. (2008). Human flourishing and moral development: Cognitive and neurobiological perspectives of virtue development. In L. Nucci & D. Narvaez (Eds.), *Handbook of moral and character education* (pp. 310–327). Oxford: Routledge.

Nesselroade, J. R. (1988). Some implications of the trait-state distinction for the study of development over the life-span: The case of personality. In P. B. Baltes, D. L. Featherman, & R. M. Lerner (Eds.), *Life-span development and behavior* (Vol. 8, pp. 163–189). Hillsdale: Erlbaum.

Nesselroade, J. R., & Molenaar, P. C. M. (2010). Emphasizing intraindividual variability in the study of development over the life span. In W. F. Overton (Ed.), *The handbook of life-span development.* Vol. 1*: Cognition, biology, methods* (pp. 30–54). Editor-in-chief: R. M. Lerner. Hoboken: Wiley.

Overton, W. F. (1973). On the assumptive base of the nature-nurture controversy: Additive versus interactive conceptions. *Human Development, 16*, 74–89.

Overton, W. F. (2010). Life-span development: Concepts and issues. In W. F. Overton (Ed), *Cognition, biology, and methods across the lifespan. Handbook of life-span development.* (Vol. 1, pp. 1–29). Editor-in-chief: R. M. Lerner. Hoboken: Wiley.

Overton, W. F. (2013). Relationism and relational developmental systems; A paradigm for developmental science in the post-Cartesian era. In R. M. Lerner and J. B. Benson (Eds.), *Advances in child development and behavior, volume 44: Embodiment and epigenesis: Theoretical and methodological issues in understanding the role of biology within the relational developmental system, Part A: Philosophical, theoretical, and biological dimensions* (pp. 24–64). London: Elsevier. Development of Character 49.

Overton, W. F. (2015). Process and relational developmental systems. In W. F. Overton & P. C. Molenaar (Eds.), *Theory and method.* Volume 1 of the *Handbook of child psychology and developmental science* (7th ed., pp. 9–62). Editor-in-chief: R. M. Lerner. Hoboken: Wiley.

Overton, W. F., & Lerner, R. M. (2014). Fundamental concepts and methods in developmental science: A relational perspective. *Research in Human Development, 11*(1), 63–73.

Overton, W. F., & Mueller, U. (2013). Meta-theories, theories, and concepts in the study of development. In R. M. Lerner, M A. Easterbrooks, & J. Mistry (Eds.), *Comprehensive handbook of psychology: developmental psychology: Vol. 6.* (pp. 19–58). Editor-in-Chief: Irving B. Weiner. New York: Wiley.

Overton, W. F., & Reese, H. W. (1981). Conceptual prerequisites for an understanding of stability–change and continuity–discontinuity. *International Journal of Behavioral Development, 4*, 99–123.

Paus, T. (2009). Brain development. In R. M. Lerner & L. Steinberg (Eds.), *Handbook of adolescent psychology* (3rd ed., pp. 95–115).

Ricco, R., & Overton, W. F. (2011). Dual systems competence ß-à procedural processing: A relational developmental systems approach to reasoning. *Developmental Review, 31*, 119–150. http://dx.doi.org/10.1016/j.dr.2011.07.005.

Riegel, K. F. (1975). Toward a dialectical theory of human development. *Human Development, 18*, 50–64.

Riegel, K. F. (1976). The dialectics of human development. *American Psychologist, 31*, 689–700.

Roberts, B. W., Walton, K. E., & Viechtbauer, W. (2006). Patterns of mean-level change in personality traits across the life course: A meta-analysis of longitudinal studies. *Psychological Bulletin, 132*(1), 1–25.

Roth, J. L., & Brooks-Gunn, J. (2003a). What is a youth development program? Identification and defining principles. In F. Jacobs, D. Wertlieb, & R. M. Lerner (Eds.), *Enhancing the life chances of youth and families: Public service systems and public policy perspectives: Vol. 2 handbook of applied developmental science: Promoting positive child, adolescent, and family development through research, policies, and programs* (pp. 197–223). Thousand Oaks: Sage.

Roth, J. L., & Brooks-Gunn, J. (2003b). What exactly is a youth development program? Answers from research and practice. *Applied Developmental Science, 7*, 94–111.

Slavich, G. M., & Cole, S. W. (2013). The emerging field of human social genomics. *Clinical Psychological Science, 1*, 331–348.

Sokol, B. W., Hammond, S., Kuebli, J., & Sweetman, L. (2015). The development of agency. In W. F. Overton & P. C. Molenaar (Eds.,) *Theory and method.* Volume 1 of development of the *Handbook of child psychology and developmental science* (7th ed.). Editor-in-chief: R. M. Lerner. Hoboken: Wiley.

Steinberg, L. (2010). A dual systems models of adolescent risk-taking. *Developmental Psychobiology, 52*, 216–224.

Susman, E., & Dorn, L. D. (2009). Puberty: Its role in development. In R. M. Lerner & L. Steinberg (Eds.), *Handbook of adolescent psychology* (3rd ed., pp. 116–151). Hoboken: Wiley.

Susman, E. J., & Dorn, L. D. (2013). Puberty: Its role in development. In R. M. Lerner, M. A., Easterbrooks, & J. Mistry (Eds.), *Handbook of psychology, Volume 6: Developmental psychology* (2nd ed., pp. 289–320). Editor-inchief: I. B. Weiner. Hoboken: Wiley.

Tobach, E., & Schneirla, T. C. (1968). The biopsychology of social behavior of animals. In R. E. Cooke & S. Levin (Eds.), *Biologic basis of pediatric practice* (pp. 68–82). New York: McGraw-Hill.

Trommsdorff, G. (2012). Development of "agentic" regulation in cultural context: The role of self and world views. *Child Development Perspectives, 6*(1), 19–26.

von Bertalanffy, L. (1933). *Modern theories of development.* London: Oxford University Press.

von Bertalanffy, L. (1968). *General systems theory.* New York: Braziller.

Whitehead, A. N. (1929/1978). *Process and reality.* Corrected edn. New York: The Free

Witherington, D. C. (2014). Self-organization and explanatory pluralism: Avoiding the snares of reductionism in developmental science. *Research In Human Development, 11*, 22–36.

4

Emerging Adulthood as a Critical Stage in the Life Course

David Wood, Tara Crapnell, Lynette Lau, Ashley Bennett, Debra Lotstein, Maria Ferris, and Alice Kuo

1 Introduction to Emerging Adulthood

The path that individuals take from dependency in childhood to independence in adulthood is now a longer and more complicated one than at any other point in history (Arnett 2014). From the mid- to late twentieth century and extending into the twenty-first century, industrial societies have experienced a surge in the concept of individualism and increased salience of self-realization and personal expression (Arnett 1998). Moreover, we have seen a dramatic increase in the number of youth seeking post-high school education, which is required for success as the economy transitions from an industrial to an information-based economy (Rifkin 2011). However, stagnation of wages for low-skilled workers and the lack of work opportunities for youth and young adults, combined with the increased costs of education and independent living, have made the pathway to independence and adulthood prolonged, complex, and varied, creating a new stage in the life course that has been labeled *emerging adulthood* (EA). While not all life course or developmental scientists agree that emerging adulthood constitutes a new developmental stage, there is agreement that social and economic forces have prolonged entry into adulthood and with significant role and developmental challenges beyond the traditional adolescent years (Cote 2014).

At the beginning of this stage, 17–18 years of age, emerging adults are generally dependent, living with their parents or caretakers, beginning to engage in romantic relationships, and attending high school. At the end of this stage, mid- to late 20s, most emerging adults live independently, are in long-term relationships, and have clear career paths ahead of them. How they traverse this life stage is dependent upon the personal, family, and social resources they possess as they enter this stage of life, dynamic and reciprocal interaction between the emerging adult and their environment, and the supports they receive during this stage. The result is that there are many pathways that youth and young adults pursue through this stage to achieve stable adulthood. For example, 40% do not

D. Wood, MD, MPH (✉)
Department of Pediatrics, ETSU College of Medicine, PO Box 70578, Johnson City, TN 37614, USA
e-mail: wooddl@etsu.edu

T. Crapnell, OTD, OTR/L • L. Lau, PhD
D. Lotstein, MD, MPH • M. Ferris, MD, PhD, MPH
A. Kuo, MD, PhD
UCLA, Department of Pediatrics, Los Angeles, CA, USA

A. Bennett, MD
Department of Pediatrics, USC, Los Angeles, CA, USA

pursue post-high school education. While 60% entered college immediately after graduating high school, many drop out or interrupt their college education with periods of work. Some 33% in this stage remain unmarried; however, 67% of them achieve stable domestic partners. Importantly, only a minority of emerging adults are employed in full-time jobs, limiting the economic opportunities they experience (U.S. Census Bureau. American Community Survey 2006).

Emerging adulthood is considered to be the *volitional years*, as it offers the most opportunity for identity exploration in the areas of love, work, and worldviews (Arnett 2000). During this time, individuals begin to develop the characteristic qualities necessary for becoming self-sufficient, engage in mature, committed relationships, assume more adult roles and responsibilities, and obtain a level of education and training that sets the foundation for work during the adult years. Characterizing emerging adulthood as a stage in the life course has proven to be beneficial to explain the social, cognitive, and psychological development that occurs during this stage. Research demonstrating continued brain development into the late 20s provides further justification for viewing emerging adulthood as a stage in the life course (Spear 2000).

2 Conceptual Framework

The Life Course Health Development (LCHD) model posits that myriad factors (e.g., biological, psychological, cultural) on multiple levels (e.g., micro, meso, macro) interact simultaneously in a transactional fashion to influence an individual's LCHD during each stage to determine a "health developmental" trajectory (see also Halfon and Forrest 2017). The Life Course Health Development (LCHD) model further posits that transitions and pivotal points in an individual's life have the potential to influence and alter an individual's developmental pathways. EA is a life stage characterized by changes in person-context cognitive, emotional, physical, and social domains, and the ultimate pathway achieved by the emerging adults during this stage is determined by the ongoing, dynamic, and reciprocal interactions between the individual and their environment. The degree of agency and role exploration that characterizes EA results in the potential for growth in intellectual and emotional functioning (Arnett 2000). EA represents a broad and diverse but fundamentally important area of consideration by virtue of the multiple avenues through which an individual's developmental trajectories and outcomes may be influenced. Important developmental challenges during EA include the continued formation of identity and values, which occur in the midst of frequent changes in personal relationships, living arrangements, vocational and educational pursuits, and social roles (Shanahan 2000).

No stage in life, other than perhaps infancy, experiences such dynamic and complex changes on the personal, social, emotional, neuroanatomical, and developmental levels. For the 10 years between 18 and 28, the vast majority of emerging adults change living situation, change their primary relationships, complete education or vocational preparation, get married, have children, and transition from adolescent/dependent roles to adult/independent roles. This occurs during often volatile emotional, neurodevelopmental, and social development. Increasing agency occurs at the same time as decreasing institutional and family supports. The theoretical framework developed by Learner and others to create the positive youth development theory nicely explains how the developmental trajectories that emerge during the period of EA are dependent upon multiple influential, bidirectional, person-context coactions. Individuals during emerging adulthood act as co-developers of their own developmental pathways, adaptively responding to different biological, social, cultural, and physical environmental contexts that they influence and are also influenced by (Learner and Overton 2008). Successfully navigating the developmental challenges inherent in EA will likely, in large part, influence the developmental trajectory of adulthood because these challenges ultimately influence the important adult outcomes of independent living, committed intimate relationships, and vocational and educational achievement. Youth and young adults with chronic disease or disabilities face additional challenges (disease management, disease complications, limitations in opportunities, etc.) in the context of these multiple domains of growth and development, which impact their pathway through this stage.

The continued positive trajectory of the emerging adult's mental health, identity formation, education achievement, social relationships, and other developmental areas is somewhat dependent on the degree to which there are matches or mismatches between the individual and his/her resources and the environmental challenges and supports. If the transition, such as school to work, provides a reasonable and developmentally appropriate challenge and the emerging adult successfully navigates that challenge, then the developmental trajectory of the emerging adult will be enhanced. In contrast, if the same transition lacks supports or is an inappropriate match for the emerging adult's abilities (e.g., an inadequate vocational program for an emerging adult with a learning disorder or lack of support for chronic disease management) and the emerging adult experiences failure, then the developmental trajectory may be impaired, resulting in significantly less achievement or developmental progression across the lifespan. A major defining characteristic of the stage of EA is that contexts are changing significantly (family to independence or romantic relationships, school to work or disconnected state, dependent living to independent living arrangements). The changes are so significant that emerging adults need substantial supports to navigate the transition successfully. Emerging adults with disabilities or chronic health conditions require more support to maximize their potential development during EA (Table 1).

Table 1 Principles of the Life Course Health Development framework

Principle	Brief description
1. Health development	Health development integrates the concepts of health and developmental processes into a unified whole
2. Unfolding	Health development unfolds continuously over the lifespan, from conception to death, and is shaped by prior experiences and environmental interactions
3. Complexity	Health development results from adaptive, multilevel, and reciprocal interactions between individuals and their physical, natural, and social environments
4. Timing	Health development is sensitive to the timing and social structuring of environmental exposures and experiences
5. Plasticity	Health development phenotypes are malleable and enabled and constrained by evolution to enhance adaptability to diverse environments
6. Thriving	Optimal health development promotes survival, enhances well-being, and protects against disease
7. Harmony	Health development results from the balanced interactions of molecular, physiological, behavioral, cultural, and evolutionary processes

The above table outlines the seven principles of the Life Course Health Development framework. These principles can be applied to the stage of emerging adulthood in a limited fashion due to the limited research literature focused on this life stage. However, conceptually, using the seven principles to view the stage of emerging adulthood can be instructive and can lead to additional research questions (see end of this article). For example, Principle 5 states that health development expressions are malleable and enable and constrain health development pathways and plasticity. According to Bogin's reserve capacity hypothesis, prolonged childhood into adolescence and perhaps emerging adulthood leads to greater biologic and social resilience in adulthood, which leads to enhanced fertility and greater longevity (Bogin 2013). Principle 4 states that health development is sensitive to life course timing and social structuring of the environment. As we described above, this is particularly true of emerging adulthood, where the interaction between age, personal development, and environment (peers, schools, social institutions, etc.) leads to multiple pathways to identify formation and academic and social achievement during this stage (Benson and Elder 2011; Benson et al. 2012).

Multiple factors can influence the life course during EA, including factors at the macro-level (historical and societal influences), meso-level (parent-child relationship, family environment, and socioeconomic status), and microlevel (individual cognitive, personality, and emotional development). The timing of these exposures during EA, which we consider a critical or sensitive period in the life course development, can significantly impact adult outcomes. For example, an emerging adult that engages in criminal activity and is convicted of a felony will suffer repercussions that will greatly diminish their chances of achieving success in relationships and work. In the sections that follow, we review the macro-, meso-, and microlevel influences occurring during EA for emerging adults generally. Next we explore the additional challenges faced by those with selected chronic health or developmental conditions including mental illness or substance abuse, diabetes, chronic renal failure, and autism, to serve as case studies of the increased complexity faced by emerging adults with chronic disease. Finally, we finish up with a set of questions and issues that are research priorities for developing an LCHD research agenda on the stage of emerging adulthood.

3 Macro-level Influences on the Trajectory of Emerging Adulthood

Emerging adulthood, like many other developmental stages, is a period in the life course that is culturally constructed and not universal (Arnett 1998, 2000). Thus, the very existence and trajectory of EA are dependent on macro-level societal expectations and influences. For many years, it was theorized that an individual transitioned from adolescence (which begins in puberty and ends in the late teens) into young adulthood. Over history and cross-culturally, the length of time during which an individual spends in adolescence has been determined by the age at which the person enters marriage or a committed relationship (Schlegel and Barry III 1991, Gilmore 1990). In fact, human life history posits that the life stage of adolescence came into existence about 75,000 years ago due to changes in human societies and cultures associated with pair bonding and living in large groups (Bogin 2013). So massive culture and reproductive change led to a change in life history with the addition of a new period of development. It is theorized by those promoting emerging adulthood as a new life stage that the same kind of massive cultural and reproductive change is happening once again and new social and cultural demands of adult life necessitate a longer and more complex prologue to adult life.

Although the functional outcome of EA, causing a delayed transition to adulthood, appears relatively novel, this practice of prolonging the transition to adulthood may be dated back to early modern English society from the 1500s to 1700s (Ben-Amos 1994). Similar to what generally occurs during EA today, individuals during that era took part in a "life cycle service" between their late teens and 20s, wherein they would engage in developing important vocational skills (e.g., a trade or craft) and marriage was often postponed until the late 20s for both men and women; adult roles and responsibilities for individuals during that era were provided only gradually, as each individual acquired the desired character qualities deemed appropriate by society (Ben-Amos 1994). It was not until industrialization in America began to emerge in the nineteenth century that the concept of individualism developed and strengthened (Rotundo 1994). The twentieth century marked the first time that an individual could obtain and gain control over the resources that would allow them to choose the timing of major life events and personal expression was valued in society (Modell 1991).

As we move forward into the twenty-first century, individualism in contemporary postindustrial society continues to strengthen, while the age at which individuals marry continues to increase, and individuals increasingly seek to pursue other life course events (Modell 1991; Alwin 1988; Bellah et al. 2007). As a reflection of these trends, recent evidence indicates that contemporary postindustrial society considers marriage status of low importance in the determination of whether or not an individual has reached adulthood; rather, societies in developed countries appear to now consider the acquisition of certain character qualities as the most important indicator of having attained adulthood, the top three character qualities of which include (1) accepting responsibility for oneself, (2) making independent decisions, and (3) assuming financial independence – all of which emphasize an individual's ability to be self-sufficient (Scheer et al. 1996; Greene et al. 1992; Arnett 1997, 1998).

4 Meso-level Influences of Life Trajectories During Emerging Adulthood

Earlier life experiences and family environment can impact one's life trajectory from childhood through EA and into adulthood. Longitudinal studies that span early childhood through EA indicate that there is both continuity and discontinuity of healthy and unhealthy paths and outcomes. (Masten et al. 2006, 2005). In this section, we will be discussing the impact of the parent-child relationship, family environment, and other sociodemographic factors, such as socioeconomic status (SES) and its influence in EA.

4.1 Earlier Parent-Child Relationships

The quality of parent-child relationships during EA is, in large part, a function of the history of early parent-child attachment experiences. Attachment theory suggests that positive bonding with an emotionally available adult during early childhood facilitates the development of the child's capacity to bond with others and respond to stressful events. A history of positive attachment experiences will ultimately provide a foundation for positive interactions with others and foster secure, lasting relationships in EA which subsequently influence the LCHD (Mikulincer M and Shaver PR 2009), whereas insecure attachments can result in mistrust or lack of security and reduced sense of self-efficacy and self-esteem. Simultaneously, social learning theory suggests that styles of family interactions learned in early and middle childhood are carried by emerging adults into adulthood (Whitbeck et al. 1994). Familiar patterns of interaction help individuals deal with new situations and have a significant influence on the emerging adult's capacity to deal with the multiple changes that occur during EA. Alternatively, inadequate parenting, disrupted family bonds, and poverty are environmental risks for childhood-onset conduct, behavioral and emotional problems, and educational underachievement that can persist into adolescence and emerging adulthood (Moffit and Caspi 2001).

Adverse events experienced in childhood such as parental divorce or alcoholism or the experience of abuse are major risk factors for the leading causes of illness and death as well as poor quality of life in adults in the USA. Disruptions in the parent relationship (e.g., divorce) can have strong, negative effects on the parent-child relationship (Aquilino 1994) causing significant emotional impact throughout the life course. Parental divorce may influence the emerging adults' ability to form stable romantic relationships and their decision to marry early or may undermine the emerging adult's financial ability to attend college (Jacquet and Surra 2001, Cherlin et al. 1998).

Importantly, parental acceptance and support for independence have been linked to higher self-esteem, individualism, and feelings of worthiness among emerging adults (Ryan and Lynch 1989). Critical to the emerging adult's achievement of independence are feeling connected, secure, understood, and loved in their families and having the willingness to call on parental resources for help in making choices in educational, relationship, living, and other changes that confront the emerging adult. Persistent connectedness to parents facilitates rather than undermines ongoing identity development in emerging adulthood (Grotevant and Cooper 1986; Ryan and Lynch 1989).

4.2 Childhood Socioeconomic Status

Socioeconomic status (SES), family supports, and the neighborhood environment all can contribute to the positive or negative life trajectory prior to and during EA (Galobardes et al. 2008; Gilman 2012; Gilman and Loucks 2012). Socioeconomic status has been identified as one of the most important health determinants throughout the life course (Miller et al. 2015). Low financial resources and all the other exposures that go along with poverty – poor schools, chaotic families, exposure to violence, and victimization – limit opportunities for growth or acquisition of other resources that enhance quality of life (Wadsworth et al. 2016; Kim et al. 2015).

In addition to being an important predictor of disease-specific morbidity and mortality in adulthood, early childhood poverty has been associated with lower adult educational attainment (Duncan and Brooks-Gunn 2000). Educational achievement has a major influence on the life trajectory, including financial stability and health in EA and onward throughout adulthood. Seventy percent of emerging adults who grow up in poverty delay enrollment in postsecondary education, in comparison to 40% who grow up in household of higher SES. Furthermore, research has indicated that individuals who delay enrollment past the age of 22 are less likely to ever enroll in postsecondary education and less likely to complete a degree (Feliciano and Ashtiani 2012). The result is that only 22% of young adults from low-income families earn college degrees, while 48% of young adults from higher-income families earn at least an associate's degree. Earning a college education results in not only higher lifetime earnings but enhancement of multiple aspects of psychosocial development (Evans and Cassells 2014).

However, while SES has been found to be predictive of educational attainment, the impact of poverty can be mitigated by a number of factors such as individual characteristics of self-efficacy and hope. Students from poor families that have high self-efficacy and a similar concept of hope for educational attainment do equally as well in school as their higher SES peers (Osgood et al. 2005). Recent research by Dweck and colleagues indicates that students' mindsets are critically linked to resilience and achievement and that they can be changed through brief interventions, leading to substantial increases in measures of resilience and achievement (Yeager and Dweck 2012). These studies suggest that in addition to SES, individual characteristics also have a large influence on outcomes of EA and that these characteristics can be influenced through individual interventions. Individual characteristics and development are discussed in the next section.

5 Microlevel Influences on the Trajectories During Emerging Adulthood

As discussed in previous sections, individualism and the qualities of character have become increasingly important in the transition to EA and ultimately reaching full adulthood in postindustrial, developed societies. Studies have shown that the ability to accept responsibility for one's self, make independent decisions, and assume financial independence are the top three most important factors in becoming an adult (Arnett 2014). In order to achieve individualism and obtain these important qualities of character, one needs to reach some degree of cognitive and psychological maturity, as well as possess some level of resilience. These individual factors are discussed in this section.

5.1 Cognitive Development

One of the identified qualities of character that is important in EA and reaching full adulthood is independent decision-making. While the ability to make independent decisions is a reflection of one's psychological and moral identity, it also has to do with cognitive maturity and the ability to weigh a variety of considerations before deciding on a choice. Recent neuroscience research indicates that brain development (particularly in the prefrontal cortex) continues well into the third decade of life, ultimately resulting in the integration and coordination of cognitions, emotion and action, and strategic executive control (Luciana et al. 2005). The continuous unfolding and acquisition of specific neurodevelopmental capacities during adolescences and EA influence the acquisition of goal directedness and future orientation that have been observed behaviorally during EA (Dahl 2004; Nelson et al. 2012; Nurmi 1999; Steinberg et al. 2006). As new capacities emerge, they are available to solve problems, delay gratification, and filter unnecessary input. With maturation of these skills, emerging adults are also more capable of reflecting on the influence of their environment and on their internal state, regulate their emotions, and use problem-solving skills to effectively compromise, which is important for the development of meaningful social interactions and personal relationships as well as in the work environment. These skills also support an emerging adult's capacity for optimally interacting with the health-care system, managing their health-care needs, and making decisions that will influence their long-term health outcomes.

However, the preceding paragraph assumes that the individual has experienced optimal neurodevelopment up to the point that they enter the stage of EA. Studies have demonstrated that exposure to chronic stress during childhood (e.g., poverty) or experiencing adverse childhood events (e.g., child maltreatment, neglect, parental divorce, parental substance abuse) may cause detrimental impact to the developing brain. For example, repeated exposure to stressful events has been associated with structural differences in specific brain regions (i.e., amygdala, hippocampus, and prefrontal cortex), which are in turn associated with functional differences in learning, memory, and aspects of executive functioning. Furthermore, preliminary studies go on to suggest that there may be sensitive periods of brain development with increased susceptibility to the effects of stress and adverse events. These environmentally induced modulations in neurodevelopment can impact an individual's cognitive development and their capacity to develop the necessary skills and relationships that will enable them to thrive.

An emerging adult, who has experienced chronic stress or adverse events earlier in childhood and adolescence and is cognitively immature, is more likely, through adverse interaction with their environment, to suffer secondary effects such as school failure, risky/impulsive behaviors, accidental injury, criminal activity, or substance misuse or overuse. These behaviors may in turn interfere with the ongoing development of an optimal pathway to adulthood. Feelings of isolation and rates of substance abuse in individuals often peak during this period as emerging adults are faced with the stresses of having to navigate societal structures that are not adequately informed or equipped to address the needs of an emerging adult population – all while their brains have yet to reach full maturation (Spear 2000). An impulsive emerging adult fueled by alcohol and despair is at high risk for suicide. It is thus apparent that multiple factors related to an individual's cognitive and emotional development may intersect and interact to multiply the likelihood of adverse or positive health outcomes in EA. It is crucial for service providers to recognize the level of cognitive maturation an emerging adult possesses and tailor their interventions and supports based on this.

5.2 Identity Formation

Identity formation is a major developmental activity during EA. Identity development, occurs in a number of dimensions: (1) psychological dimension, or ego identity via a sense of temporal-spatial continuity and its concomitants; (2) the personal dimension, or a behavioral and character repertoire that differentiates the individuals; and (3) the social dimension, or recognized roles within a community. These components come together during the stage of identity formation (adolescence and EA) and stabilization (EA and young adulthood), and once the identity is considered stable, this is when a relatively firm sense of ego identity is developed, behavior and character become stabilized, and community-sanctioned roles are acquired (2002).

Identity formation during adolescence was thought to be a critical milestone in adolescence; however, it has been recognized that in certain societal contexts, identity formation continues beyond adolescence. In the postindustrial society, with the prolongation of educational and vocational attainment, prolongation of identity exploration in the three main areas of love, work, and worldviews into the 20s has become the norm. Identity formation is critical in EA, as it has direct implications on psychological and moral identity and in achieving the three qualities of character deemed as important in the transition to adulthood.

5.3 Resilience in Emerging Adulthood

Resilience is an individual's capacity to adapt to change in healthy and flexible ways during stressful events (Catalano et al. 2004). Resilience can be measured in various ways, including internal adaption (e.g., well-being, happiness, or self-concept) or external adaption (academic achievement, relationship development) to adverse circumstances, such as how well a person navigates and achieves the developmental tasks presented by the external world (e.g., educational achievement, stable work/career, marriage, etc.). Resiliency in adolescence and young adulthood is higher among youth with higher intellectual resources, optimistic future orientation, the presence of caring relationships with positive adult role models, and opportunities to succeed and serve the community. Emerging adulthood is a particularly important stage in the life course to understand resilience because the important changes in functional capacity, educational achievement, and social roles are large and varied and have a significant influence on life course outcomes.

Key individual characteristics that predict resilience during EA are goal-directed motivation and planfulness about the future. In addition, adult support and mentorship are important factors that help promote resilience (Miller GE 2015; Masten et al. 2005; Arnett 2005). Furstenberg, Brooks-Gunn, and others studied young women who became pregnant during adolescence and found that a small proportion with positive adult relationships had dramatic change in trajectory for the better (Furstenberg 2002). Masten, studying a cohort of low-income youth (beginning at ages 8–12) over a 20-year period, found that a number of factors predict competence in EA including higher intellectual capacity, higher parenting quality, and higher SES (Masten and Coatsworth 1998). When they examined resilience between the 10- and 20-year follow-up, they found that youth doing well in EA was predicted from doing well 10 years earlier. In the context of high adversity, childhood IQ was particularly an important moderator and predictor of resilience. During EA, individuals who were doing well from high-adversity backgrounds had significant personal resources in intelligence and personal competence and a history of receiving high-quality parenting (Masten et al. 2004).

6 Trajectories During Emerging Adulthood for Emerging Adults with Chronic Health Condition

Chronic health conditions can significantly impact the developmental trajectory of emerging adults during this life stage. Many types of chronic conditions, including those that impact physical, intellectual, or emotional functioning, may undermine the assumption of adult roles by the emerging adult, undermine success in school, impair the transition to work, and make living independently more of a challenge. Eighteen percent of youth aged 12–17 in the USA are defined as having a special health-care need, meaning they have a chronic physical, medical, emotional, or developmental condition that requires a more intensive use of health-care and related services. Emerging adults with chronic conditions are at risk for a number of problems during transition to adulthood, including experiencing gaps in needed medical and related services and gaps in health insurance (Lotstein et al. 2008, Reiss et al. 2005). Below we review the impact of several specific chronic conditions on the growth trajectory during emerging adulthood.

6.1 Autism Spectrum Disorders (ASDs)

For youth with autism spectrum disorders (ASDs) and their families, the transition from adolescence to emerging adulthood is a time of uncertainty and loss of entitlement to many services that were available while in the public school system under the Individuals with Disabilities Education Act (IDEA). In comparison to childhood, young adults with autism often experience a dearth of appropriate supports and opportunities. Leaving high school is associated with deterioration in ASD symptom presentation, increase in maladaptive behaviors, and worsening family functioning (Taylor and Seltzer 2010, 2011a, b). Many persons with ASD are able to work successfully within the community (Garcia-Villamisar et al. 2000; Mawhood and Howlin 1999); however, the majority experience difficulty securing meaningful employment (Eaves and Ho 2008; Howlin et al. 2004; Newman et al. 2011). A recent study indicated that only 58% have ever worked for pay. In addition, it was found that only one in five individuals ever lived independently (Roux et al. 2015). Even among those employed, their jobs tended to be low level and low income (Cimera and Cowan 2009; Eaves and Ho 2008; Howlin et al. 2004). Jobs often ended prematurely because of social or behavioral difficulties or other work-related difficulties (Mawhood and Howlin 1999).

Young adults on the autism spectrum are reported to experience difficulties in assuming other important adult roles and responsibilities, including attaining postsecondary education and living independently (Roux et al. 2015). A number of studies (Billstedt et al. 2005; Gillespie-Lynch et al. 2012; Howlin et al. 2004) have found that having an IQ of around 70 seemed to be a critical cutoff point for better outcome (e.g., level of independence). A number of comorbid conditions can complicate the trajectory for youth with intellectual disability through adolescence and EA, such as seizure disorder, which substantially increase in prevalence from childhood through adolescence into adulthood. Adults with ASD and related conditions are more vulnerable to anxiety and depression which can require specific treatments (Skokauskas and Gallagher 2010; White et al. 2009). The majority of young adults with ASD remain dependent on parents for support in living, recreation, and occupational situations. The availability of appropriate resources, services, and supports for the individuals with ASD and their families is key for successful transition into adulthood and better outcomes throughout adult life. The following elements are important for high-quality transition services and associated with improved young adult outcomes: (1) individualized services that reflect the strengths of the individual, (2) positive career development and early work experiences, (3) collaboration and interagency involvement, (4) family supports and expectations, (5) fostering self-determination and independence, (6) social and employment-related skill instruction, and (7) establishment of job-related supports. Therefore, outcomes for emerging adults with ASD could be improved if social and institutional supports available through adolescence continued into adulthood.

6.2 Type 1 Diabetes Mellitus (DM)

The study of emerging adults with type 1 DM has elucidated the potential challenges facing emerging adults with diabetes and other chronic health conditions that have significant self-management burden. Emerging adults with type 1 diabetes face extensive behavioral demands in order to maintain their health, including the necessity for precisely scheduled daily insulin injections, blood glucose monitoring, dietary monitoring, regular physical exercise, and the management of DM-related complications. In early adulthood, frequent changes in roles, living situations, educational routines, jobs, friendships, and romantic relationships are common and can undermine the routines and the resolve needed to maintain metabolic control (Anderson and Wolpert 2004).

The developmental tasks of emerging adulthood may be at odds with maintaining the intensive self-care that is required of those with type 1 diabetes and vice versa. For example, the tasks of establishing autonomy and prevailing egocentrism may be associated with the emerging adult not wanting to follow medical advice or advice of his or her family (Masten et al. 1995). Heightened concern for peer acceptance or the establishment of intimate relationships is characteristic of this period of development. Emerging adults may be reluctant to admit to their significant others that they have type 1 diabetes or any other chronic condition that puts them at risk for being rejected (Madsen et al. 2002). Moreover, the major cognitive developmental milestone during the stage of emerging adulthood is the ability to think abstractly (Erikson 1994). Those who have not yet reached this developmental milestone may struggle with taking responsibility to maintain good disease management and understanding the consequences of poor disease management. Lastly, increased rates of drinking, illicit drug use, or other high-risk behaviors may disrupt the emerging adults' lifestyle and negatively impact self-care management of diabetes, resulting in (Madsen et al. 2002) lack of control of diabetes and the resulting physical and mental consequences of hypo- or hyperglycemia, which undermine emerging adults' abilities to perform in school, maintain relationships, or keep employment.

As has been demonstrated in other chronic childhood conditions, the transition from pediatric- to adult-centered medical care for youth with DM is associated with a decline in DM control (Busse et al. 2007; Oeffinger et al. 2006). Adverse health-related outcomes documented in the young adult population with diabetes include a decline in disease self-care behaviors and an increased risk for diabetes-related complications (Bryden et al. 2001; Fredericks et al. 2010; Yeung et al. 2008). In addition, emerging adults with diabetes are at higher than average risk for psychosocial morbidity including social delays and isolation, impaired social competence, and emotional problems such as depression (Helgeson et al. 2007). As in the case in ASD, additional support for an emerging adult with DM during the transition to adult medical care has been shown to help decrease the adverse outcomes seen with usual practice. For example, DM transition programs that include introductions to new adult care providers or intensive care coordination have been found to be protective (Holmes-Walker et al. 2007).

6.3 Chronic Kidney Disease

Chronic kidney disease (CKD) is a condition characterized by disease progression, significant cardiovascular morbidity, growth failure, neurocognitive impairment, and impaired quality of life changes (Sarnak 2003; Copelovitch et al. 2011; Gerson et al. 2006; McKenna et al. 2006). CKD is divided into five stages based on glomerular filtration rate, with stage 1 being the mildest form and stage 5 the worst form, also called end-stage kidney disease (ESKD), requiring renal replacement therapy (dialysis or transplant) (Hogg et al. 2003). The prevalence of pediatric CKD is unknown as it may be silent in early stages. The prevalence of pediatric ESKD is 15 cases per million population (Saran et al. 2015). African-Americans and Latinos are disproportionately affected by CKD in part due to a higher incidence of glomerular conditions (Ferris et al. 2006). While the 10-year survival for adolescent-onset ESKD is 80–85% (much higher than adult-onset ESKD patients), this still represents a 30-fold increase in mortality compared to the general US adolescent population. Survival is better for younger adolescents, males, Caucasians, Asians, and transplant recipients (2006). However, emerging adults with CKD achieve adult milestones (e.g., employment, marriage) less frequently than their healthy peers (Bartosh et al. 2003).

The burden of care directly correlates with the stage of CKD. Based on the mean number of unique medications, those with CKD stages 1–4 take 6.2 ± 4 of medications, those with peritoneal dialysis (CKD 5) take 8.5 ± 2 medications, those with kidney transplant (CKD 5) take 9.7 ± 4.2 medications, and those on hemodialysis (CKD 5) take 11.3 ± 2.1 (So et al. 2011). The complexity of care also include procedures such as self-catheterization several times per day, fluid and dietary restrictions, blood pressure measurements daily, and injections (erythropoiesis-stimulating agents once to thrice weekly, growth hormone daily, or insulin several times per day). The life course of pediatric-onset CKD-ESKD varies by etiology and age at onset of this condition, but once they reach ESKD, most patients share the same comorbidities (hypertension, anemia, acidosis, metabolic bone disease, and growth delay). Patients with greater level of CKD have a decreased sense of self-worth, perceive a poor future, and feel limited in their physical and psychosocial capacities to have the same potential and opportunity as their healthy peers.

While most children and adolescent patients with ESKD will receive a kidney transplant, they likely will experience dialysis prior to receiving an organ. The most common cause of kidney transplant rejection in adolescents and emerging adults is treatment nonadherence (Andreoni et al. 2013). Adherence among adolescents is compromised by poor understanding and poor consequence recognition leading to an inconsistent commitment to the treatment regimens. Once the kidney transplant is lost, patients return to dialysis and likely will not receive another kidney transplant for many years. As in adult patients, cardiovascular disease (CVD) accounts for a majority of deaths in patients with pediatric-onset CKD, but unlike adults, pediatric-onset CKD patients rarely demonstrate symptomatic atherosclerosis (Shroff et al. 2011). Lastly, survivors of pediatric-onset CKD are at greater risk for malignancies and post-transplant diabetes mellitus (Koukourgianni et al. 2010).

Patients who transfer to adult-focused services without transition preparation and support appear to be at greater risk to lose their kidney transplant (Watson 2000, 2005). The international societies of internal medicine and pediatric nephrology have published position statements and policies to promote health-care transition preparation (Watson 2005; Watson et al. 2011). Strategies to increase patient autonomy, health-care transition, and self-management are needed to achieve successful outcomes at the time of transfer to adult-focused providers.

6.4 Mental Health and Substance Use

Emerging adulthood is a time of increased experimentation with tobacco, drugs, and alcohol (Schulenberg et al. 2004; Schulenberg and Maggs 2002), increasing from rates of 12.2% in adolescence to 40.2% in young adulthood for cigarette smoking, from 10.7% to 41.9% for binge drinking, from 11.2% to 20.3% for illicit drug use, and from 2.6% to 14.9% for heavy alcohol use. While cigarette, alcohol, and drug use are normative during adolescence and emerging adulthood, a number of factors predict excessive use rather than experimentation including genetic (e.g., family history of alcohol abuse), biological (e.g., early puberty timing), family (e.g., low parental monitoring), school (e.g., low grade average, school failure), peer (e.g., peer substance use), and youth personality and psychopathology (e.g., depression) factors (Cicchetti 1999). However, the pattern of use/abuse of these substances is influenced by the experience during the stage of EA. For example, increasing responsibility, work, and marriage all are associated with decreased use of these substances (Masten et al. 1999; Bachman et al. 2014). Again, there is great heterogeneity in the trajectories followed by individuals with regard to substance use during this period, all influenced by the multiplicity of factors listed above.

Among young adults, 13.7% experience serious mental illness such as major depressive disorders, schizophrenia, and bipolar disorder (AmericanPsychiatricAssociation 2013). The neuropsychological pathology that has onset during EA has many of the predisposing factors related to family adversities, such as social disadvantage, divorce, dysfunctional parenting, multiple family changes/moves, and peer group choices. The expanded independence and self-reliance during EA may be difficult to handle for youth with preexisting emotional or social challenges or poor attachment. The decrease in supports from school or family during EA may be even further destabilizing, leading to increased emotional and interpersonal difficulties. Young people with serious mental health conditions have difficulty with impulse control and self-regulation (Walker and Gowen 2011). Their apparent immaturity reflects a delay in social and emotional development and undermines progress toward goals in education, relationships, independence in health, and health-care management.

Three-quarters of lifetime cases of mental, emotional, and behavioral disorders begin by age 24 (Kessler et al. 2005). In emerging adults with social, emotional, and behavioral disorders, much higher risk is associated with onset in early adolescence versus onset in late adolescence (Mofitt and Caspi 2001). Dysfunctional family environments and participation in deviant peer group increase the likelihood of early-onset delinquency followed by a long trajectory of social, emotional, and behavioral problems. Youth with later onset of social, emotional, and behavioral problems are more commonly from relatively healthy family backgrounds and more likely to desist from delinquency by age 23 (Roisman et al. 2004). Similar patterns can be seen for major psychiatric disorders such as depression, with early-onset mood disorders being representative of more severe recurrent forms of mood disorders arising from increased severity and complexity of family and biologic risk factors (Fergusson and Woodward 2002) and later-onset disorders reflecting lower levels of risk factors in childhood.

7 Protective and Risk Factors That Impact Emerging Adulthood

The supports, opportunities, and experiences that occur during the stage of EA greatly influence the ultimate outcome of this stage and the ensuing life trajectory into young adulthood. As discussed in this chapter, critical influences during EA include mentoring relationships, socioeconomic supports, and educational and vocational opportunities. Emerging adulthood typically is accompanied by an increase in agency/independence and decrease in social and institutional support (e.g., schools and family), such that most individuals have more choice in day-to-day activities and life decisions. This increase in choice may result in greater success which will likely contribute to well-being. However, increased freedom can result in poor choices (e.g., drug use, criminal activity) that have a negative impact on the developmental trajectory as well (Schulenberg and Maggs 2002; Schulenberg et al. 2004). For example, many relationships and other aspects of life are so unstable during EA that important and powerful negative experiences can occur such as date rape, school failure, and substance addiction. These experiences can have a lasting, if not lifetime, detrimental impact on the developmental and mental health trajectory of the emerging adult. Similarly, many potential powerful positive influences can occur during this period in life (e.g., marriage, educational achievement, mentoring) that can enhance the developmental and mental health trajectory. Therefore, experiences both distal (early childhood) and proximal (during emerging adulthood) can influence, either positively or negatively, the developmental and mental health trajectory of the emerging adult (Miller et al. 2015).

Practical supports during EA provided by families include financial support for education, transportation, independent living, health insurance, and other necessities. The primary determinant of parental support are the level of parental resources. Emerging adults with wealthier parents and those with fewer siblings receive more financial support for education (Steelman and Powell 1991). Divorced parents provide less financial support than parents with intact marriages (Cooney and Uhlenberg 1992). Support from families by parents and grandparents during EA is also provided in the form of guidance or advice, information, and emotional support. Parents of emerging adults may also help the emerging adult negotiate the health-care system, formulate and carry out educational and vocational goals, and acquire leases for apartments and even provide advice for intimate relationships. In short, continued social and financial connection to parents with adequate emotional and financial resources can be a very significant factor in the positive life trajectory during emerging adulthood (Aquilino 2005). Previous studies have found a high correlation between improved EA outcomes and adolescent hope in the future (Bennett 2014). Hope is a form of personal capital that protects youth from social, emotional, and behavioral disorders and correlates with and predicts the rates of many outcomes, including academic achievement, delay of initiation of early sexual activity, and lower likelihood of violent behavior. Hope requires a sense of self-efficacy and knowledge of alternate outcomes. Hope is reflected in adolescent and young adult goals as they reflect and make ongoing assessments of their current and future selves. Individual goals and aspirations relate to the sense of control an individual feels in relation to a particular domain.

Positive youth development (PYD) programs are approaches that provide supports to adolescents and emerging adults to achieve social, emotional, behavioral, and moral competence, foster self-efficacy, a clear and positive identity, and belief in the future; and reinforce pro-social norms (Catalano et al. 2004). Positive development approaches involve a paradigm shift from targeting the risk factors to enhancing the assets and protective factors. The emphasis on hope, empowerment, and well-being resonates with youth and mental health professionals. The PYD approach outlined above suggests that effective programs to support EA would include an individualized approach supporting young people to identify and move toward personally meaningful goals. This begins with envisioning a positive future identity ("Who do I want to become?"). Pursuing goals promotes a sense of purpose, and making progress toward those goals contributes to building feelings of efficacy, empowerment, and self-determination, enhancing the individual's ability to act as the primary causal agent in pursuing personally meaningful goals (Silbereisen and Lerner 2007).

A PYD perspective further suggests that youth and emerging adults will benefit from learning specific strategies for increasing and maintaining interpersonal support from positive peers, family, providers, and people in the community (Guerra and Bradshaw 2008). Young people can learn specific steps and skills that can help them increase the quality and the extent of their interpersonal networks, as well as the amount of emotional, instrumental, and informational support available to them. Using a PYD perspective suggests that the development of assets is an important recovery-oriented outcome in and of themselves, as well as a mediator of longer-term outcomes related to education, employment, mental health, and general quality of life. Indeed, a review of the available research on community-based programs and interventions for EA reveals a common focus on personal asset building (Lerner 2014). Also consistent with the PYD perspective is that many of the programs and interventions include a focus on changing the meso-environment of youth so that it encourages young people to develop or express strengths and assets.

8 Services and Supports

As we better understand the limits of and issues related to EA, it is imperative that we review and revise policy and current social and medical services and supports so they optimally address the current and future needs of individuals during this life stage. Current medical, mental health, and social service delivery models are geared toward either child or adult populations. In other words, individuals generally seek child-serving services between the ages of 0 and 18, and they are subsequently transferred directly to adult-serving services. However, the various biobehavioral and sociocultural factors discussed above make this direct transition from child to adult-centered care ill-suited for optimally addressing the nuances and challenges that individuals may face during EA. For example, an adult-centered medical doctor may regularly treat patients with fixed habits and lifestyles, who may already suffer from a variety of chronic health conditions. However, many such chronic health conditions in adults represent a culmination of experiences from an individual's earlier years, which may not yet be apparent during EA. It is thus strongly recommended that EA service providers reorient themselves using a prevention-based paradigm and familiarize themselves with the possible antecedents to social, emotional, and medical conditions so that they may make health-care or social service recommendations to minimize risk factors and to maximize strengths and assets to facilitate development along optimal health trajectories. EA presents a unique opportunity for service providers to intervene and influence an individual's LCHD before significant social, emotional, and medical pathology fully develops, utilizing existing knowledge of the skills and capacities associated with EA to inform services and interventions.

In addition to training service providers to reorient their approach to care and become more sensitive to antecedents of chronic health conditions in adulthood, the multifactorial nature of the LCHD model suggests that it would be important for service providers to consider horizontal (i.e., cross sector) and longitudinal (i.e., across the lifespan) service integration. Specifically, the current model posits that myriad factors (e.g., biological, psychological, cultural) on multiple levels (e.g., micro, meso, macro) interact simultaneously in a transactional fashion to influence an individual's LCHD and overall health trajectory. However, most current training models which emphasize specialization in their independent fields and opportunities for cross-disciplinary case conceptualization and collaboration with regard to service delivery – particularly with respect to preventive care, which may be of special importance when considering EA as a sensitive period of development – tend to be rare. Such specialization in service delivery may result in service fragmentation. Additionally, adult service providers generally do not work in tandem with child service providers as individuals transition from one care setting to the next, consequently resulting in potential gaps in service delivery and care, which may be exacerbated as individuals work to rebuild rapport with their new service providers. Moreover, health, mental health, social service, and education professionals rarely collaborate to create comprehensive models across the EA stage. Clearly, the current service delivery infrastructure does not adequately support the needs and challenges unique to emerging adult populations. It is thus important to recognize emerging adults as a unique population requiring additional and specialized skills of service providers and the creation of specific pathways for transition which support continuity of care.

The larger sociopolitical and cultural contexts may also facilitate or create challenges which impact service and intervention efforts directed at emerging adults. The majority of individuals in developed nations transitioning through EA, for instance, may be classified as "digital natives," individuals who have been brought up in environments where exposure to digital technology may be normative and who are therefore familiar with computers and the Internet. As emerging adults increasingly turn to digital and mobile solutions to support and enhance their daily routines, it behooves service providers to creatively explore ways of engaging emerging adult populations using technology. Use of social networks, such as Instagram, Twitter, and Facebook, to advance primary prevention efforts, increase awareness of public health issues, and provide basic health and psychological education affords service providers the opportunity to outreach to unprecedented numbers and populations. Use of text messaging may also be effective as a way of engaging with digital native emerging adult populations and promoting engagement and adherence by emerging adults or to promote youth development programs. Also, as service providers keep pace with technological advancements, they may even begin to explore novel methods of service delivery and intervention using digital or Internet-based platforms, which may increase "buy-in" and potentially preventive service utilization, among digitally native emerging adult populations. For example, service providers might potentially leverage the data that digitally native emerging adults might collect as part of the "quantified self" movement (e.g., pedometer information, weight, blood pressure, etc.) in an effort to inform their ongoing care efforts.

On the other hand, due to clinical billing practices and regulations, as well as patient privacy concerns and regulations (e.g., Health Insurance

Portability and Accountability Act, HIPAA), current service delivery models often tend to operate in a fragmented and siloed fashion, which in turn may limit the ability of service providers to develop a holistic treatment plan to address each individual's needs. Further complicating this fragmentation is the restricted access to health records once an individual turns 18 years of age, when parents who may have been primarily responsible for managing their child's health-care needs no longer are able to access their child's medical records (unless explicit permission is granted by the child, who is now an emerging adult). Depending on each family's cultural context and the relationship between the emerging adult and his or her parents, this transition may be a cause for significant stress and/or strife between family members as they work to renegotiate previously familiar boundaries. Mothers of children with diabetes, for example, have indicated feeling increased stress as their children transitioned from pediatric to adult care, particularly if they perceived that their children were not managing their health-care condition as well as they had been when it was previously under greater parent control (Allen et al. 2011). Such stress might result in familial conflict and dysfunction which could subsequently interfere with the emerging adult's willingness or ability to adequately access services. One potential solution to overcoming the issue of patient privacy may be to implement public health programs and tools to educate and empower individuals with respect to managing and taking an active role in their own care. However, it is important to underscore the need for larger, overall systems to change in order to support service providers in working together with individuals and their families to ensure continuity and comprehensiveness of services and health-related information during the transition.

Finally, the implementation of health-care policies may have important implications for service and intervention delivery with an emerging adult population. With the introduction of the Patient Protection and Affordable Care Act of 2010 (ACA), for example, individuals may now remain on their parents' health insurance plans until they turn 26 years of age. While this theoretically affords emerging adults the opportunity to develop the necessary skills for interacting with the health-care system and managing their own care, research indicates that emerging adults frequently perceived themselves as being at lower risk for health problems and the financial burden of health insurance as lacking in value. Consequently, emerging adults may opt for high-deductible catastrophic insurance which generally costs less compared to other health insurance plans, but translates to fewer opportunities for interaction with the health service sector and fewer opportunities for service providers to intervene early during an individual's LCHD trajectory prior to the onset of chronic adult disease. Importantly, research indicates that despite preventive maintenance health visits being mandatory under the ACA, emerging adults were less likely to request health maintenance visits. Thus, it may be important for public health efforts to determine the underlying factors associated with this diminished utilization of health services by emerging adults and subsequently develop health literacy programs to promote prevention mindedness and service utilization in emerging adults.

9 Recommendations for Research Priorities

The following is a list of issues in life course research that are critical for better understanding the positive supports and challenges that influence the trajectory of development of emerging adults organized along the macro-, meso-, micro-framework.

Macro Issues

- What community supports in emerging adulthood enhance health development into adulthood and improve outcomes for an emerging adult with specific health, mental health, and developmental conditions? Is there an "early intervention model" to optimize outcomes for EA? What model should be used for an emerging adult with chronic health, mental health, and developmental conditions?

- What are the historical, economic, and cultural influences on the meaning of EA, adaptation, and maladaptation to the stage and expectations for normative transitions? How have these changed over time? How are they different for an emerging adult with social, health, mental health, and developmental problems?
- How have the delays in marriage/relationship commitment impacted adult life trajectories?
- What are the racial and ethnic differences for how these factors interact to support development during EA?
- How has the information economy and the increased demands for education impacted the life course for youth in upper, middle, and lower socioeconomic strata? Are there regional variations in these outcomes and how can they be improved?

Meso Issues

- Earlier childhood development and family environment are predictors of adult outcomes, but it is unclear how optimizing health development can be achieved with supports during EA.
- What is the interaction between health and social system supports, family supports, youth abilities, cognitive and psychological maturity, and EA outcomes for an emerging adult with and without mental or physical disabilities?
- How can the different support systems be integrated to provide seamless services to youth and emerging adults with significant physical, mental health, or intellectual disabilities?
- Using the model below from the work of Masten et al. (2005), how do these different resources, supports, and personal characteristics interact to promote optimal development during EA? (Fig. 1)
- What factors promote resilience for youth during EA who lack family supports?
- What is the role of extended families in support for EA?
- How can studies of conditions and processes that influence development during EA inform educational/vocational/EA support policies?
- How can data be gathered across this stage in the lifespan given that emerging adults leave school and have many changes in living arrangements, education, relationships, and work?

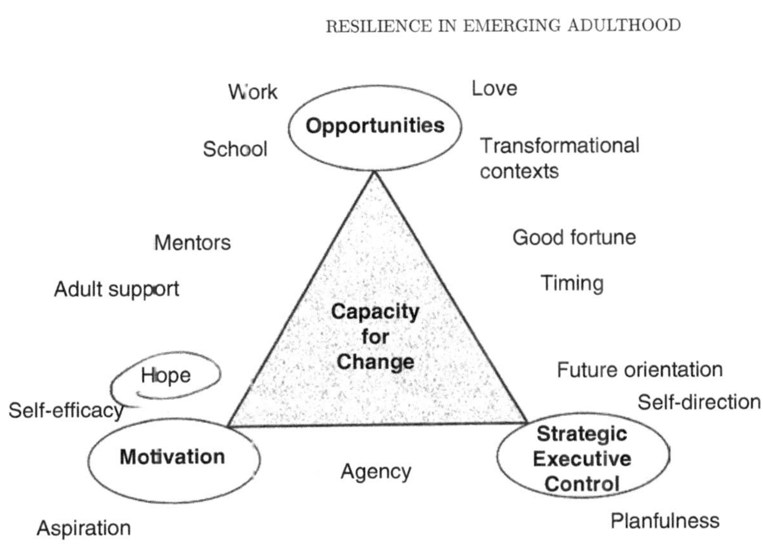

Fig. 1 Moving toward resilience: a model of positive change in emerging adulthood

Micro Issues

- To what degree is cognitive, social, physical, moral, and spiritual development mediated during emerging adulthood? How are these developmental pathways impacted by chronic health, mental health, and developmental conditions?
- How can we optimize the person-context match to promote development during EA with and without chronic health, mental health, and developmental conditions?
- What is the impact of positive turning points in EA compared to early life stages on life trajectories into adulthood?
- During EA, exploration of new experiences is normative. Is more exploration better or worse and for which activities is it better or worse? How is this equation different for an emerging adult with chronic health, mental health, and developmental conditions?
- Do emerging adults with particular health conditions, such as diabetes, spina bifida, solid organ transplant, or cancer survivorship, experience sharply downward trajectories during EA, and what supports are effective to prevent these sharply downward trajectories?
- How does brain development progress during EA? What is the impact of brain development on the factors that influence the developmental trajectory during EA such as executive control (planfulness, future orientation), motivation, self-efficacy, and hope?

References

Allen, D., Channon, S., Lowes, L., Atwell, C., & Lane, C. (2011). Behind the scenes: The changing roles of parents in the transition from child to adult diabetes service. *Diabetic Medicine, 28*(8), 994–1000.

Alwin, D. F. (1988). From obedience to autonomy changes in traits desired in children, 1924–1978. *Public Opinion Quarterly, 52*, 33–52.

American Psychiatric Association. (2013). *Diagnostic and statistical manual of mental disorders*. Arlington: American Psychiatric Publishing.

Anderson, B. J., & Wolpert, H. A. (2004). A developmental perspective on the challenges of diabetes education and care during the young adult period. *Patient Education and Counseling, 53*, 347–352.

Andreoni, K. A., Forbes, R., Andreoni, R. M., Phillips, G., Stewart, H., & Ferris, M. (2013). Age-related kidney transplant outcomes: Health disparities amplified in adolescence. *JAMA Internal Medicine, 173*, 1524–1532.

Aquilino, W. S. (1994). Impact of childhood family disruption on young Adults' relationships with parents. *Journal of Marriage and the Family, 56*, 295–313.

Aquilino, W. S. (2005). Impact of family structure on parental attitudes toward the economic support of adult children over the transition to adulthood. *Journal of Family Issues, 26*, 143–167.

Arnett, J. J. (1997). Young People's conceptions of the transition to adulthood. *Youth & Society, 29*, 3–23.

Arnett, J. J. (1998). Learning to stand alone: The contemporary American transition to adulthood in cultural and historical context. *Human Development, 41*, 295–315.

Arnett, J. J. (2000). Emerging adulthood: A theory of development from the late teens through the twenties. *American Psychologist, 55*, 469.

Arnett, J. J. (2005). The developmental context of substance use in emerging adulthood. *Journal of Drug Issues, 35*, 235–254.

Arnett, J. J. (2014). *Emerging adulthood: The winding road from the late teens through the twenties*. New York: Oxford University Press.

Bachman, J. G., O'malley, P. M., Schulenberg, J. E., Johnston, L. D., Bryant, A. L., & Merline, A. C. (2014). *The decline of substance use in young adulthood: Changes in social activities, roles, and beliefs*. New York: Psychology Press.

Bartosh, S. M., Leverson, G., Robillard, D., & Sollinger, H. W. (2003). Long-term outcomes in pediatric renal transplant recipients who survive into adulthood. *Transplantation, 76*, 1195–1200.

Bellah, E. R. N., Bellah, R. N., Tipton, S. M., Sullivan, W. M., Madsen, R., Swidler, A., Sullivan, W. M., & Tipton, S. M. (2007). *Habits of the heart: Individualism and commitment in American life*. Berkeley: University of California Press.

Ben-Amos, I. K. (1994). *Adolescence and youth in early modern England*. New Haven: Yale University Press.

Bennett, A. (2014). Finding hope in hopeless environments. *International Journal of Child Health And Human Development, 7*, 313.

Benson, J. E., & Elder, G. H. (2011). Young adult identities and their pathways: A developmental and life course model. *Developmental Psychology, 47*, 1646–1657.

Benson, J. E., Johnson, M. K., & Elder, G. H. (2012). The implications of adult identity for educational and work attainment in young adulthood. *Developmental Psychology, 48*(6), 1752.

Billstedt, E., Gillberg, C., & Gillberg, C. (2005). Autism after adolescence: Population-based 13-to 22-year follow-up study of 120 individuals with autism diagnosed in childhood. *Journal of Autism and Developmental Disorders, 35*, 351–360.

Bogin, B. (2013). Chapter 2, Childhood, adolescence and longevity: A chapter on human Evolutionary life history. In B. Hewlett (Ed.), *Adolescent identify: Evolutionary, cultural and developmental perspectives*. New York: Routledge.

Brody, G. H., et al. (2013). Is resilience only skin deep? Rural African Americans' socioeconomic status–related risk and competence in preadolescence and psychological adjustment and Allostatic load at age 19. *Psychological Science*. doi:10.1177/0956797612471954.

Bryden, K. S., Peveler, R. C., Stein, A., Neil, A., Mayou, R. A., & Dunger, D. B. (2001). Clinical and psychological course of diabetes from adolescence to young adulthood a longitudinal cohort study. *Diabetes Care, 24*, 1536–1540.

Busse, F., Hiermann, P., Galler, A., Stumvoll, M., Wiessner, T., Kiess, W., & Kapellen, T. (2007). Evaluation of patients' opinion and metabolic control after transfer of young adults with type 1 diabetes from a pediatric diabetes clinic to adult care. *Hormone Research in Pædiatrics, 67*, 132–138.

Catalano, R. F., Berglund, M. L., Ryan, J. A., Lonczak, H. S., & Hawkins, J. D. (2004). Positive youth development in the United States: Research findings on evaluations of positive youth development programs. *The Annals of the American Academy of Political and Social Science, 591*, 98–124.

Cherlin, A. J., Chase-Lansdale, P. L., & Mcrae, C. (1998). Effects of parental divorce on mental health throughout the life course. *American Sociological Review, 63*(2), 239–249.

Cicchetti, D., et al. (1999). *A developmental psychopathology perspective on drug abuse. Drug abuse: Origins & interventions* (pp. 97–117). Washington, DC: American Psychological Association, xxiii, 492 pp.

Cimera, R. E., & Cowan, R. J. (2009). The costs of services and employment outcomes achieved by adults with autism in the us. *Autism, 13*, 285–302.

Cooney, T. M., & Uhlenberg, P. (1992). Support from parents over the life course: The adult Child's perspective. *Social Forces, 71*, 63–84.

Copelovitch, L., Warady, B. A., & Furth, S. L. (2011). Insights from the chronic kidney disease in children (Ckid) study. *Clinical Journal of the American Society of Nephrology, 6*, 2047–2053.

Cote, J. E. (2014). The dangerous myth of emerging adulthood: An evidence-based critique of a flawed developmental theory. *Applied Developmental Science, 18*(4), 177–188.

Dahl, R. E. (2004). Adolescent brain development: A period of vulnerabilities and opportunities. Keynote address. *Annals of the New York Academy of Sciences, 1021*, 1–22.

Duncan, G. J., & Brooks-Gunn, J. (2000). Family poverty, welfare reform, and child development. *Child Development, 71*, 188–196.

Eaves, L. C., & Ho, H. H. (2008). Young adult outcome of autism Spectrum disorders. *Journal of Autism and Developmental Disorders, 38*, 739–747.

Erikson, E. H. (1994). *Identity: Youth and crisis*. New York: Ww Norton & Company.

Evans, G. W., & Cassells, R. C. (2014). Childhood poverty, cumulative risk exposure, and mental health in emerging adults. *Clinical Psychological Science, 2*(3), 287–296.

Feliciano, C., & Ashtiani, M. (2012). *Postsecondary educational pathways of low-income youth: An analysis of add health data*. Irvine: Uc/Accord.

Fergusson, D. M., & Woodward, L. J. (2002). Mental health, educational, and social role outcomes of adolescents with depression. *Archives of General Psychiatry, 59*, 225–231.

Ferris, M. E., Gipson, D. S., Kimmel, P. L., & Eggers, P. W. (2006). Trends in treatment and outcomes of survival of adolescents initiating end-stage renal disease care in the United States of America. *Pediatric Nephrology, 21*, 1020–1026.

Fredericks, E. M., Dore-Stites, D., Well, A., Magee, J. C., Freed, G. L., Shieck, V., & James Lopez, M. (2010). Assessment of transition readiness skills and adherence in pediatric liver transplant recipients. *Pediatric Transplantation, 14*, 944–953.

Furstenberg, F. F. (2002). How it takes thirty years to do a study. In *Looking at lives: American longitudinal studies of the twentieth century* (pp. 37–57).

Galobardes, B., Lynch, J. W., & Smith, G. D. (2008). Is the Association between childhood socioeconomic circumstances and cause-specific mortality established? Update of a systematic review. *Journal of Epidemiology and Community Health, 62*, 387–390.

Garcia-Villamisar, D., Ross, D., & Wehman, P. (2000). Clinical differential analysis of persons with autism in a work setting: A follow-up study. *Journal Of Vocational Rehabilitation, 14*, 183–185.

Gerson, A. C., Butler, R., Moxey-Mims, M., Wentz, A., Shinnar, S., Lande, M. B., Mendley, S. R., Warady, B. A., Furth, S. L., & Hooper, S. R. (2006). Neurocognitive outcomes in children with chronic kidney disease: Current findings and contemporary endeavors. *Mental Retardation and Developmental Disabilities Research Reviews, 12*(3), 208–215.

Gillespie-Lynch, K., Sepeta, L., Wang, Y., Marshall, S., Gomez, L., Sigman, M., & Hutman, T. (2012). Early childhood predictors of the social competence of adults with autism. *Journal of Autism and Developmental Disorders, 42*, 161–174.

Gilman, S. E. (2012). The successes and challenges of life course Epidemiology: A commentary on Gibb, Fergusson and Horwood (2012). *Social Science & Medicine, 75*, 2124–2128.

Gilman, S. E., & Loucks, E. B. (2012). Invited commentary: Does the childhood environment influence the Association between every X and every Y in adulthood? *American Journal of Epidemiology, 176*, 684–688.

Gilmore, D. D. (1990). *Manhood in the making: Cultural concepts of masculinity*. New Haven: Yale University Press.

Greene, A., Wheatley, S. M., & Aldava, J. F. (1992). Stages on Life's way Adolescents' implicit theories of the life course. *Journal of Adolescent Research, 7*, 364–381.

Grotevant, H. D., & Cooper, C. R. (1986). Individuation in family relationships. *Human Development, 29*, 82–100.

Guerra, N. G., & Bradshaw, C. P. (2008). Linking the prevention of problem behaviors and positive youth development: Core competencies for positive youth development and risk prevention. *New Directions for Child and Adolescent Development, 2008*, 1–17.

Halfon, N., & Forrest, C. B. (2017). The emerging theoretical framework of life course health development. In N. Halfon, C. B. Forrest, R. M. Lerner, & E. Faustman (Eds.), *Handbook of life course health-development science*. Cham: Springer.

Helgeson, V. S., Snyder, P. R., Escobar, O., Siminerio, L., & Becker, D. (2007). Comparison of adolescents with and without diabetes on indices of psychosocial functioning for three years. *Journal of Pediatric Psychology, 32*, 794–806.

Hogg, R. J., Furth, S., Lemley, K. V., Portman, R., Schwartz, G. J., Coresh, J., Balk, E., Lau, J., Levin, A., & Kausz, A. T. (2003). National Kidney Foundation's kidney disease outcomes quality initiative clinical practice guidelines for chronic kidney disease in children and adolescents: Evaluation, classification, and stratification. *Pediatrics, 111*, 1416–1421.

Holmes-Walker, D., Llewellyn, A., & Farrell, K. (2007). A transition care Programme which improves diabetes control and reduces hospital admission rates in young adults with type 1 diabetes aged 15–25 years. *Diabetic Medicine, 24*, 764–769.

Howlin, P., Goode, S., Hutton, J., & Rutter, M. (2004). Adult outcome for children with autism. *Journal of Child Psychology and Psychiatry, 45*, 212–229.

Jacquet, S. E., & Surra, C. A. (2001). Parental divorce and premarital couples: Commitment and other relationship characteristics. *Journal of Marriage and Family, 63*, 627–638.

Kessler, R. C., Berglund, P., Demler, O., Jin, R., Merikangas, K. R., & Walters, E. E. (2005). Lifetime prevalence and age-of-onset distributions of Dsm-iv disorders in the National Comorbidity Survey Replication. *Archives of General Psychiatry, 62*, 593–602.

Kim, P., Neuendorf, C., Bianco, H., & Evans, G. W. (2015). Exposure to childhood poverty and mental health symptomatology in adolescence: A role of coping strategies. *Stress and Health, 32*, 494–502.

Koukourgianni, F., Harambat, J., Ranchin, B., Euvrard, S., Bouvier, R., Liutkus, A., & Cochat, P. (2010). Malignancy incidence after renal transplantation in children: A 20-year single-Centre experience. *Nephrology Dialysis Transplantation, 25*, 611–616.

Lerner, R. M. (2014). Developmental science, developmental systems, and contemporary theories of human development. In *Handbook of child psychology*. New York: Wiley and Sons.

Lotstein, D. S., Inkelas, M., Hays, R. D., Halfon, N., & Brook, R. (2008). Access to care for youth with special health care needs in the transition to adulthood. *Journal of Adolescent Health, 43*, 23–29.

Luciana, M., Conklin, H. M., Hooper, C. J., & Yarger, R. S. (2005). The development of nonverbal working memory and executive control processes in adolescents. *Child Development, 76*, 697–712.

Madsen, S. D., Roisman, G. I., & Collins, W. A. (2002). The intersection of adolescent development and intensive intervention: Age-related psychosocial correlates of treatment regimens in the diabetes control and complication trial. *Journal of Pediatric Psychology, 27*, 451–459.

Masten, A. S., & Coatsworth, J. D. (1998). The development of competence in favorable and unfavorable environments: Lessons from research on successful children. *American Psychologist, 53*, 205.

Masten, A. S., Coatsworth, J. D., Neemann, J., Gest, S. D., Tellegen, A., & Garmezy, N. (1995). The structure and coherence of competence from childhood through adolescence. *Child Development, 66*, 1635–1659.

Masten, A. S., Hubbard, J. J., Gest, S. D., Tellegen, A., Garmezy, N., & Ramirez, M. (1999). Competence in the context of adversity: Pathways to resilience and maladaptation from childhood to late adolescence. *Development and Psychopathology, 11*, 143–169.

Masten, A. S., Burt, K. B., Roisman, G. I., Obradovic, J., Long, J. D., & Tellegen, A. (2004). Resources and resilience in the transition to adulthood: Continuity and change. *Development and Psychopathology, 16*, 1071–1094.

Masten, A. S., Roisman, G. I., Long, J. D., Burt, K. B., Obradović, J., Riley, J. R., Boelcke-Stennes, K., & Tellegen, A. (2005). Developmental cascades: Linking academic achievement and externalizing and internalizing symptoms over 20 years. *Developmental Psychology, 41*, 733.

Masten, A. S., Burt, K. B., & Coatsworth, J. D. (2006). Competence and psychopathology in development. D. Cicchetti, C. Dante, & J. Donald (Eds). *Developmental psychopathology: Risk, disorder, and adaptation* (Vol. 3, 2nd ed., pp. 696–738). Hoboken: John Wiley & Sons Inc, xvi 944 pp.

Mawhood, L., & Howlin, P. (1999). The outcome of a supported employment scheme for high-functioning adults with autism or Asperger syndrome. *Autism, 3*, 229–254.

Mckenna, A. M., Keating, L. E., Vigneux, A., Stevens, S., Williams, A., & Geary, D. F. (2006). Quality of life in children with chronic kidney disease—Patient and caregiver assessments. *Nephrology Dialysis Transplantation, 21*, 1899–1905.

Mikulincer, M., & Shaver, P. R. (2009). The attachment and behavioral systems perspective on social support. *Journal of Social and Personal Relationships, 26*(1), 7–19.

Miller, G. E., Yu, T., Chen, E., & Brody, G. H. (2015 Aug 18). Self-control forecasts better psychosocial outcomes but faster epigenetic aging in low-Ses youth. *Proceedings Of The National Academy Of Sciences., 112*(33), 10325–10330.

Modell, J. (1991). *Into One's own: From youth to adulthood in the United States, 1920–1975*. Berkeley: University of California Press.

Moffitt, T. E., & Caspi, A. (2001). Childhood predictors differentiate life-course persistent and adolescence-limited antisocial pathways among males and females. *Devcelopment and Psychopathology, 13*, 355–375.

Nelson, C. A., Thomas, K. M., & De Haan, M. (2012). *Neuroscience of cognitive development: The role of experience and the developing brain*. Hoboken: John Wiley & Sons.

Newman, L., Wagner, M., Knokey, A.-M., Marder, C., Nagle, K., Shaver, D., & Wei, X. (2011). *The post-high school outcomes of young adults with disabilities up to 8 years after high school: A Report from the National Longitudinal Transition Study-2 (Nlts2). Ncser 2011–3005*. Washington, DC: National Center For Special Education Research.

Nurmi, J.-E. (1999). 15 self-definition and mental health during adolescence and young adulthood. In J. Schulenberg, J. L. Maggs, & K. Hurrelmann (Eds.), *Health risks and developmental transitions during adolescence* (p. 395). New York: Cambridge University Press.

Oeffinger, K. C., Mertens, A. C., Sklar, C. A., Kawashima, T., Hudson, M. M., Meadows, A. T., Friedman, D. L., Marina, N., Hobbie, W., & Kadan-Lottick, N. S. (2006). Chronic health conditions in adult survivors of childhood cancer. *New England Journal of Medicine, 355*, 1572–1582.

Osgood, D. W., Ruth, G., Eccles, J. S., Jacobs, J. E. & Barber, B. L. (2005). *Six paths to adulthood: Fast starters, parents without careers, educated partners, educated singles, working singles, and slow starters*. na.

Reiss, J. G., Gibson, R. W., & Walker, L. R. (2005). Health care transition: Youth, family, and provider perspectives. *Pediatrics, 115*, 112–120.

Rifkin, J. (2011). *The Thired industrial revolution*. New York: St. Martin's Press.

Roisman, G. I., Aguilar, B., & Egeland, B. (2004). Antisocial behavior in the transition to adulthood: The independent and interactive roles of developmental history and emerging developmental tasks. *Development and Psychopathology, 16*, 857–871.

Rotundo, E. A. (1994). *American manhood: Transformations in masculinity from the revolution to the modern era*. New York: Basic Books.

Roux, A. M., Shattuck, P. T., Rast, J. E., Rava, J. A., & Anderson, K.,. A. (2015). *National autism indicators report: Transition into young adulthood*. Philadelphia: Life Course Outcomes Research Program/A.J. Drexel Autism Institute/Drexel University.

Ryan, R. M., & Lynch, J. H. (1989). Emotional autonomy versus detachment: Revisiting the vicissitudes of adolescence and young adulthood. *Child Development, 60*(2), 340–356.

Saran, R., Li, Y., Robinson, B., Ayanian, J., Balkrishnan, R., Bragg-Gresham, J., Chen, J., Cope, E., Gipson, D., & He, K. (2015). US renal data system 2014 annual data Report: Epidemiology of kidney disease in the United States. *American Journal of Kidney Diseases: The Official Journal of the National Kidney Foundation, 65*, A7.

Sarnak, M. J. (2003). Cardiovascular complications in chronic kidney disease. *American Journal of Kidney Diseases, 41*, 11–17.

Scheer, S. D., Unger, D. G., & Brown, M. B. (1996). Adolescents becoming adults: Attributes for adulthood. *Adolescence, 31*, 127.

Schlegel, A., & Barry Iii, H. (1991). *Adolescence: An anthropological inquiry*. New York: Free Press.

Schulenberg, J. E., & Maggs, J. L. (2002). A developmental perspective on alcohol use and heavy drinking during adolescence and the transition to young adulthood. *Journal of Studies on Alcohol, Supplement No. 14*, 54–70.

Schulenberg, J. E., Sameroff, A. J., & Cicchetti, D. (2004). The transition to adulthood as a critical juncture in the course of psychopathology and mental health. *Development and Psychopathology, 16*, 799–806.

Shanahan, M. J. (2000). Pathways to adulthood in changing societies: Variability and mechanisms in life course perspective. *Annual Review of Sociology, 26*, 667–692.

Shroff, R., Weaver, D. J., & Mitsnefes, M. M. (2011). Cardiovascular complications in children with chronic kidney disease. *Nature Reviews Nephrology, 7*, 642–649.

Silbereisen, R. K., & Lerner, R. M. (2007). *Approaches to positive youth development*. Los Angeles/London: Sage.

Skokauskas, N., & Gallagher, L. (2010). Psychosis, affective disorders and anxiety in autistic Spectrum disorder: Prevalence and Nosological considerations. *Psychopathology, 43*, 8–16.

So, T.-Y., Bradley Layton, J., Bozik, K., Farrington, E., Gipson, P. E., Gibson, K., Primack, W., Conley Iii, W., Gipson, D. S., & Ferris, M. (2011). Cognitive pharmacy services at a pediatric nephrology and hypertension clinic. *Renal Failure, 33*, 19–25.

Spear, L. P. (2000). The adolescent brain and age-related behavioral manifestations. *Neuroscience & Biobehavioral Reviews, 24*(4), 417–463.

Steelman, L. C., & Powell, B. (1991). Sponsoring the next generation: Parental willingness to pay for higher education. *American Journal of Sociology, 96*(5), 1505–1529.

Steinberg, L., Dahl, R., Keating, D., Kupfer, D. J., Masten, A. S., & Pine, D. S. (2006). The study of developmental psychopathology in adolescence: Integrating affective neuroscience with the study of context. In D. Cicchetti & D. Cohen (Eds.), *Handbook of developmental psychopathology* (Vol. 2, pp. 710–741). New York: Wiley.

Taylor, J. L., & Seltzer, M. M. (2010). Changes in the autism behavioral phenotype during the transition to adulthood. *Journal of Autism and Developmental Disorders, 40*, 1431–1446.

Taylor, J. L., & Seltzer, M. M. (2011a). Changes in the mother–child relationship during the transition to adulthood for youth with autism Spectrum disorders. *Journal of Autism and Developmental Disorders, 41*, 1397–1410.

Taylor, J. L., & Seltzer, M. M. (2011b). Employment and post-secondary educational activities for young adults with autism Spectrum disorders during the transition to adulthood. *Journal of Autism and Developmental Disorders, 41*, 566–574.

Wadsworth, M. E., et al. (2016). Poverty and the development of psychopathology. In: M. E. Wadsworth, G. W. Evans, K. Grant, J. S. Carter, & S. Duffy (Eds.), *Development and psychopathology. Volume Four. Risk, resilience, and intervention*, Ch 8 (pp. 215–237). Hoboken: John Wiley & Sons.

Walker, J. S., & Gowen, L. K. (2011). *Community-based approaches for supporting positive development in youth and young adults with serious mental health conditions*. Portland: Research and Training Center for Pathways to Positive Futures, Portland State University.

Watson, A. R. (2000). Non-compliance and transfer from Paediatric to adult transplant unit. *Pediatric Nephrology, 14*, 469–472.

Watson, A. R. (2005). Problems and pitfalls of transition from Paediatric to adult renal care. *Pediatric Nephrology, 20*, 113–117.

Watson, A. R., Harden, P., Ferris, M., Kerr, P. G., Mahan, J., & Ramzy, M. F. (2011). Transition from pediatric to adult renal services: A consensus statement by the international society of nephrology (Isn) and the international pediatric nephrology Association (Ipna). *Pediatric Nephrology, 26*, 1753–1757.

Webster, B. H., Jr., & Bishaw, A. (2006). *U.S. Census Bureau, American Community Survey Reports, ACS-02, Income, Earnings, and Poverty Data From the 2005 American Community Survey*. Washington, DC: U.S. Government Printing Office.

Whitbeck, L., Hoyt, D. R., & Huck, S. M. (1994). Early family relationships, intergenerational solidarity, and support provided to parents by their adult children. *Journal of Gerontology, 49*, S85–S94.

White, S. W., Oswald, D., Ollendick, T., & Scahill, L. (2009). Anxiety in children and adolescents with autism Spectrum disorders. *Clinical Psychology Review, 29*, 216–229.

Yeager, D. S., & Dweck, C. S. (2012). Mindsets that promote resilience: When students believe that personal characteristics can be developed. *Educational Psychologist, 47*(4), 302–314.

Yeung, E., Kay, J., Roosevelt, G. E., Brandon, M., & Yetman, A. T. (2008). Lapse of care as a predictor for morbidity in adults with congenital heart disease. *International Journal of Cardiology, 125*, 62–65.

5

A Life Course Health Development Perspective on Oral Health

James J. Crall and Christopher B. Forrest

1 Introduction

1.1 Life Course Health Development Concepts and Principles

Life Course Health Development(LCHD) is a conceptual framework that helps to explain how health develops over an individual's lifetime and emphasizes the need to treat health development as a long-term investment, beginning early and continuing throughout life (Halfon and Hochstein 2002). LCHD provides a powerful approach to understanding diseases and conditions and how risk factors, protective factors, critical life experiences, and environments affect long-term health and disease outcomes. LCHD also can help examine and explain how health and disease patterns, particularly health disparities, develop across populations and over time (Halfon and Hochstein 2002; Ben-Shlomo and Kuh 2002; Keating and Hertzman 1999).

J.J. Crall (✉)
Division of Public Health and Community Dentistry, University of California Los Angeles (UCLA) School of Dentistry, Los Angeles, CA, USA
e-mail: jcrall@dentistry.ucla.edu

C.B. Forrest
Applied Clinical Research Center, Children's Hospital of Pennsylvania, Philadelphia, PA, USA

Efforts to relate the life course perspective or life course theory to the field of maternal and child health (Fine and Kotelchuck, 2010) have emphasized the following key concepts:

Pathways or Trajectories Health pathways or trajectories are constructed and modified throughout the life span. While individual trajectories vary, general patterns can be predicted for populations and communities based on social, economic, and environmental exposures and experiences. A life course does not reflect a series of discrete steps or stages, but rather an integrated, dynamic, and continuous set of exposures and experiences. The set of possible trajectories that a person can experience is constrained by evolutionary forces and is highly determined by exposure to various environmental contexts.

Importance of Early Life Exposures Early experiences can markedly influence an individual's future health development. Of particular salience are exposures that occur prenatally (i.e., exposures in utero) and intergenerationally (i.e., factors related to the health of the mother prior to conception). While adverse events and exposures can have an impact at any point in a person's life course, the impact may be greatest at specific critical or sensitive periods when developing biological systems are most readily modified (e.g., during fetal development, in early childhood, during adolescence).

Cumulative Impact Cumulative experiences also can influence an individual's future health and development, even though any individual experience may not impact health development. For example, individuals may adapt with minimal impact to each episode of stress; however, the cumulative impact of multiple stresses over time (also referred to as "weathering" or "allostatic load") may have a profound direct impact on health development by altering biological function and human behavior.

Risk and Protective Factors Throughout the life span, protective factors improve health and contribute to health development, while risk factors diminish health and make it more difficult to reach full health potential. Moreover, pathways are changeable, and risk and protective factors are not limited to individual behavioral patterns or receipt of health-care and social services, but also include factors related to family, neighborhood, community, and social policy.

The LCHD theoretical framework (presented more thoroughly in Chap. 2) incorporates and expands these concepts into a robust explanatory synthesis of how health in individuals and populations is produced and modified. In this chapter, we use the LCHD principles to guide our review of oral health development. The Table 1 illustrates each LCHD principle's relevance to oral health.

1.2 Previous Efforts to Apply Life Course Concepts to Oral Health

The multifactorial etiology of oral conditions, their chronic nature and occurrence over the life span, and inherent features of their expression make oral health well suited to studies which seek to apply life course concepts. For example, Nicolau and colleagues (Nicolau et al. 2007) have highlighted several features that make oral conditions amenable to life course epidemiological studies, the first of which is their observability—i.e., once these conditions develop, they are readily detectable during assessments as opposed to conditions that resolve or go unnoted if study participants fail to report them. A second feature relates to their being cumulative conditions, which allows for comparisons of the degree of disease development among individuals so that, rather than all who develop the disease being enumerated together, distinctions can be made among them with respect to the extent or severity of their disease. Third, oral conditions can be reliably measured and validly diagnosed without sophisticated or costly technology. Fourth, these conditions are moderately prevalent; thus, the required sample size for cohort studies is manageable. And, finally, oral health conditions have a public health importance that makes their study justifiable on both ethical and economic grounds.

Despite growing interest in using life course concepts as the basis for various oral health-related scientific studies, robust applications have been rather limited. A PubMed search conducted as part of the literature review for this chapter using the terms "life course and oral health" yielded over 500 citations. However, a substantial portion of the publications examined in this and other literature searches were found to have one or more of the following limitations: studies focused on a single condition, used cross-sectional data, or analyzed a relatively narrow portion of the life span, studies were based on relatively small sample sizes, and studies were predicated on retrospective analyses that frequently relied on recall of rather distant events.

Furthermore, efforts to examine oral health from the perspective of LCHD concepts and principles have not been pursued. Therefore, the goals of this chapter are to (a) examine the concept of oral health and major oral diseases and conditions from a LCHD perspective using the key concepts and principles noted in the table, (b) assess what is (and what is not) known about the development of oral health and its impact on general health and well-being across the life course, and (c) offer recommendations for future research. In light of the evidence-based literature shortcomings noted in the preceding paragraph, assessments of what is known about applications of life course research approaches to studies of oral health are limited to research publications consistent with the life course epidemiology

Table 1 Life Course Health Development principles

	Principle	Brief description	Oral health illustrations
1	Health Development	Health development integrates the concepts of health and developmental processes into a unified whole. Health enables adaptation to the environment, task execution, participation in desired activities, and attainment of thriving. Development refers to the mechanisms by which health changes over time. Health development, then, comprises trajectories of health assets and integrated sets of health resources that emerge as a result of a person's continuous and relational interactions with their environments.	Oral health is not merely the absence of oral diseases. Instead, oral health refers to the capacity to adapt to ubiquitous environmental and microbial challenges, maintaining the robustness of teeth and other structures in the mouth, and oral health development refers to the pathways and trajectories of change of these assets over the life course.
2	Unfolding	Health development unfolds continuously over the lifespan, from conception to death, and is shaped by prior experiences and environmental interactions. For human health development, there are four major functional phases: (1) *generativity*, preconception and prenatal period; (2) *acquisition of capacity*, the early years; (3) *maintenance of capacity*, the middle years; and (4) *managing decline*, the later years. Each is conceptually distinct but can be overlapping.	Prenatal conditions can predispose developing teeth to elevated risk of early childhood caries, which is in turn a risk factor for caries later in life, which can lead to tooth loss and associated negative impacts on oral and overall health.
3	Complexity	Health development results from adaptive, multilevel, and reciprocal interactions between individuals and their physical, natural, and social environments. There is a dynamic interplay between individual and multiple physical, biochemical, psychological, social, and cultural networks which enable adaptation and individual robustness. Each level is both a part and a whole, nested and hierarchically aligned to optimize health development.	Oral health is strongly influenced by nutritional intake and changes in the microbiome. These effects in turn impact health development of individuals as well as their energy levels, healing, behavior, and cognitive development.

(continued)

Table 1 (continued)

	Principle	Brief description	Oral health illustrations
4	Timing	Health development is sensitive to the timing and social structuring of environmental exposures and experiences. Time-specific health development pathways refer to biological embedding that occurs during sensitive or critical periods, when developing systems are most alterable, and exogenous and endogenous influences can result in different adaptive responses. Socially structured pathways link experiences and exposures in ways that create recursive and mutually reinforcing patterns of risk, protection, and promotion.	Oral cancers result from the dynamic interaction of genetic, physical, biochemical, psychological, behavioral, social, and cultural factors. Risk for these conditions is highest for individuals who use alcohol, use tobacco, are exposed to human papilloma virus or Epstein-Barr virus, or are exposed to x-radiation before the age of 50 years
5	Plasticity	Health development phenotypes are systematically malleable and enabled and constrained by evolution to enhance adaptability to diverse environments. Heredity transmits evolutionary signals through genetic, epigenetic, behavioral, and symbolic dimensions, which establish health phenotypes that depending on environmental circumstances may or may not be selected and optimized to produce desirable outcomes. At the microlevel, a range of strategies introduce variable types and levels of plasticity to optimize adaptability from the molecular to the behavioral level. At a macrolevel, strategies organize health development phases and life stages into functional entities.	The human jaw developed over millennia among our human ancestors who spent hours each day chewing their food. The interaction between chewing of tough food and bone development may have been responsible for the lack of malocclusion observed in the hominid fossil record. Today a softer diet has contributed to smaller jaws and smaller teeth in modern humans, leading to the large numbers of individuals with malocclusion and need for orthodontic treatment.
6	Thriving	Optimal health development promotes survival, enhances well-being, and protects against disease. Health development can also be perturbed to create suboptimal states that are precursors to fully formed disease—so-called endophenotypes that represent intermediate phase transitions toward a fully manifest phenotypic expression of a disease or disorder.	Diabetes perturbs oral health development by increasing risk for periodontal disease, which when present causes pain, chewing difficulties, and tooth loss. Dry mouth, often a symptom of undetected diabetes, can cause sores, ulcers, infections and tooth decay. Smoking makes these problems worse. Conversely, reducing diabetes risk and reducing or eliminating smoking can promote oral health.
7	Harmony	Health development results from the balanced interactions of molecular, physiological, behavioral, cultural, and evolutionary processes. Genetic modulations that occur in molecular time frames measured in nanoseconds are linked to biochemical modulation measured in milliseconds, homeostatic mechanisms measured in seconds to days, social norms that evolve over years and decades, cultural processes that change from years to centuries, and ecological processes that until recently took millennia. Harmonization of these processes produces rhythms and variability that characterize health. Loss of coordination of these processes results in less robustness of the human system with negative consequences.	Analysis of the DNA from ancient humans has demonstrated shifts in oral bacterial species ecology following dietary pattern changes and reductions in the diversity of the oral ecosystem, a possible factor in the rise of dental caries and periodontal disease in modern humans whose oral health may be better matched to circumstances in our evolutionary history than to modern environments.

standard and LCHD framework. Furthermore, because of the diverse nature of the major oral health-related conditions noted above, assessments are largely limited to "dental conditions" (i.e., dental caries, periodontal diseases, and tooth loss), with limited additional examples pertaining to craniofacial abnormalities, oral cancers, or temporomandibular joint dysfunction.

2 Conceptualizing Oral Health and Overview of Major Conditions

2.1 Conceptualizing Oral Health

Concepts and definitions of oral health have varied over time, often paralleling broader conceptualizations of health. Concepts of how oral health changes over time also often parallel more general paradigms. For example, many recent concepts of oral health have been based on the biopsychosocial model, which focuses on how the integration of various aspects of biological, psychological, and social domains influence individuals' health in different contexts and over time (Borrell-Carrio et al. 2004).

The US Surgeon General's Report on Oral Health (SGROH), issued in 2000, and ensuing initiatives have emphasized two major themes regarding the concept of oral health—i.e., oral health means much more than healthy teeth, and oral health is integral to general health (US Department of Health and Human Services 2000). Interestingly, the SGROH embraced the World Health Organization (WHO) definition of oral health as "a state of being free from mouth and facial pain, oral and throat cancer, oral infection and sores, periodontal (gum) disease, tooth decay, tooth loss, and other diseases and disorders that limit an individual's capacity in biting, chewing, smiling, speaking, and psychosocial wellbeing." This definition espoused by both the WHO and SGROH is deficient in that it does not positively define what oral health is, but rather presents the concept as the absence of detrimental conditions or disorders. Conflating oral health and oral disorders is contrary to the WHO definition of overall health which states that health is more than just the absence of disease and represents a state of complete physical, mental, and social well-being. Researchers working to develop measures related to oral health and its impact on quality of life also have concluded that health and disease are different domains of human experience, which vary both over time and among individuals, and are dependent on context (Locker and Slade 1994; Gregory et al. 2005).

A recent development in the conceptualization and definition of oral health has emerged from the FDI World Dental Federation in late 2016. According to the new FDI definition, "Oral health is multifaceted and includes the ability to speak, smile, smell, taste, touch, chew, swallow, and convey a range of emotions through facial expressions with confidence and without pain, discomfort, and disease of the craniofacial complex. The core elements of oral health in the FDI framework are as follows: *disease and condition status* refers to a threshold of severity or a level of progression of disease, which also includes pain and discomfort; *physiological function* refers to the capacity to perform a set of actions that include, but are not limited to, the ability to speak, smile, chew, and swallow; and *psychosocial function* refers to the relationship between oral health and mental state that includes, but is not limited to, the capacity to speak, smile, and interact in social and work situations without feeling uncomfortable or embarrassed." (Glick et al. 2016).

LCHD theoretical principles conceptualize health as an emergent set of integrated assets that enable adaptation and pursuit of meaning and happiness, reflect broader notions of the impact of various health determinants over time, and consider health in a more positive context (see Table 1). Applying LCHD concepts, individuals with disease (e.g., diabetics or persons living with AIDS) can also be considered healthy if they have developed assets which enable adaptation to their environment, task execution, participation in desired activities, and an ability to thrive; health and disease are distinct, albeit interrelated concepts.

LCHD builds and expands upon the basic tenets of the biopsychosocial and other ecological models and establishes a conceptual foundation for a future era of health care that moves beyond systems focused on management of acute and chronic diseases and conditions to systems whose focus is on optimizing lifelong health for individuals and populations (Halfon et al. 2014). Using LCHD concepts and principles to conceptualize and define oral health has the potential to move practitioners, researchers, policy makers, and the public beyond their historical limited focus on the physical form and function of structures in and surrounding the oral cavity and the clinical consequences of oral/dental diseases to a new paradigm—one which fully embraces LCHD tenets and the development of more robust LCHD-based policies and systems for optimizing the oral health of individuals and populations.

2.2 Major Oral Health-Related Diseases and Conditions

Clinical conditions that have major significance with respect to oral health in terms of prevalence, impact on health, development and well-being, and economic considerations include *dental diseases and their consequences* (dental caries, periodontal diseases, tooth loss), *craniofacial developmental disorders* (e.g., cleft lip, cleft palate, malocclusion), *oral cancers* (including pharyngeal and salivary gland cancers), and *facial pain* (distinct from dental pain) generally associated with temporomandibular joint and muscular disorders. Brief overviews of these conditions are provided below.

Dental Conditions Despite significant progress during the latter portion of the twentieth century, *dental caries (tooth decay)* remains the most common chronic disease of childhood and a major cause of tooth loss in children and adults. In the United States, approximately 25% of 2–5-year-olds and over 50% of 6–8-year-old children experience dental caries in their primary teeth, and over 50% of 12–15-year-olds and 67% of 16–19-year-olds experience caries in their permanent teeth (Dye et al. 2011a). Although substantial declines in the average number of teeth and tooth surfaces affected by caries have been documented in recent decades, particularly in developed countries, according to the WHO, the prevalence of tooth decay in school-age children globally ranges from 60% to 90% (WHO, The World Oral Health Report 2008).

Significant disparities in childhood caries experience also persist. On average, US children from lower-income households and children of color are three to five times more likely than their white more affluent counterparts to experience caries and exhibit more severe forms of tooth decay (Dye et al. 2011a; Vargas et al. 1998). Of interest from a LCHD perspective, many children from high-risk population groups do not exhibit severe forms of dental caries, presumably because the balance between individual's risk and protective factors (e.g., diet, toothbrushing habits, fluoride exposure, oral microflora or other unidentified characteristics) is conducive to maintaining a healthy dentition (Feathersone 2000).

Caries affects dentate individuals across the life span (Fig. 1), with over 90% of US adults with natural teeth experiencing dental caries in their permanent teeth (Dye et al. 2011a, b). According to the WHO (WHO, The World Oral Health Report, 2008) nearly 100% of dentate adults globally are affected by dental caries, making it the most prevalent chronic condition of people worldwide. From a life course perspective, early childhood caries can have a profound deleterious lifelong effect on an individual's dentition status, as ECC often is a precursor of caries and its consequences in adults.

Periodontal disease mainly results from infections and inflammation of the gingiva (gums) and bone that surround and support the teeth. In its early stage, called gingivitis, the gums can become swollen and red and may bleed. In its more serious form, called periodontitis, the gums can pull away from the teeth, bone can be lost, and teeth may loosen or even fall out. Thirty percent of US adults 30+ years of age have moderate periodontal disease, and 8.5% have severe periodontitis (Thornton-Evans 2013). Males, older adults, Black and Hispanic adults, current smokers, and those with lower incomes and less education are more likely to have moderate or severe

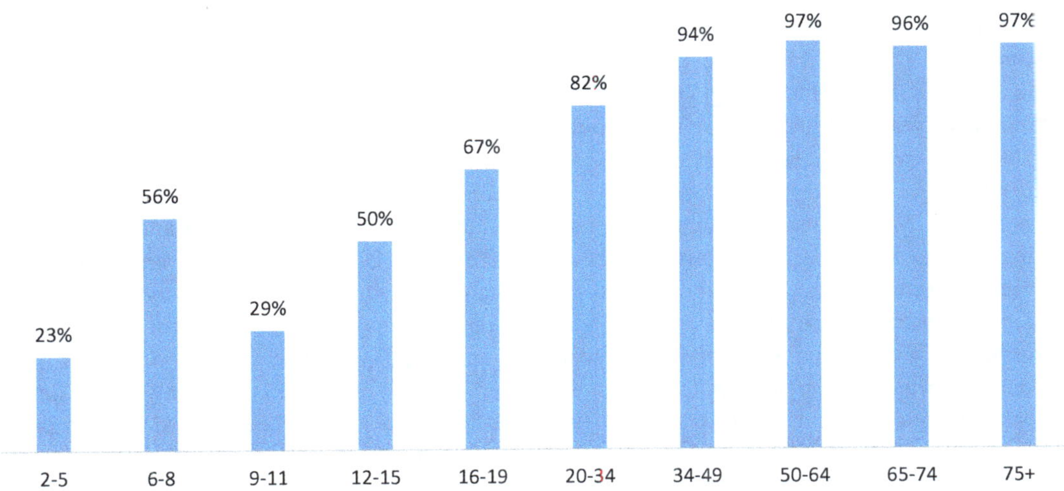

Fig. 1 Proportion of the US population with caries experience (percentages for 2–5- and 6–8-year-olds reflect the percentage of individuals with caries experience in primary teeth; for ages 9 and above, percentages reflect the percentage with caries experience in permanent teeth) by age (years) (Data Source: National Health and Nutrition Examination Survey, 2011–2012. National Center for Health Statistics, CDC)

periodontal disease (Thornton-Evans 2013). Globally, severe periodontal disease is found in 15–20% of adults aged 35–44 years and increases in prevalence with advancing age (WHO, The World Oral Health Report 2008).

Dental caries and periodontal disease are the primary reasons for *tooth loss* (Dye et al. 2011b; Thornton-Evans 2013) which in its more severe forms (loss of multiple teeth) can have negative psychological, social, nutritional, and physical effects. A person's quality of life is diminished as a result of tooth loss due to reductions in their ability to chew and speak and reduced social interactions and self-esteem (US Department of Health and Human Services 2000; Hollister & Weintraub 1993; Brennan et al. 2008). National survey data indicate that approximately 50% of US adults have lost at least one tooth. Approximately 5% of US adults overall and 25% of adults aged 65+ are completely edentulous (have no natural teeth) (Dye et al. 2011b). Worldwide, about 30% of people aged 65–74 have no natural teeth, with considerable disparities across countries (WHO, The World Oral Health Report 2008).

Total US spending for dental services has been relatively flat at approximately $111 billion since 2010 (Wall 2013). The bulk of dental care spending is related to diagnosis, prevention and treatment of dental caries and periodontal disease, and treatment related to removal and replacement of lost teeth.

Craniofacial Conditions Craniofacial defects such as *cleft lip and cleft palate (CLP)* are among the most common of all birth defects. The US incidence of cleft palate is 6 per 10,000 live births, and the incidence for cleft lip with or without cleft palate is 11 per 10,000 live births (Center for Disease Control and Prevention (CDC) 2014). CLP can occur as an isolated condition or may be a component of an inherited disease or syndrome. Cleft lip and cleft palate are thought to be caused by a combination of genes and other factors, such as things the mother comes in contact with in her environment, what the mother eats or drinks, or certain medications she uses during pregnancy. Maternal smoking, alcohol use, steroid use, and anticonvulsants are associated with increased risk for cleft lip and palate (Kohli and Kohli 2012). The incidence of CLP also varies by race, with Asians and Native Americans having higher rates and African-Americans having lower rates. According to the Centers for Disease Control and Prevention

(CDC), in the United States, cleft lip and palate is the third most common birth defect, and health expenditures are approximately eight times higher in the first 10 years of life for children with clefting than for those without (Boulet et al. 2009).

Malocclusion Misalignment or abnormal positioning of the teeth or an incorrect relation between the teeth in the upper and lower jaws—is neither a disease nor a life-threatening condition. Nevertheless, growing numbers of people seek and undergo orthodontic treatment, often because of esthetic concerns and other quality of life issues (Liu et al. 2009). Although children make up the majority of orthodontic patients, adults increasingly are seeking treatment for malocclusion and now comprise one-fifth of all orthodontic patients in the US. Orthodontic services account for approximately one-eighth of US dental care expenditures (Agency for Healthcare Research and Quality 2015).

Oral Cancers Approximately 45,000 Americans and over 450,000 people worldwide are diagnosed each year with cancers that affect the mouth and/or pharynx. Oral cancers comprise 85% of all head and neck cancers and have relatively high mortality rates (5-year survival = 63%) (The Oral Cancer Foundation 2015; American Cancer Society 2015). Oral cancer occurrence rates are significantly higher for males than for females (except in American Indians/Alaska Natives) and higher for black males than for white males up to age 70. Oral cancer rates increase with age, increase more rapidly after age 50, and peak between ages 70 and 80 (Fig. 2) (Ram et al. 2011). Extensive case-control and longitudinal studies have implicated tobacco and alcohol as major risk factors for oral cancer. Human papillomavirus, syphilis, oro-dental factors, dietary deficiencies, chronic candidiasis, and viruses also have been shown to be significantly associated with oral cancer (Ram et al. 2011). Findings of a recent study (Jacobson et al. 2012) suggest that oral cancers may be among the most costly forms of cancer to treat in the United States.

Facial Pain Associated with Temporoman dibular Joint Disorders The most common cause of facial pain is a group of conditions called temporomandibular joint and muscle disorders (TMJD). These disorders cause recurrent or chronic pain and dysfunction in the jaw joint and its associated muscles and supporting tissues. TMJD are the second most commonly occurring musculoskeletal condition resulting in pain and disability (after chronic low back pain), affecting

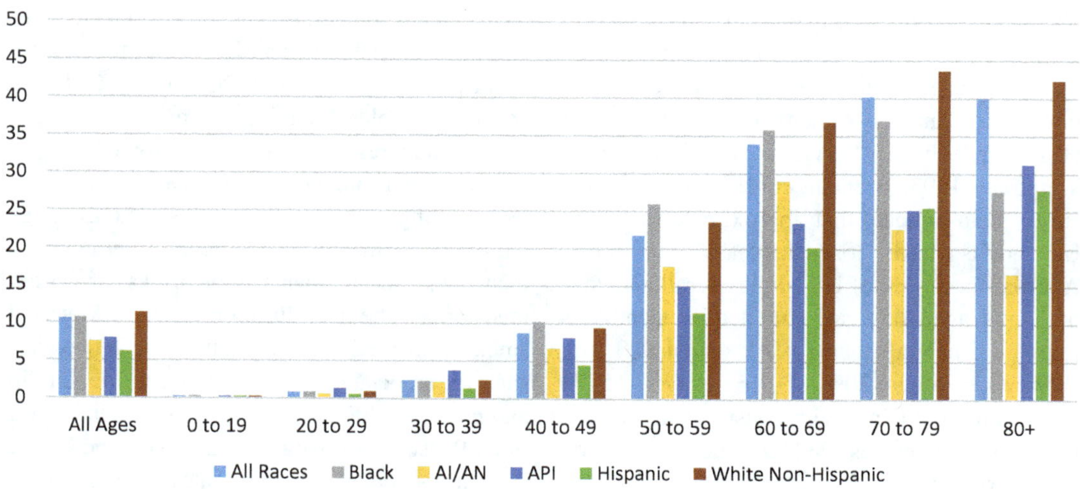

Fig. 2 Incidence of oral cancer cases per 100,000 among different age and racial groups (Data Source: Oral Cancer Incidence by Age, Race and Gender, 2009. National Institute of Dental and Craniofacial Research)

approximately 5–12% of the population, with an annual cost estimated at $4 billion. About half to two-thirds of those with TMJD seek treatment; among those seeking treatment, approximately 15% develop chronic TMJD (NIDCR 2003).

3 Evolution of Oral Health Paradigms

The evolution of concepts regarding oral health and associated analytical models designed to measure oral health in the aggregate and its various components have paralleled the evolution of general health concepts, albeit frequently with a variable time lag. Ancient theories and hypotheses have given way to more scientifically grounded concepts reflecting changing scientific paradigms, initially based on biomedical models of disease causation, followed by biopsychosocial models that attempted to incorporate a wider range of factors influencing health and, more recently, Life Course Health Development. The following section provides a broad overview of that progression, focusing primarily on concepts regarding dental conditions.

3.1 Changing Concepts of Dental Disease: From Worms to Germs to Chronic Disease Terms

Tooth Worm Theory The concept of a tooth worm which according to prevailing popular beliefs caused caries and periodontitis existed in diverse cultures across the ages and, despite being labeled by medical doctors as superstition during the time of the Enlightenment, persisted in some cultures into the twentieth century. Numerous popular "therapies" were applied to eradicate the tooth worm, including fumigations with henbane seeds, magical formulas, and oaths (Gerabek 1999).

Chemo-Parasitic and Focal Infection Theories In 1890, W.D. Miller (an American dentist and the first oral microbiologist), building on Pasteur's discovery that bacteria can ferment sugars into lactic acid, formulated the chemo-parasitic theory of caries. This theory held that tooth decay is caused by acids, produced by oral bacteria following fermentation of ingested sugars, which lead to loss of mineral from teeth (demineralization) (Miller 1890). Miller's second major contribution was the focal infection theory, which hypothesized that oral microorganisms or their products have a role in the development of a variety of diseases in sites removed from the oral cavity, including brain abscesses, pulmonary diseases, and gastric problems (Miller 1891). Later work by Keyes in the 1960s led to explanations of the mechanisms by which dental caries develops based on the interaction of cariogenic bacteria in biofilm/dental plaque and dietary substrates that lead to acid production, which in turn leads to demineralization of tooth structure (illustrated in the Venn diagram in Fig. 5).

Concept of Caries as a Specific and Transmissible Infection The concept of dental caries being infectious and transmissible is based on the biomedical model of disease causation, and grew out of well-designed rodent studies performed by Keyes (Keyes 1960) showing that caries only developed in rodents when they were caged with or ate the fecal pellets of groups of caries-active rodents. Further proof emerged when certain streptococci isolated from caries lesions in hamsters, unlike other types of streptococci, caused rampant decay in previously caries-inactive animals (Fitzgerald and Keyes 1960). The bacteria, later identified as *Streptococcus mutans* (SM), gave rise to the concept of caries being due to a specific infection with mutans streptococci (MS), a concept that has gained wide support within the field of caries microbiology (Fejerskov 2004). Subsequent studies conducted from the mid-1970s through the 1990s demonstrated that infants acquire MS from their mothers and that MS can colonize the mouths of infants even before teeth erupt (Berkowitz 2006).

Conceptualizing Caries as a Complex, Chronic Disease More recently, Featherstone (Feathersone 2000) used a modification of the chronic disease model, referred to as the "caries balance," to describe caries as a dynamic process that depends on the balance between constellations of risk factors (e.g., high levels of cariogenic bacteria, reduced salivary function, cariogenic dietary practices, tooth structure anomalies) and protective factors (e.g., salivary components and flow, exposure to fluorides, anti-cariogenic dietary components). Although the caries balance concept highlights the importance of risk factors and protective factors and the potential for dynamic changes over time, published examples generally depict factors related to biomedical models rather than broader biopsychosocial models.

The shift from conceptualizing dental caries based on biomedical models to models based on biopsychosocial theory represents a relatively recent paradigm change. These newer models recognize that caries expression not only depends on the complex interplay between saliva, dietary habits, and many biological determinants related to biofilm composition and metabolism; it also depends on those factors acting in concert with innumerable other biological, behavioral, and social factors acting at the level of individuals and populations. In summarizing the implications of this paradigm shift, Fejerskov (Fejerskov 2004) highlighted the following:

> By appreciating that dental caries belongs to the group of common diseases considered as 'complex' or 'mulifactorial' such as cancer, heart diseases, diabetes, and certain psychiatric illnesses, we have to realize that there is no simple causation pathway. It is not a simplistic problem such as 'elimination of one type of microorganism', or a matter of improving 'tooth resistance'. Complex diseases cannot be ascribed to mutations in a single gene or to a single environmental factor. Rather they arise from the concerted action of many genes, environmental factors, and risk-conferring behaviors. ... [This concept also] explains why dental caries has to be controlled lifelong if a functional dentition is to be maintained.
>
> These new concepts explain why . . . several of the 'old' recommended preventive programs are no longer effective. It is of course not because the agents we used in prevention are no longer efficacious. They just become ineffective because the caries incidence rate has changed as the environment has changed.

This brief overview highlights changes in popular and scientific concepts regarding the etiology of common dental diseases and methods for preventing or minimizing their consequences over time. Nevertheless, the persistence of relatively high levels of dental disease in sizeable segments of the population and substantial disparities within and across populations serve to highlight the limitations of traditional concepts and approaches.

3.2 Common Risk Factors, Social Determinants, and Ecological Models

Common Risk Factors As noted above, there is growing recognition that major oral health-related conditions are complex (multifactorial), chronic conditions whose occurrence and severity across the lifespan depend on interactions of a broad array of biological, behavioral, social, and environmental factors, which also are implicated in other chronic diseases and conditions as indicated in Fig. 3 (Fejerskov 2004; Sheiham and

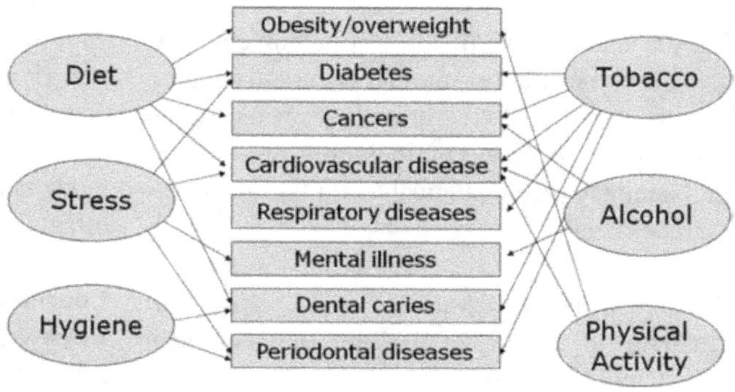

Fig. 3 Common risk factor model of oral disease and other chronic diseases (Source: Tomar 2012)

Watt 2000; Larson et al. 2008; Tomar 2012). We now realize that different types of organisms are involved in the etiology of dental caries and periodontal diseases and that the ecology of the oral microbiome is influenced by an array of common biological and biopsychosocial factors. We recognize that craniofacial disorders are caused by developmental disturbances that occur in utero and are influenced by genetic and environmental factors. We know that oral cancers result from mutations in genes that control cell behavior and are influenced by exposure to carcinogens (most notably tobacco) and biological factors, including viruses and fungi. Evidence also indicates that risk factors implicated in TMJD include poor alignment of teeth, stress, parafunctional habits, arthritis, trauma, and structural developmental abnormalities.

Cumulative Impact of Multiple Social Determinants Larson et al. (Larson et al. 2008) highlighted the cumulative impact of multiple social risk factors (limited parental education, low family income, single-parent household, race, being uninsured, family conflict, poor maternal mental health, living in an unsafe neighborhood) on various aspects of children's health, including their oral health. As shown in Fig. 4, the percentage of parents who reported that their children had suboptimal oral health and other indicators of poor health rises with increases in the number of prevailing social risk factors, with the relationship between social risk factors and poor oral health demonstrating the steepest linear gradient. The proportion reporting less than very good teeth ranged from 14% for children with no social risk factors to 64% for children with ≥6 social risk factors. Analyses that controlled for child age, gender, and number of children in the household showed an almost 11-fold increase in the odds for less than very good teeth in children with ≥6 versus no social risks, underscoring the importance of social structure to healthy development.

Ecological Models of Caries and Periodontal Disease Figure 5 depicts a multidimensional

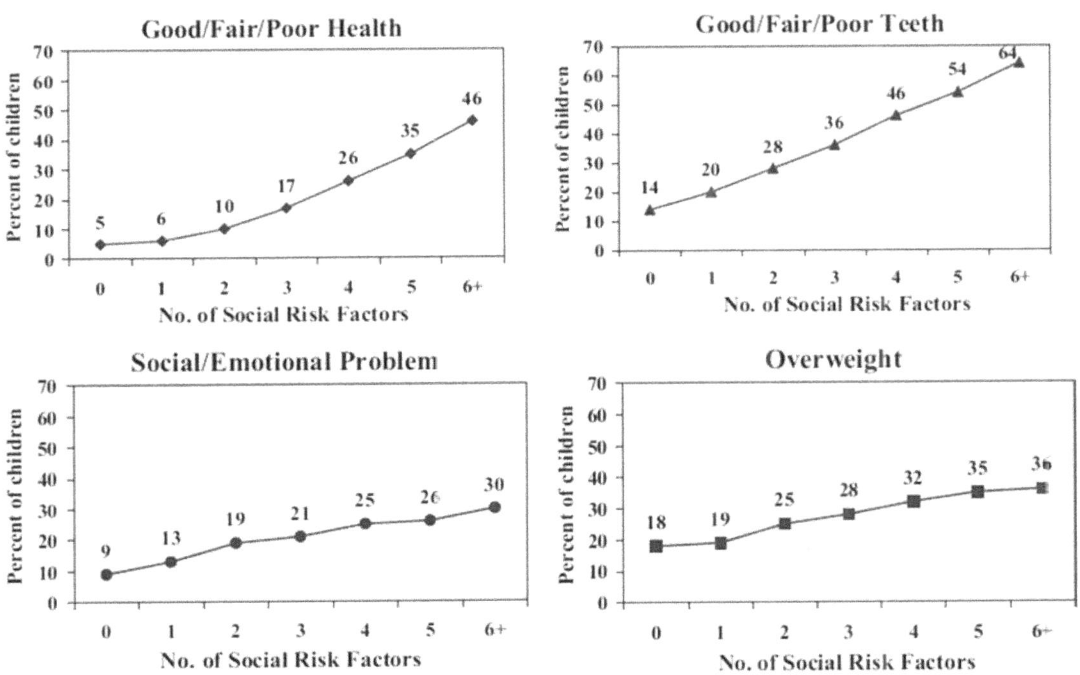

Fig. 4 Percentage of children in worse health by number of social risk factors (Source: Larson et al. 2008)

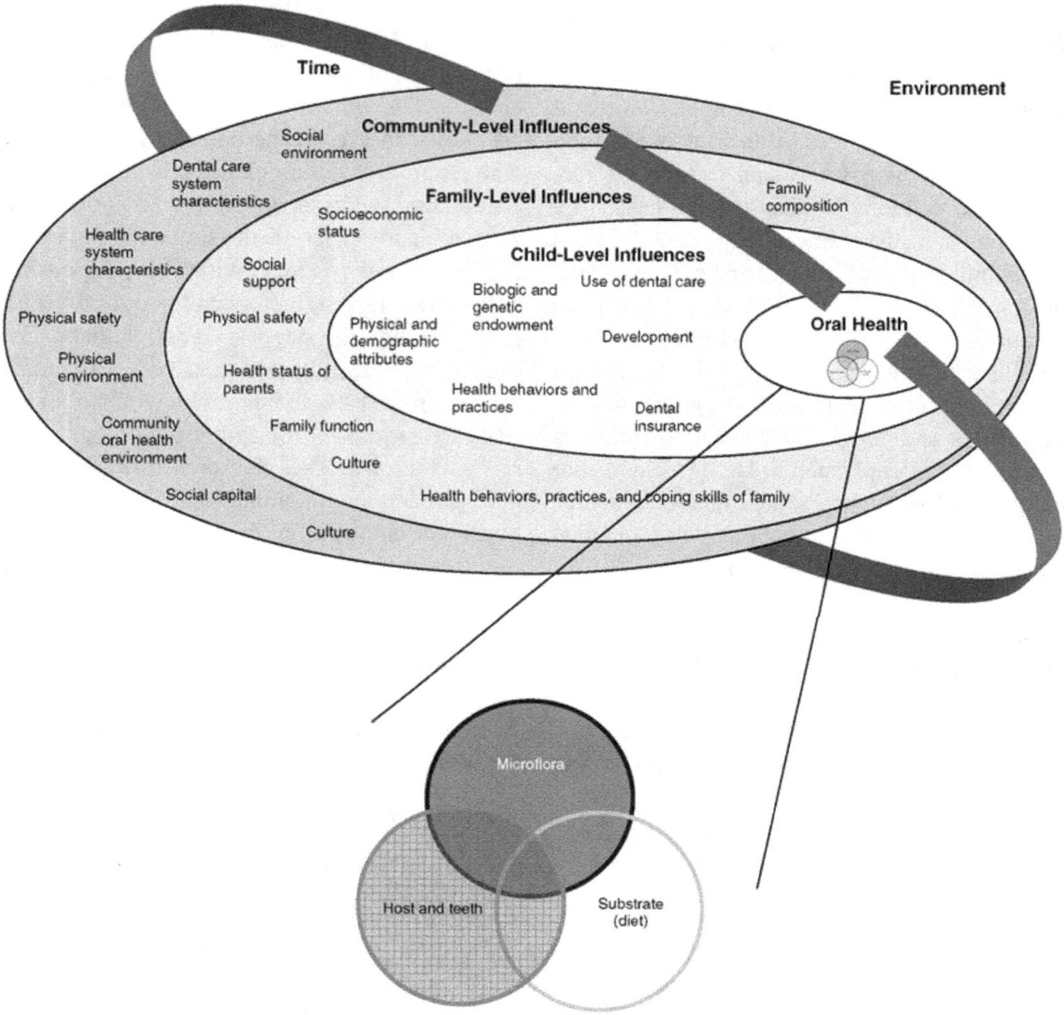

Fig. 5 Influences on children's oral health: a conceptual model (Source: Fisher-Owens et al. 2007)

ecological model for childhood dental caries, enumerating an array of biopsychosocial influences (including six child-level, eight family-level, and eight community-level influences identified in the literature) in addition to the Keyes classic biological triad model and the influence of environmental factors and time (Fisher-Owens et al. 2007). The bulk of published studies underlying ecological models such as this have study design limitations similar to those identified in conducting the literature review for this chapter. Accordingly, their utility with respect to LCHD studies lies in helping to identify disease correlates and generate hypotheses, not in establishing oral disease or health development pathways.

Ecological models like the one shown in Fig. 5 have been used to design a variety of caries-risk assessment instruments. However, most caries-risk assessment instruments include only a subset of the broad range of influences depicted in the Fisher-Owens model and generally have not undergone extensive validity testing (Quinonez and Crall 2009).

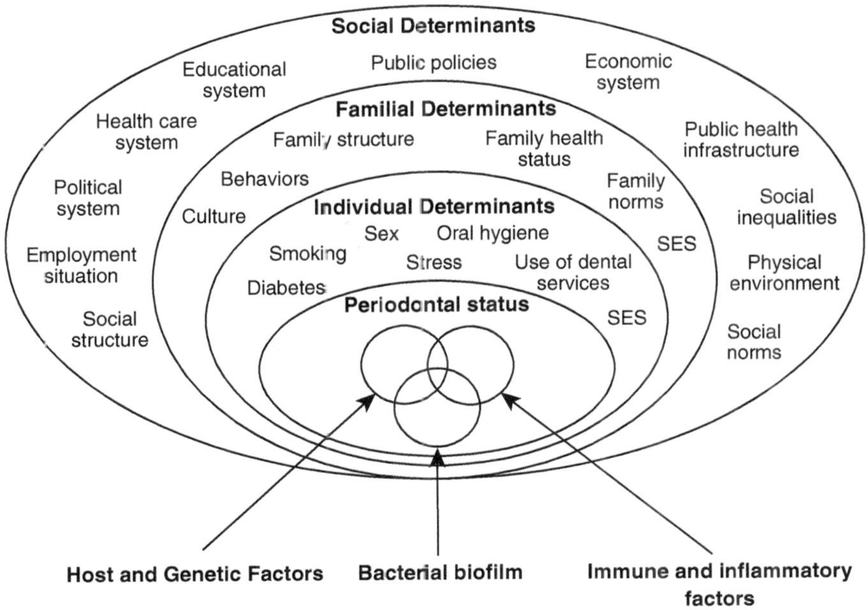

Fig. 6 Social determinants of oral health and disease in US men (Source: Tomar 2012)

Figure 6 depicts an ecological conceptual model for periodontal disease using a framework similar to the Fisher-Owens et al. model for childhood caries (Tomar 2012). In this case, the biological model emphasizes the interactions among host and genetic factors, bacteria associated with periodontal disease (different and distinct from cariogenic bacteria), and immune and inflammatory factors—reflecting a different pathogenic mechanism for periodontal disease than for dental caries. Constellations of individual, familial, and social influences are identified within categories of social, behavioral, and contextual factors in this model.

Ecological models like those shown in Figs. 5 and 6 are useful for depicting the complex array of etiological factors that potentially influence disease development, but are of limited value for explaining disease mechanisms or pathways as they do not explicitly incorporate developmental mechanisms or time into the frameworks. LCHD principles address these gaps by building on ecological models, adding time dimensions and developmental pathways to the models.

4 Research Applications of Life Course Concepts to Oral Health

4.1 Life Course Epidemiology

Life course epidemiology adds the time dimension to disease causation models, moving beyond the limitations of models such as those shown in the preceding section which depict an unspecified, essentially cross-sectional interplay among nested layers of environmental and individual factors. According to Kuh and Ben-Shlomo (Ben-Shlomo and Kuh 2002), "Life course epidemiology is defined as 'the study of long-term effects on chronic disease risk of physical and social exposures during gestation, childhood, adolescence, young adulthood and later adult life. It seeks to understand causal links between exposures and outcomes, taking into consideration the importance of time (duration) and timing in the disease development." In a recent paper on concepts and theoretical models of life course epidemiology and its relevance to chronic oral conditions, Nicolau et al. (Nicolau et al. 2007) noted that "The life course approach to studying chronic disease etiology is not merely a collection of longitudinal data or the use of a particular study design or analytical method. Rather, the unique feature of this approach is a theoretical framework which assumes and tests a temporal ordering of exposure variables and their interrelationship with a specific outcome." The following section provides several examples of applications of life course epidemiology to studies of chronic oral diseases and conditions.

4.2 Oral Health Trajectories: Dunedin Cohort Studies

A number of studies published since the turn of the twenty-first century have begun to more fully embrace life course research methodologies and examine a broader array of life course influences. Foremost among them from the standpoint of assessing changes in oral health status over time and the influence of socioeconomic influences beginning in early childhood is the Dunedin Multidisciplinary Health and Development Study—a longitudinal investigation of health and behavior in a complete birth cohort of study members born in Dunedin, New Zealand, between April, 1972 and March, 1973. Findings of several Dunedin studies are summarized below.

Poulton et al. (Poulton et al. 2002) assessed a number of health outcomes, including dental caries, dental plaque scores, gingival bleeding, and periodontal disease status in a cohort of 1000 26-year-old Dunedin Study subjects whose socioeconomic status (SES) had been documented at birth and at ages, 3, 5, 7, 9, 11, 13, and 15 years. All dental health measures at age 26 years showed a graded relation with childhood SES. As SES increased, the amount of plaque and gingival bleeding and the proportion of individuals with periodontal disease and decayed surfaces decreased. The adverse influence of low childhood socioeconomic status was seen after controlling for infant health and contemporaneous adult SES. Additionally, the results showed that low adult SES had a significant effect on poor adult dental health after controlling for low childhood SES. The authors concluded that their "findings document that the social gradient in health—which has been amply documented among middle-aged and older adults—actually emerges in childhood. Whereas clinical and research interest in the social gradient has been generated mostly by studies of adults, the findings from this study suggest that the social gradient can be scrutinised in paediatric and adolescent populations as well. Further, whereas most studies of the social gradient have narrowed their attention to specific diseases, such as cardiovascular diseases, we document that the social gradient is far more ubiquitous and troubling. Low social class adversely affects many areas of people's health, including their physical, dental and mental health" (Poulton et al. 2002). This finding concerning children's dental health is highly noteworthy because there are few pediatric conditions that show a substantial SES gradient, which raises the possibility that body systems that develop rapidly and dramatically during childhood, such as the structures and physiological systems of the oral cavity, are more vulnerable to, and perhaps dependent on, environmental exposures.

Thomson et al. (2004) analyzed data on 789 Dunedin Study subjects at ages 5 and 26 years to investigate whether adult oral health status is influenced by (a) childhood socioeconomic advantage or disadvantage (controlling for childhood oral health) or (b) oral health in childhood (controlling for childhood socioeconomic advantage or disadvantage) and whether oral health in adulthood is affected by changes in SES. With respect to the question of whether poor adult oral health is predicted by socioeconomic disadvantage in childhood, after controlling for childhood oral health, analyses revealed that oral health inequalities present at age 5 years were also apparent at age 26 years when the early childhood SES categories were used, suggesting that early socioeconomic inequalities in a number of important oral health indicators do persist well into the third decade of life. Concerning the question of whether poor adult oral health is predicted by poor oral health in childhood, after controlling for childhood socioeconomic status, the evidence was unequivocal regarding dental caries: having high caries disease experience early in life predicted having greater disease experience in adulthood, other factors being equal. The pattern was not as clear with respect to periodontal disease, however. Finally, in examining the impact of individuals' SES at ages 5 and 26, Thomson and colleagues (Thomson et al. 2004) found that, for nearly all oral health indicators, a clear gradient for disease severity and prevalence was observed across socioeconomic trajectory groups in the following ascending order: "high (at age 5)–high (at age 26)," "low–high" (upwardly mobile), "high–low" (downwardly mobile), and "low–low." These findings led the authors to conclude that adult oral health is predicted by not only childhood socioeconomic advantage or disadvantage but also by oral health in childhood. Changes in socioeconomic advantage or disadvantage between ages 5 and 26 were associated with differing levels of oral health in adulthood. Also of interest from the standpoint of LCHD is the possibility that oral health may represent a sentinel system, with early manifestations of disease serving as a harbinger for elevated risk of other chronic diseases (e.g., obesity, diabetes).

Broadbent et al. (2008) investigated longitudinal patterns of caries experience in a birth cohort of 955 Dunedin Study subjects in order to identify and describe developmental trajectories of caries experience in the permanent dentition using data collected from dental examinations at ages 5, 9, 15, 18, 26, and 32 years. Three caries experience trajectory classes were identified: "high" (15% of subjects), "medium" (43%), and "low" (42%) with respect to decayed, missing, and filled (tooth) surfaces (DMFS). All trajectories were relatively linear, although the higher trajectories were more "S-shaped" (Fig. 7). This effect disappeared following adjustment for the number of unaffected surfaces remaining at each age, suggesting that, among individuals following a similar caries trajectory, the caries rate is relatively constant across time. This finding is

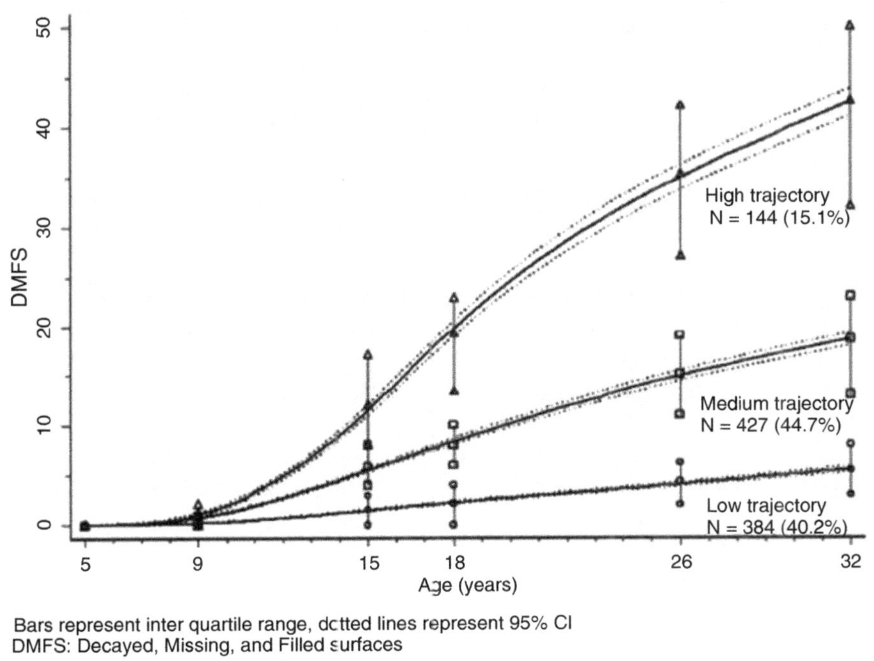

Fig. 7 Trajectory patterns of dental caries experience in the permanent dentition to the fourth decade of life (Source: Broadbent et al. 2008)

consistent with observations by Fejerskov (2004) that the caries incidence rate in a group of individuals appears fairly constant throughout life if no special efforts to control lesion progression are made. Broadbent et al. (2008) concluded that these results did not support the commonly held belief among dentists that childhood and adolescence are periods of special risk for dental caries or that caries "immunity" may be acquired during late adolescence or early adulthood. In fact, other studies have reported that ECC is one of the most reliable predictors of elevated risk of caries experience later in life.

Crocombe et al. (2011) also analyzed data from 833 participants in the Dunedin Study to assess the impact of dental visiting trajectory patterns on clinical oral health and oral health-related quality of life measures. Information on the use of dental services was collected at ages 15, 18, 26, and 32. Dental visiting trajectories were significantly associated with both measures of self-reported oral health and three of the four dental clinical indicators. The regular dental attendance group had less than half the mean number of missing teeth, a lower mean DMFS score, and a lower mean decayed surfaces (DS) than those defined as "opportunists" and "decliners." The regular group had the lowest mean Oral Health Impact Profile (OHIP-14) score and was nearly twice as likely as opportunists and decliners to report that they had better-than-average oral health. Low SES and being dentally anxious were associated with worse health outcomes for all outcome variables, while "poor plaque trajectory" and smoking were associated with worse outcomes for all variables except filled surfaces (FS). The influence of dental visiting trajectory on clinical oral health outcomes was much higher at lower SES levels than higher SES levels, leading the authors to conclude that improving dental visiting behavior among people of lower SES would improve clinical oral health outcomes more and have a greater reduction of oral health impacts than it would for people of higher SES.

A number of additional studies of shorter duration and/or employing retrospective methods of data collection (which may be subject to some degree of recall bias) have been conducted in other countries, most notably Brazil, Norway, the United Kingdom, and Hong Kong (Lu et al. 2011; Holst; Peres et al. 2011; Mason et al. 2006). Collectively, these studies generally affirm the findings from analyses conducted as part of the Dunedin Study, with some variation that likely reflects varying levels of SES (particularly poverty) and differences in the types of oral health-care systems and programs available across countries. Many of these studies are limited to adolescents (starting at age 15) or adults. An exception is the work of (Holst and Schuller 2011) which examined different birth cohorts in Norway and found that the health environment in childhood was important for adults' oral health during most of the twentieth century. Attention from parents and the local environment lead to better oral health outcomes in adulthood. Social status measured by length of education also was associated with choices leading to better oral health. Regular dental visits were important especially for the eldest birth cohort. Good oral health behaviors early and during adulthood were important for oral health.

The studies summarized in this section represent advances in our understanding of the impacts of various influences on oral health over the life course. Interest in using a life course perspective to study various aspects of oral health has grown steadily in recent times. Main lines of pursuit include investigations of critical periods and accumulation of risk models, which have shed light on the importance of early life experiences, oral health trajectories, and the importance of social determinants to oral and general health (Heilman et al. 2015). However, it is worth noting that life course epidemiology only reflects the principles of LCHD (see Table 1) in a very limited way, primarily with respect to LCHD Principle 3 (Complexity: multidimensional person-environmental interactions) and LCHD Principle 5 (Timing: health is highly sensitive to timing and social structuring of environmental exposures).

4.3 Relating Oral Health, General Health, and Quality of Life

Summarizing what is known about the influences of oral health and oral health problems on life course outcomes, general health and overall quality of life is a daunting challenge that goes beyond the scope of this chapter. In lieu of attempting such a synopsis, the reader is referred initially to the US Surgeon General's Report on Oral Health (US Department of Health and Human Services 2000) for a broad introduction to the literature. Chapters of that extensively researched and widely vetted document are summarized below.

Chapter of the SGROH examines multiple linkages between oral and general health, noting that the mouth and the face reflect signs and symptoms of health and disease that can serve as an adjunct for diagnosis for some conditions. Diagnostic tests using oral cells and fluids—especially saliva—are available to detect drug abuse, hormonal changes, and specific diseases, and more are being developed. The mouth also is a portal of entry for pathogens and toxins, which can affect the mouth and, if not cleared by the many defense mechanisms that have evolved to protect the oral cavity, may spread to the rest of the body. Recent epidemiologic and experimental animal research provides evidence of possible associations between oral infections—particularly periodontal disease—and diabetes, cardiovascular disease, and adverse pregnancy outcomes. The review in Chapter of the SGROH also highlights the need for an aggressive research agenda to better delineate the specific nature of these associations and the underlying mechanisms of action.

Chapter of the SGROH looks at the impact of oral health problems on quality of life and includes examples of the kinds of questionnaires used to measure oral-health-related quality of life. Oral health generally is highly valued by society and individuals, and the chapter begins with a brief description of the reflections of those values in myth and folklore concerning facial appearance and the meaning of teeth. It then explores dimensions beyond the biological and the physical to examine how oral diseases and disorders can interfere with the functions of daily living, including participation in work or school, and what is known about their psychosocial impacts and economic costs. The deleterious effects of facial disfigurement and tooth loss may be magnified in modern societies that celebrate youth and beauty. Self-reported impacts of oral conditions on social functions include limitations in communication, social interactions, and intimacy. Additional research on oral-health-related quality of life is recommended to permit further exploration of the dimensions of oral health and well-being.

Sheiham (2005) also has provided a commentary on the relationships among oral health, general health, and quality of life. Many of the points highlighted in this commentary relate to LCHD Principle 1 (Health Development) that health is an emergent property and that oral health is a component of and contributes to overall health. Sheiham's summary ultimately reiterates the SGROH's call for cessation of "the compartmentalization involved in viewing the mouth separately from the rest of the body, noting that oral health affects general health by causing considerable pain and suffering and by altering what people eat, their speech, and their quality of life and well-being."

Additional excerpts from Sheiham's commentary include the following. "Oral health also has an effect on other chronic diseases, and failure to tackle social and material determinants and incorporate oral health into general health promotion means that millions suffer intractable toothache and poor quality of life, and end up with few teeth.

Oral diseases are the most common of the chronic diseases and are important public health problems because of their prevalence, their impact on individuals and society, and the expense of their treatment. The general determinants of oral diseases are known and include risk factors common to a number of chronic diseases: diet, inadequate hygiene practices, smoking, alcohol, risky behaviors causing injuries, and stress. Moreover, effective methods are available to prevent or reduce the impact of major oral diseases.

Oral health affects people physically and psychologically and influences how they grow, enjoy life, look, speak, chew, taste food and socialize, as well as their feelings of social well-being. Severe caries detracts from children's quality of life: they experience pain, discomfort, disfigurement, acute and chronic infections, and eating and sleep disruption as well as higher risk of hospitalization, high treatment costs and loss of school days with the consequently diminished ability to learn. Caries affects nutrition, growth and weight gain. Children of three years of age with nursing caries weigh about 1 kg less than control children because toothache and infection alter eating and sleeping habits, dietary intake and metabolic processes. Disturbed sleep affects glucocorticoid production. In addition, there is suppression of hemoglobin from depressed erythrocyte production.

Chronic diseases such as obesity, diabetes and caries are increasing in developed and developing countries, with the implication that quality of life related to oral health, as well as general quality of life, may deteriorate. Because oral and other chronic diseases have determinants in common, more emphasis should be on the common risk factor approach. The key concept underlying future oral health strategies is integration with this approach, a major benefit being the focus on improving health conditions in general for the whole population and for groups at high risk, thereby reducing social inequities."

5 Relating Oral Health and LCHD Concepts

5.1 Relating Oral Health Research Findings to Key LCHD Concepts

Pathways and Trajectories Analyses based on the Dunedin prospective, longitudinal birth cohort studies have distinguished three oral health trajectory groupings (high, medium, low) that emerge as early as age 5, remain relatively constant over time, and exhibit increasing divergence through the third decade of life. Authors of the Dunedin Study acknowledge that aggregating their findings into three trajectory 'groups' is an analytical convenience that may mask the heterogeneity of individuals within each group. To that point, LCHD suggests that a focus on intraindividual trajectories rather than on "group" means may prove more insightful because it allows for careful ascertainment of temporal exposure-outcome relationships and allows the analysis to take advantage of the diversity and complexity of these interactions rather than masking variability by aggregation into a few classes. Classes assume homogeneity of persons within a group, an assumption that is generally not supported. Little if any investigations of intraindividual change with detailed ascertainment of exposure and outcome over time have been reported in the dental/oral health literature.

Additional Dunedin cohort studies have examined the effect of SES in childhood and adulthood on adult oral health, and the effect of early childhood oral health on adult oral health, and found that the highest oral health trajectories are exhibited by those who have higher SES and better oral health in childhood; the lowest trajectories are found in those who have low SES and poor oral health in childhood; and those whose SES changed (either upwardly or downwardly) between childhood and adulthood fall between the other two trajectories. Oral health-care utilization and other personal, family, and community factors (e.g., oral hygiene, diet, dental anxiety, emphasis placed on oral health within one's family or community) also appear to exert influences on oral health trajectories throughout the life course.

Early Programming Evidence concerning the impact of early programming on oral health over the lifespan is less well defined, in part because many studies focus on adolescents or adults. Developmental disturbances that result in structural anomalies of tooth structure represent one documented example of early programming influences that can increase risk for dental disease (Targino et al. 2011). Findings from studies conducted by Holst and Schuller (2011) and Alm (Alm et al. 2008) suggest that good oral hygiene habits, including the use of fluoride toothpaste, established in early childhood provide a foundation for a low risk of proximal caries in adolescents. Evidence for the influence of less direct influences such as low birth weight is more equivocal, but represents an area of growing research interest (Nicolau et al. 2007). Evidence of intergenerational programming has been documented, particularly with respect to maternal-child oral health relationships (Shearer and Thomson, 2010; Shearer et al. 2011).

Critical or Sensitive Periods Some evidence, including studies cited above, supports the critical or sensitive period hypothesis with respect to the impact of various influences during fetal, early childhood, and later stages on life course oral health development and the determinants of oral health disparities. The importance and etiological mechanisms of disturbances arising during the prenatal period on craniofacial developmental problems such as cleft lip and/or cleft palate have been extensively documented. However, much remains to be elucidated with respect to the effects of different influences, at different times, on other oral health-related conditions (dental caries, periodontal disease, cancer, TMJD) (Hallqvist et al. 2004).

Cumulative Impact Substantial evidence also exists to support the hypothesis that the impact of major oral health-related conditions is a function of cumulative experiences or episodes of disease over time. Clearly, it is well established that dental caries is a chronic, cumulative disease and that the caries status of an individual develops and is subject to biological, behavioral, social, and environmental influences over time. Caries occurs at any stage in life, provided that an individual has susceptible teeth (and surfaces) remaining (Broadbent et al. 2008). The same case can be made for periodontal disease and tooth loss resulting from caries and periodontal diseases (Shearer et al. 2011; Watt 2007).

Risk and Protective Factors Considerable evidence has been compiled with respect to the biological and, to a lesser extent, behavioral risk and protective factors for major dental conditions (see Figs. 5 and 6). The influence of genetic, epigenetic, family, community, social, and environmental risk factors, in individual populations or across populations, is less well documented and understood.

5.2 Gaps in Knowledge Concerning Oral Health from a LCHD Perspective

Researchers involved in studying life course influences on oral health have identified a number of gaps in the current knowledge base. Using the lens of the LCHD principles, we have compiled research needs for future studies on oral health:

- Evaluate the contribution of social isolation, social relationships, and social support to oral health.
- Obtain more information on the economic, political, social, and environmental causes of individual behaviors related to oral health.
- Increase the number of longitudinal studies assessing the long-term effects of early childhood caries (ECC) and treatment on the health and quality of life of preschool children.
- Longitudinal studies are needed in order to obtain more knowledge about causative factors and the possible relationships between dental caries and overweight/obesity in children.
- Conceptual work that articulates a definition of oral health motivated by the LCHD principles is needed.
- Theoretical explanations for health inequalities are limited and biased due to the types of data collected in modern epidemiological studies, which are geared toward identifying and quantifying risk factors for disease and intended as a basis for description (of disease), not explanation (of causal pathways). This raises questions about the validity of current explanations. Current epidemiological approaches are widely criticized for neglecting broad social factors and failing to dig below the surface into issues such as how differ-

ent social class groups live their lives and what factors influence their lifestyle decisions. Current explanations are based largely on what epidemiological researchers can see and measure; factors that are harder to assess (such as culture), but which may be critically important to advancing our understanding of social inequalities in health, are frequently neglected.

- Epidemiologists have largely persisted in the use of disease-based measures to assess inequalities in health and oral health. The most significant advance to our understanding of social inequalities in health may come from the creation of a data set that measures oral health as defined by the FDI or oral-health-related quality of life.
- To date there is no research exploring how members of the population understand and account for inequalities in oral health, which remains a significant omission as it could offer promising new insights.
- Further research is needed to clarify the apparently differing oral health beliefs, attitudes, and practices of lower and higher SES groups.
- Much work remains to be done to establish which biological, social, and environmental factors are determinants of oral health or disease and which are merely markers, "proxies," or confounders.
- The process by which social stratification translates to poor oral health beginning in earliest childhood, especially for groups at higher risk for disease, is not well understood.
- There is a need for future research to move beyond traditional risk factors and more closely examine the impact of the social environment on oral health beliefs, behavior, and outcomes.
- A number of oral health problems have been shown to be associated with other health conditions (e.g., low birth weight, cardiovascular disease, respiratory disease); however, the demonstration of actual causal connections or pathways, such as the bidirectional relationship between diabetes and periodontal disease, has been modest.

5.3 Recommendations for Research and Policy Priorities

The knowledge gaps noted above give rise to a number of recommendations for research priorities to better understand oral health life course influences and policy changes to help reduce the impact of oral health problems and reduce oral health inequalities, which can be summarized as follows:

- Greater support for longer-term longitudinal oral health life course studies with detailed and frequent data collection to allow for the construction of intraindividual trajectories
- Replication of true oral health life course studies in different populations to assess whether findings apply across diverse settings
- Greater emphasis on research delineating relationships among oral health determinants to identify causal pathways
- Greater emphasis on identifying and addressing broader influences on oral health (i.e., family, community, social, and environmental influences)

6 Summary

This chapter has outlined major concepts embodied in the Life Course Health Development framework, examined evidence relating various aspects of major oral health-related conditions to this framework, and produced recommendations for advancing research and policy concerning oral health. LCHD provides a highly useful approach for understanding oral health determinants, disparities, and influences on general health and well-being and for advancing knowledge, policies, and programs to optimize health across individuals and populations.

References

Agency for Healthcare Research and Quality. 2015. Dental Services Mean and Median Expenses per Person With Expense and Distribution of Expenses by Source of Payment: United States, 2012. Medical Expenditure

Panel Survey Household Component Data. Generated interactively. (3 Mar 2015).

Alm, A., et al. (2008). Oral hygiene and parent-related factors during early childhood in relation to approximal caries at 15 years of age. *Caries Research, 42*(1), 28–36.

American Cancer Society. (2015). Cancer Facts & Figures 2015. Atlanta: American Cancer Society.

Ben-Shlomo, Y., & Kuh, D. (2002). A life course approach to chronic disease epidemiology: Conceptual models, empirical challenges and interdisciplinary perspectives. *International Journal of Epidemiology, 31*, 285–293.

Berkowitz, R. J. (2006). Mutans steptococci: Acquistion and transmission. *Pediatric Dentistry, 28*, 106–109.

Borrell-Carrio, F., Suchman, A. L., & Epstein, R. M. (2004). The biopsychosocial model 25 years later: Principles, practice, and scientific inquiry. *Annals of Family Medicine, 2*, 576–582.

Boulet, S. L., Grosse, S. D., Honein, M. A., & Correa-Villasenor, A. (2009). Children with orofacial clefts: Health care use and costs among a privately insured population. *Publ Health Reports, 124*, 447–453.

Brennan, D. S., Spencer, A. J., & Roberts-Thomson, K. F. (2008). Tooth loss, chewing ability and quality of life. *Quality of Life Research, 17*, 227–235.

Broadbent, J. M., Thomson, W. M., & Poulton, R. (2008). Trajectory patterns of dental caries experience in the permanent dentition to the fourth decade of life. *Journal of Dental Research, 87*, 69–72.

Center for Disease Control and Prevention (CDC). (2014). Prevalence (number of cases) of cleft lip and cleft palate. Available at: http://www.nidcr.nih.gov/DataStatistics/FindDataByTopic/CraniofacialBirthDefects/PrevalenceCleft%20LipCleftPalate.htm.

Crocombe, L. A., et al. (2011). Dental visiting trajectory patterns and their antecedents. *Journal of Public Health Dentistry, 71*(1), 23–31.

Dye, B. A., Thornton-Evans, G., Li, X., & Iafolla, T. J. (2015a). *Dental caries and sealant prevalence in children and adolescents in the United States, 2011a–2012. NCHS data brief, no 191*. Hyattsville: National Center for Health Statistics.

Dye, B. A., Thornton-Evans, G., Li, X., & Iafolla, T. J. (2015b). *Dental caries and tooth loss in adults in the United States, 2011b–2012. NCHS data brief, no 197*. Hyattsville: National Center for Health Statistics.

Feathersone, J. B. D. (2000). The science and practice of caries prevention. *Journal of the American Dental Association (Chicago, IL), 131*, 887–899.

Fejerskov, O. (2004). Changing paradigms in concepts on dental caries: Consequences for oral health care. *Caries Research, 38*, 182–191.

Fine, A., & Kotelchuck, M. (2010). *Rethinking MCH: The life course model as an organizing framework*. Washington, DC: US Department of Health and Human Services, Health Resources and Services Administration, Maternal and Child Health Bureau.

Fisher-Owens, S. A., Gansky, S. A., Platt, L. J., et al. (2007). Influences on children's oral health: A conceptual model. *Pediatrics, 120*, e510–e520.

Fitzgerald, R. J., & Keyes, P. H. (1961). Demonstration of the etiologic role of streptococci in experimental caries in the hamster. *Journal of the American Dental Association (Chicago, IL), 61*, 9–19.

Gerabek, W. E. (1999). The tooth-worm: Historical aspects of a popular medical belief. *Clin Oral Invest, 3*, 1–6.

Glick, M., et al. (2016). A new definition for oral health developed by the FDI World dental federation opens the door to a universal definition of oral health. *Journal of the American Dental Association (Chicago, IL), 147*, 915–917.

Gregory, J., Gibson, B., & Robinson, P. G. (2005). Variation and change in the meaning of oral health related quality of life: A 'grounded' systems approach. *Social Science & Medicine, 60*, 1859–1868.

Halfon, N., & Hochstein, M. (2002). Life course health development: An integrated framework for developing health, policy, and research. *The Milbank Quarterly, 80*, 433–479.

Halfon, N., Larson, K., Lu, M., Tullis, E., & Russ, S. (2014). Lifecourse health development: Past, present and future. *Maternal and Child Health Journal, 18*, 344–365.

Hallqvist, J., et al. (2004). Can we disentangle life course processes of accumulation, critical period and social mobility? An analysis of disadvantaged socio-economic positions and myocardial infarction in the Stockholm heart epidemiology program. *Social Science & Medicine, 58*(8), 1555–1562.

Heilman, A., et al. (2015). Oral health over the life course. In C. Burton-Jeangros, S. Cullati, & A. Sacker (Eds.), *A life course perspective on health trajectories and transitions [Internet]*. Cham (CH): Springer. doi:10.1007/9783319204840_3.

Hollister, M. C., & Weintraub, J. A. (1993). The association of oral status with systemic health, quality of life, and economic productivity. *Journal of Dental Education, 57*(12), 901–912.

Holst, D., & Schuller, A. A. (2011). Equality in adults' oral health in Norway. Cohort and cross-sectional results over 33 years. *Community Dent Oral Epidemiol, 39*(5), 488–497. doi:10.1111/j.1600-0528.2011.00624.x.

Jacobson, J. J., et al. (2012). The cost burden of oral, oral pharyngeal, and salivary gland cancers in three groups: Commercial insurance, Medicare, and Medicaid. *Head & Neck Oncology, 4*, 15.

Keating, D. P., & Hertzman, C. (1999). *Developmental health and the wealth of nations : Social, biological, and educational dynamics*. New York, NY: Guilford Press.

Keyes, P. H. (1960). The infectious and transmissible nature of experimental dental caries. *Archives of Oral Biology, 1*, 304–320.

Kohli, S. S., & Kohli, V. S. (2012). A comprehensive review of the genetic basis of cleft lip and palate. *J Oral Maxillofac Pathol., 16*, 64–72. doi:10.4103/0973-029X.92976.

Larson, K., Russ, S. A., Crall, J. J., & Halfon, N. (2008). Influence of multiple social risks on children's health. *Pediatrics, 121*, 337–344.

Liu, Z., et al. (2009). The impact of malocclusion/orthodontic treatment need on the quality of life: A systematic review. *The Angle Orthodontist, 79*, 585–591.

Locker, D., & Slade, G. (1994). Association between clinical and subjective indicators of oral health status in an older adult population. *Gerodontology, 11*, 108–114.

Lu, H. X., et al. (2011). Trends in oral health from childhood to early adulthood: A life course approach. *Community Dentistry and Oral Epidemiology, 39*(4), 352–360.

Mason, J., et al. (2006). How do factors at different stages of the lifecourse contribute to oral-health-related quality of life in middle age for men and women? *Journal of Dental Research, 85*(3), 257–261.

Miller, W. D. (1890). *The micro-organisms of the human mouth*. Philadelphia: S.S. White Publishing Co..

Miller, W. D. (1891). The human mouth as a focus of infection. *Dental Cosmos, 33*, 689–706.

Nicolau, B., et al. (2007). Life-course epidemiology: Concepts and theoretical models and its relevance to chronic oral conditions. *Community Dentistry and Oral Epidemiology, 35*(4), 241–249.

NIDCR. (2003). Prevalence of TMJD and its signs and symptoms; Available from: http://www.nidcr.nih.gov/DataStatistics/FindDataByTopic/FacialPain/PrevalenceTMJD.htm.

Peres, M. A., et al. (2011). The influence of family income trajectories from birth to adulthood on adult oral health: Findings from the 1982 Pelotas birth cohort. *American Journal of Public Health, 101*(4), 730–736.

Poulton, R., et al. (2002). Association between children's experience of socioeconomic disadvantage and adult health: A life-course study. *Lancet, 360*(9346), 1640–1645.

Quinonez, R., & Crall, J. J. (2009). Caries-risk assessment in early childhood. In J. H. Berg & R. Slayton (Eds.), *Early childhood oral health*. Hoboken: Wiley-Blackwell.

Ram, H., Kumar, H., Konwar, R., Bhatt, M. L. B., & Mohammad, S. (2011). Oral cancer: Risk factors and molecular pathogenesis. *J Maxillofac Oral Surg, 10*, 132–137.

Shearer, D. M., & Thomson, W. M. (2010). Intergenerational continuity in oral health: A review. *Community Dentistry and Oral Epidemiology, 38*(6), 479–486.

Shearer, D. M., et al. (2011). Maternal oral health predicts their children's caries experience in adulthood. *Journal of Dental Research, 90*(5), 672–677.

Sheiham, A. (2005). Oral health, general health and quality of life. *Bulletin of the World Health Organization, 83*(9), 644–644.

Sheiham, A., & Watt, R. G. (2000). The common risk factor approach: A rational basis for promoting oral health. *Community Dentistry and Oral Epidemiology, 28*, 399–406.

Targino, A. G. R., et al. (2011). The relationship of enamel defects and caries: A cohort study. *Oral Diseases, 17*(4), 420–426.

The Oral Cancer Foundation. (2015). Oral cancer facts. Available at: http://www.oralcancer.org/facts/.

Thomson, W. M., et al. (2004). Socioeconomic inequalities in oral health in childhood and adulthood in a birth cohort. *Community Dentistry and Oral Epidemiology, 32*, 345–353.

Thornton-Evans, et al. (2013). Periodontitis among adults aged > United States, 2009–2010. *MMWR, 62*(3), 129–135.

Tomar, S. L. (2012). Social determinants of oral health and disease in US men. *Journal of Mens Health, 9*, 113–119.

U.S. Department of Health and Human Services. (2000). Oral Health in America: A Report of the Surgeon General. Rockville: U.S. Department of Health and Human Services, National Institute of Dental and Craniofacial Research, National Institutes of Health.

Vargas, C. M., Crall, J. J., & Schneider, D. A. (1998). Sociodemographic distribution of pediatric dental caries: NHANES III, 1988-1994. *Journal of the American Dental Association (1939), 129*(9), 1229–1238.

Wall, T., & Vujicic M. (2014). No growth in U.S. dental spending in 2013. Health policy Institute research brief. American Dental Association. December 2014. Available from: http://www.ada.org/~/media/ADA/Science%20and%20Research/HPI/Files/HPIBrief_1214_4.ashx.

Watt, R. G. (2007). From victim blaming to upstream action: Tackling the social determinants of oral health inequalities. *Community Dentistry and Oral Epidemiology, 35*(1), 1–11.

WHO, The World Oral Health Report 2003. (2008). Continuous improvement of oral health in the 21st century–the approach of the WHO global oral health Programme. *Community Dent Oral Epidemiol, 31*(s1), 3–24.

6

Life Course Health Development Outcomes After Prematurity: Developing a Community, Clinical, and Translational Research Agenda to Optimize Health, Behavior, and Functioning

Michael E. Msall, Sarah A. Sobotka, Amelia Dmowska, Dennis Hogan, and Mary Sullivan

Definitions Late preterm infants (LPIs) $34^{0/7}$–$36^{6/7}$ week infants; moderate preterm infants (MPI) $32^{0/7}$–$33^{6/7}$ week infants; very preterm infants (VPI) $28^{0/7}$–$31^{6/7}$ weeks; extreme preterm infants (EPI) $<28^{0/7}$ weeks; cerebral palsy (CP); normal birth weight (NBW) ≥2500 g; low birth weight (LBW) 1500–2499 g; very low birth weight (VLBW) 1000–1499 g; extremely low birth weight (ELBW) <1000 g; *IQ* = intelligence quotient; *ID* = intellectual disability

1 Introduction

National vital statistics from 2013 estimate that the rate of preterm birth (<37 weeks of gestation) involves approximately 1 in 10 infants in the United States each year (Hamilton et al. 2015). An estimated 68 per 1000 US live births, over 270,000 annually, are born at late preterm gestation (34–36 weeks). Currently, 28 per 1000 US live births, more than 100,000 infants annually,

M.E. Msall, MD (✉)
Developmental and Behavioral Pediatrics University of Chicago, Comer and LaRabida Children's Hospitals, Chicago, IL, USA

JP Kennedy Research Center on Intellectual and Developmental Disabilities, University of Chicago Comer Children's Hospital, Section of Developmental and Behavioral Pediatrics, 950 East 61St Street, SSC Room 207, Chicago, IL 60637, USA
e-mail: mmsall@peds.bsd.uchicago.edu

S.A. Sobotka, MD, MS • A. Dmowska, BA
Section of Developmental and Behavioral Pediatrics, University of Chicago Comer Children's Hospitals, Chicago, IL, USA

D. Hogan, PhD
Sociology and Demography, Population Research and Training Center, Brown University, Providence, RI, USA

M. Sullivan, PhD, RN
University of Rhode Island, College of Nursing, Women and Infants Hospital, Providence, RI, USA

are born <34 weeks of gestation, and 56,000 are born at very low birth weight status (<1500 g). These infants have high risks for long-term neurodevelopmental disabilities such as intellectual disability (ID), blindness, sensorineural hearing loss, and cerebral palsy (CP). There are several biomedical causes for these high rates of preterm birth, such as the role of assisted reproductive technologies increasing the rate of multiple births (twins, triplets, or quadruplets) and maternal age. Teenage pregnancy, also a risk factor for prematurity, has instead been decreasing over the past decade (Hamilton et al. 2015; The March of Dimes Data Book for Policy Makers 2012). However, it is very critical to remember that both very preterm infants (VPI) and extreme preterm infants (EPI) are heterogeneous, and our understanding of causal pathways that lead to successful interventions is at an early scientific stage (Rubens et al. 2014). For example, the same factors that create the biological risk in the mothers for prematurity may be the same factors that influence the inflammatory, hormonal, and neurochemical regulators that influence the mothers' caregiving capacity once their premature infant is born. Therefore, ascribing causality to biomedical, behavioral, or neuro-regulatory factors is difficult and does not allow for the complex systems understanding required to advance life course-oriented prevention and intervention strategies. In addition, despite increased access to prenatal care, there still remain limitations on our ability to prevent all moderate and late preterm birth (Requejo et al. 2013).

Estimates of the economic impact of prematurity typically factor in acute care medical costs, early childhood intervention expenditures, long-term special education, special health care, and disability costs. A report released by the Institute of Medicine in 2007 estimated that the economic burden associated with preterm birth was at least \$26.2 billion in 2005, equivalent to \$51,600 per infant born preterm. These estimates included \$16.9 billion in medical care costs, \$1.9 billion in maternal delivery costs, \$611 million for early intervention services, \$1.1 billion for special education services, and \$5.7 billion in lost household and labor market productivity (Preterm Birth: Causes, Consequences, and Prevention 2007). Importantly, each premature/LBW baby costs employers an average of \$54,149 in payments for newborn medical care during the first year of life, about twelve times that of an uncomplicated newborn (Preterm Birth: Causes, Consequences, and Prevention 2007). In addition to medical care, children born preterm are more likely to experience learning and behavior disabilities later in life, often resulting in poor test scores, grade repetition, and increased utilization of special education services. The Institute of Medicine estimates the costs of special education at \$2200 per year per child (Preterm Birth: Causes, Consequences, and Prevention 2007), though for children with major neurodevelopmental disabilities, the special cost per child can exceed \$50,000 per academic year.

High-quality early childhood intervention programs, however, may minimize the later need for special education and drastically reduce these additional costs (Aron and Loprest 2012). Model programs like the Infant Health Development Program (IHDP) are successful in improving educational, behavioral, and life course outcomes for preterm infants experiencing poverty, thereby decreasing children's need for special education (Aron and Loprest 2012). Economic modeling estimates the impact of comprehensive early intervention services on long-term special education costs as having a direct savings of \$2.60 for every dollar invested in early intervention, early childcare services, and Early Head Start (Dmowska et al. 2016). When considering costs incurred from school dropouts, reentry to school, and additional weight on mental health-care services and the criminal justice system, the savings would likely double (Dmowska et al. 2016). Increased access to comprehensive family-centered early intervention services, therefore, may substantially reduce special education costs for children born preterm as well as long-term behavioral and social health costs.

There have been dramatic improvements in long-term survival for infants born premature and low birth weight, but developmental outcomes are far from optimized. Survival has increased dramatically with the regionalization of neonatal intensive care and the application of obstetrical and neonatal biomedical interventions for optimizing growth, lung maturity, cardiopulmonary functioning, and infection control. Overall, these efforts resulted in decreased rates of major neurodevelopmental disabilities in survivors in the 1980s and 1990s from 25–40% to 15–25%. For those born with extreme prematurity (<28 weeks of gestation) and extremely low birth weight status (<1000 g), survival has increased dramatically from <50% to >80%. However, there remain high rates of cognitive impairment and intellectual disability (ID), with over 50% of survivors requiring special education services.

Growing inequality in the United States hits families with young children very hard. Close to 50% of children younger than 5 are growing up in households living below 200% of the poverty level. Research shows that families with this level of income do not have the economic, social, educational, and community assets they need to support optimal health development (Crouter and Booth 2014). So many of the 8% premature babies, who start off life with higher levels of inherent vulnerabilities, are increasingly facing a family, social, and community landscape that cannot support their optimal development.

In addition, there is increased recognition that both moderate and late preterm births (32–36 weeks of gestation), which account for over 8% of live births or approximately 325,000 children yearly, have increased risk for long-term health, developmental, and behavioral challenges (Table 1). In spite of these biomedical advances, environmental and social conditions that can deleteriously affect the health and well-being of these already vulnerable children have not only improved in the United States; there are some indications that they have in fact worsened. Additionally, there are major gaps in accessing comprehensive family supports and quality health, early childhood, and educational and community experiences for recent cohorts of children at the highest biomedical and social risks.

The purpose of this paper is to apply a life course health development perspective in order to identify factors that promote more optimal health and developmental trajectories and the mechanisms that underlie resilience for children with prematurity from a life course health development perspective. We will describe some research findings about the role of social and environmental factors among VPI and EPI survivors in aggravating or moderating neonatal risks for suboptimal developmental and behavioral outcomes. We will also discuss available evidence from longitudinal studies of preterm children at psychosocial disadvantage and what lessons can be learned from the bidirectional impacts of prematurity and poverty. Longitudinal studies will be evaluated for health, disability, and community outcome trajectories for children with prematurity across preschool, middle childhood, adolescent, and young adult epochs. Our review will highlight important opportunities on a community level for systematically optimizing population-based prevention strategies for individuals with the double jeopardy of prematurity and social adversity and the long-term impact of failing to optimize these outcomes.

1.1 Approach

Two frameworks will inform our analysis. The first framework will be the International Classification of Functioning, Disability, and Health (ICF) model (World Health Organization

Table 1 Life course impact of prematurity

Weeks gestation	Children special health-care needs	Major neurodevelopmental disability	Educational supports	Behavioral disorders
<28	50%	20%	50%	20%
28–31	40%	15%	40%	15%
32–36	30%	10%	25%	10%
37+	20%	5%	15%	5%

Morse et al. (2009), Allen et al. (2011), Stephens and Vohr (2009), B. Vohr (2013), Saigal and Doyle (2008)

2007), which we will use to comprehensively describe the diverse outcomes occurring in preterm survivors. This framework goes beyond dichotomous classification of impairments (e.g., cerebral palsy, yes or no; intellectual disability, yes or no) and instead describes a spectrum of functioning at body structure and body function levels. For example, activities in whole-person tasks include running, reading, and dancing and participation in children's roles with peers including being on a team; participating in church, temple, or mosque; or meeting friends for a movie.

The second framework will be the *life course health development (LCHD) model,* which holds that the trajectories of children are influenced by the dynamic interaction of multiple risk, protective, and promoting factors, especially during sensitive periods of health development. From the standpoint of fetal development, due to critical human brain development in the second and third trimesters, a focus on premature infants must consider complex maternal, placental, and fetal dynamic interactions. Likewise, infant, toddler, and childhood periods of development are indelibly influenced by multilevel, multidirectional, transactional, and long-lasting interactions and critically emphasize the importance of timing. Using a LCHD framework to analyze the origins and impact of prematurity and the opportunities to optimize health development outcomes suggest the following considerations:

- Children who are born prematurely are assumed to be more developmentally vulnerable and are potentially more sensitive to a wide range and nested array of dynamic interacting influences.
- Because the alterations in evolutionarily influenced and developmentally determined adaptive mechanisms are well documented, lags in developmental processes, as well as catch-up and feed-forward processes that are specific to premature infants, may influence the nature and dynamic of their health and developmental trajectories.
- Understanding how the caregiving environment of premature infants interacts with emerging developmental capacities and how different types of exposures, levels of support, and adversity influence these emergent developmental trajectories is important if specific and targeted interventions are to be designed to modify developmental pathways based on specific risk profiles to shift the health and developmental curves for the entire population of premature infants.
- In order to implement a broader approach to improve the health and developmental outcomes of diverse preterm populations, it is important to determine what is known about the special development vulnerabilities of premature infants, how that vulnerability manifests (timing, context, specific risks), and whether the mechanisms involved are phase or period specific, modifiable, or one of cumulative risk.

2 Framing Our Inquiry and Agenda

On a population level, it is important to acknowledge the diversity of both the underlying causes and life course effects of prematurity and the gaps in proactive and comprehensive medical, developmental, and behavioral supports. This is occurring within the context of recognizing that current community systems are under-resourced to systematically audit barriers and facilitators to home visiting, medical homes, early interventions, parenting supports, and coordinated services for children with special health-care needs (CSHCN). In particular, we must go from a crisis-oriented response system for the few with the severest impairments to an optimization system for all at risk for less than optimal health development.

To address these systemic needs, the following themes will be highlighted that require increased research and policy efforts:

- We must better understand the role of and need to engage mothers and other caregivers in developmentally optimizing interactions from the neonatal period through school entry. This includes how they gain and utilize their knowledge about their child's health and development, as well as how to optimally serve as their child's first teacher and advocate. This requires understanding ways that early parent involvement and developmental activities can be part of everyday childcare tasks.

- We must explore how social environments are best tailored to maximally support positive growth, child regulatory behaviors, and developmental competencies. This includes how all children can access comprehensive preschool services and how health, developmental, and behavioral competencies are measured, monitored, and accounted for from birth to kindergarten entry. In keeping with a two-generation model of optimizing health development, close attention to caregiver physical and behavioral health and supports that help vulnerable children access quality childcare and early child education have the potential to ensure that children's social-emotional, communicative, and cognitive competencies are supported so that children enter kindergarten healthy and ready to learn.
- We must clarify the roles that preconception maternal, physical, and behavioral health play on maternal and child vulnerabilities and on epigenetic programming. This includes a better understanding of how maternal mental health stressors (depression, anxiety, isolation, and violence) increase vulnerability of children when they do not receive quality early childhood social, learning, and behavioral supports.
- We must determine the optimum and appropriate role and function of community outreach strategies that promote parental physical and behavioral health, child development, and social competencies.
- We should pursue evidence-based strategies to promote resiliency and positive adult health trajectories which include independent living, employment, and family formation while minimizing physical risk factors that increase early-onset adult chronic diseases (e.g., cardiac, pulmonary, mental illness, substance abuse) (Figs. 1 and 2).

Our cases illustrate how the interaction of positive home, preschool, and educational supports can increase thriving and reduce adverse long-term adult health conditions.

3 Risk Factors for Poor Birth Outcomes

3.1 Social Risks

An important determinant of preterm birth is social risk. Social risk factors include suboptimal home and community environments. Poverty, domestic violence, drug addiction, crime, hunger, and poor-quality housing are some of the features of social risks (Holzmann and Jørgensen 2001). Mothers who live in adverse environments often experience multiple stressors and are prone to nutritional deficiency, suboptimal prenatal care, single parenthood, and frequent tobacco and alcohol use compared to mothers from non-poor backgrounds (Jiang 2015). Several studies have also shown that rates of marijuana, cocaine, tobacco, and alcohol use are higher for women who are unmarried, unemployed, and have less than a college education, indicating that substance abuse and poverty are closely related (Huston 1991). It has been suggested that the prevalence of substance abuse, illicit drug use, and smoking among women from impoverished or low SES background is largely due to the sense of helplessness, low self-esteem, difficulties coping with stress, and pressure from coping with difficult financial situations in everyday living (Huston 1991; Weitzman et al. 2002).

When mothers receive late prenatal care (or not at all), the opportunity to identify and intervene on maternal reproductive complications or health problems that jeopardize fetal growth is limited. Also, late or no prenatal care decreases the chances of maternal access to educational and support services (such as counseling, community health, and education services) (The March of Dimes Data Book for Policy Makers 2012).

3.2 Race and Social Disadvantage

Race in the United States is closely related to SES; thus, it is not surprising to see racial discrepancies in preterm births (Table 2). African-American infants are more than 1.5 times likely than whites to be born preterm and 2.5 times likely to be very premature than their white peers

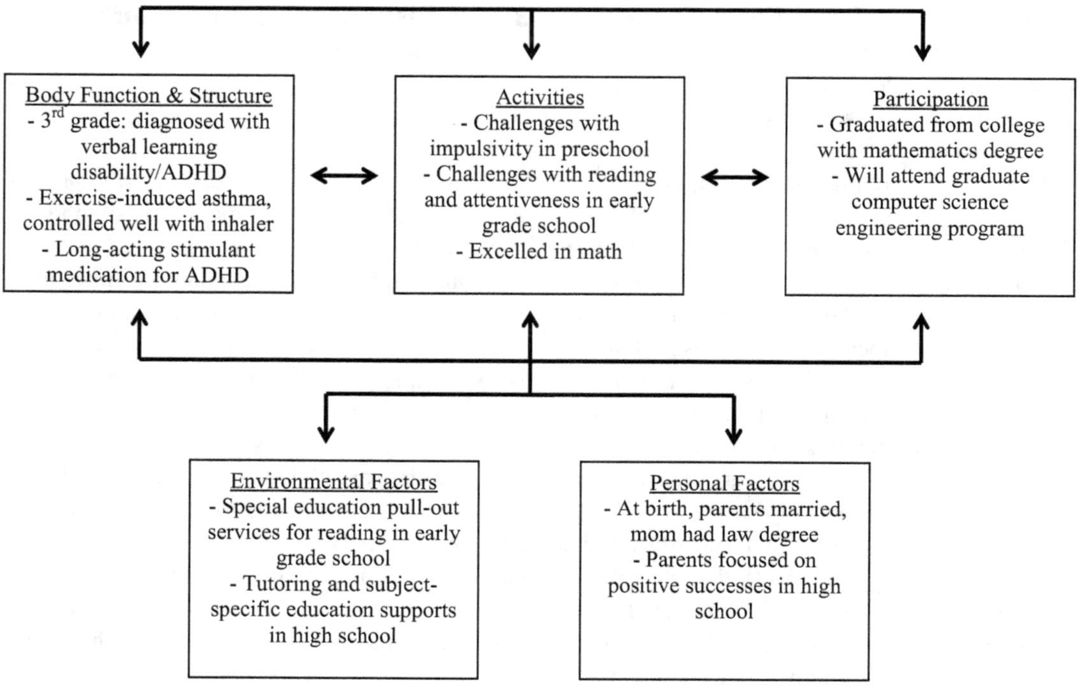

Fig. 1 Case 1. James was born late preterm at 34 weeks of gestation due to preeclampsia. His parents were married and mother completed law school. She had some challenges with impulsivity in preschool, and reported significant job-related stressors during pregnancy. The immediate newborn period was complicated by immature lungs leading to respiratory distress syndrome; however, ultimately James was discharged at 38 weeks of gestational age without a need for oxygen in the home. He was enrolled in full-day daycare and preschool since the age of 2 years. James was found to have some challenges with impulsivity in preschool, which his parents addressed with occupational and behavioral therapies. He entered kindergarten without an Individualized Education Program and in early grade school was found to struggle with reading and inattentiveness. He received a formal diagnosis of verbal learning disability and ADHD in third grade. James received special education pull-out services for reading and language arts and was starting on a long-acting stimulant medication for ADHD with the guidance of a Developmental and Behavioral Pediatrician. James received tutoring and subject-specific special education supports throughout high school. His parents focused on his positive successes, such as his strong performance in math. James went to college and pursued a math and engineering program. His adult health is complicated by exercise-induced asthma, well-controlled on an inhaler

(The March of Dimes Data Book for Policy Makers 2012). These data on preterm birth rates correlate with disparities in wealth distribution, with African-American families experiencing the lowest 3-year average median income (2003–2005) among US racial groups (Income, Poverty, and Health Insurance Coverage in the United States: 2005–2006). These data on higher rates of prematurity in women experiencing social disadvantage from poverty and minority status also hold across both developing and developed countries. The role of maternal health, educational, behavioral, and social competencies during her own childhood and how they impact on her child's health and development require systematically measuring both maternal and child allostatic load. These data can help understand what factors promote positive adaptations.

4 Prematurity and Developmental Outcomes

Prematurely born infants have long-term vulnerabilities on multiple outcomes, including physical and developmental health, behavioral and adaptive well-being, as well as social functioning. Over the past decade, much has been learned

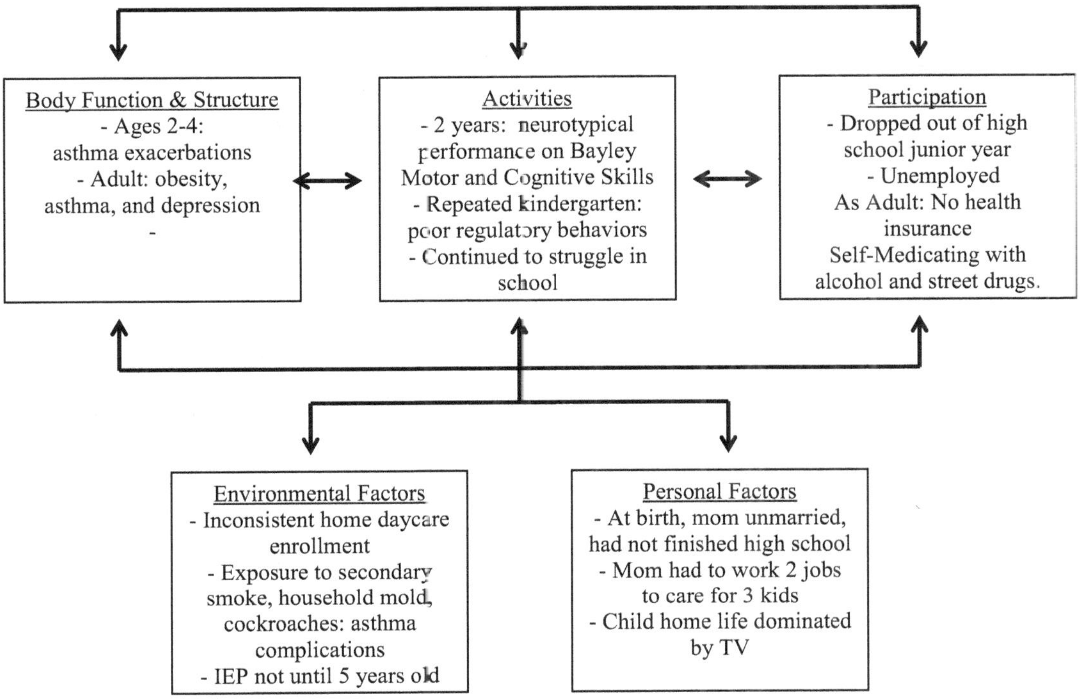

Fig. 2 Case 2. Michael was born at 28 weeks due to pre-eclampsia and preterm labor. His mother was unmarried and did not finish high school. His NICU course was complicated by intubation for the first 4 weeks of life, but he did not experience additional medical complications and was able to be slowly transitioned to room air and oral feedings. At 2 years of age, he tested within age appropriate range on the Bayley Scales of Toddler Development. Between ages 2 and 4, he experienced asthma exacerbations complicated by environmental exposures to secondary tobacco smoke, household mold, and cockroach infestation and was hospitalized about 2–3 times a year. Until the age of 5 years, Michael was enrolled in inconsistent home daycare programs and did not receive early intervention services because he was considered less than 30% delayed and thereby was deemed not eligible for services. He enrolled in kindergarten at age 5 years. However, he had to repeat kindergarten due to poor regulatory behaviors, which interfered with learning. Throughout his early childhood education, he continued to struggle in school. His home life was largely dominated by television watching while his mom worked two jobs to help care for him and his two siblings. In school he was supported by an Individual Education Plan, but did not access pharmacotherapies for ADHD. He dropped out of high school in his junior year. His adult health is complicated by obesity, asthma, and depression. Because of unemployment, he does not have health insurance. His state has not expanded Medicaid access

in the management of preterm infants and the interventions required to stabilize their immature organ system functioning.

Table 2 Rate (%) of preterm birth by maternal race and trimester of first prenatal visit

Trimester of first prenatal visit	Non-Hispanic black	Non-Hispanic white	Hispanic
First	14.7	8.3	9.7
Second	17.6	10.2	10.0
Third	16.0	10.0	10.0
None	33.4	21.7	19.8

Lang and Iams (2009)

4.1 Cerebral Palsy and Neurosensory Impairment

Table 3 highlights rates of CP and neurodevelopmental disabilities in early childhood among extremely preterm cohorts born into the medical era, which had both prenatal maternal corticosteroid and surfactant replacement interventions available. These studies demonstrate that, despite common misconceptions, the overwhelming majority of children who survive extreme prematurity do not experience CP. These data

Table 3 Major neurodevelopmental disabilities at age 2 years among survivors of ELBW in the 1990s

Study	Sample	% CP	% DD	% HI	% VI
Schmidt et al. (1996–1998)	$N = 944$ 500–999 g	12	27	2	2
Mikkola et al. (1996–1998)	$N = 206$ <1000 g	14	9	4	2.6
Vohr et al. (1993–1998)	$N = 2291$ 22–26 weeks	19	30	2	2
	$N = 1494$ 27–32 weeks GA	11.6	26	1	0.7
Wood et al. (1995)	$N = 283$ 22–25 weeks GA	16	30	2	2
Doyle et al. (1997)	$N = 170$ 500–999 g	11	22	1.8	2.4
Mestan et al. (1998–2001)	$N = 138$ 27.4 weeks GA	9.5	27.3	0.8	1.5
Shankaren et al. (1993–1999)	$N = 246$; ≤750 g ≤24 weeks; API ≤3	30	46	5	5
Wilson-Costello et al. (1990–1998)	$N = 417$ 500–999 g	14	26	7	1
Fily et al. (1997)	$N = 545$ <33 weeks GA	9	4.7	0.8	0.2

DD developmental disability as defined as mental developmental index < 70, *HI* hearing impairment, *VI* visual impairment
AP1 Apgar 1 min
GA gestational age

complement population registries, which dramatically highlight the increased rate of CP among preterm survivors with decreasing gestational age. In Sweden, EPI have rates of CP at 71 per 1000, VPI 40 per 1000, and LPI (32–36 weeks) 6.4 per 1000, compared to term births at 1.1 per 1000 (Himmelmann and Uvebrant 2014).

Although there are many types of CP with varying degrees of difficulty with motor control and higher cortical function, the two most common types among preterm survivors are spastic diplegia and spastic hemiplegia. These CP syndromes affect the motor control of lower extremities (diplegia) or one side of the body (hemiplegia) and increase risks for communicative, perceptual, learning, and attention disorders (Allen et al. 2011). However, an examination of these broader outcomes for recent VPI and EPI cohorts at ages 5–8 years has not occurred in large United States regional or multicenter cohorts. Furthermore, functional measures of gross motor, manual ability, and communication activities offer more detailed descriptions of performance in everyday activities than topographical classifications of CP.

Over the past decade, there has been an increased appreciation of a wider range of motor challenges that have been characterized as developmental coordination disorders. A developmental coordination disorder is defined by acquisition and execution of coordinated motor skills below what would be expected at a given chronologic age. Difficulties are manifested as clumsiness, slowness, and inaccuracy of performance of motor skills. These motor skill deficits persistently interfere with activities of daily living appropriate to the chronologic age (*Diagnostic and Statistical Manual of Mental Disorders: DSM-5* 2013). A systematic analysis of 14 studies of children <33 weeks of gestation and <1501 g demonstrated 41% had mild developmental coordination disorder (characterized by motor standard scores 1–2 standard deviations below the mean) and 19% had moderate developmental coordination disorder (≥2 standard deviations below the mean) (Williams et al. 2010).

The second column in Table 3 reviews rates of developmental disability. These studies demonstrated rates of cognitive disability ranging between 9 and 46% among those EPI and 5% when VPI and EPI were combined. It must be emphasized that their early cognitive disabilities do not fully capture long-term educational impact.

Among ELBW survivors, there are high rates of neurosensory impairments. Severe hearing impairment ranges from 1% to 7%. This is also substantially higher than the 1 per 1000 rate in term infants. Another neurodevelopmental disability after prematurity is visual loss or blindness caused by retinopathy of prematurity (ROP). This disorder primarily affects premature infants weighing 1250 g or less and those born before 31 weeks of gestation. ROP in the current era of neonatology reaches its severest stages in those who are most immature and medically fragile. Severe visual impairment occurs in 1–2% of <27-week preemies, 20–40 times higher than in term infants. In a multicenter study on cryosurgery for ROP, increased severity of ROP was linked to motor, self-care, and communicative disability at kindergarten entry (Msall et al. 2000). Children with severe ROP, but with favorable visual acuity, had a motor disability rate of 5% compared to 43% of children with severe ROP and unfavorable visual acuity (eyesight worse than 6.4 cycles per degree on Teller Cards includes legal and total blindness). In this cohort, neonatal risk factors for severe disability involving multiple motor, self-care, and communicative domains included severe ROP, gestational age <27 weeks, birth weight <750 g, and poverty as reflected by the absence of private health insurance. A protective factor associated with a significant risk reduction for severe disability was African-American race. In middle childhood, children with severe ROP had substantial differences in cognitive and educational outcomes (Msall et al. 2004). Children with severe ROP and unfavorable visual status had a 3 in 5 chance of ID (57%) and a 3 in 5 chance of needing special education services. Children with severe ROP and favorable visual skills had a 1 in 5 chance of ID (22%) and a 1 in 4 chance of needing special education. More than 4 in 5 children with unfavorable vision (84%) but less than half of children with favorable vision (48%) were below grade level in school performance. Lower socioeconomic status (SES) and minority status were associated with lower-grade performance and utilization of special education services across both visual outcome groups. Table 3 also highlights that over 95% of extremely preterm survivors do not experience blindness.

4.2 Cognitive Outcomes

The assessment of cognitive outcomes can focus on three related domains: intelligence testing, achievement testing, and neuropsychological testing. The latter includes evaluation of specific higher cortical processes such as executive function, working memory, and information processing. Assessment of toddlers and young children combines precursors of verbal and nonverbal intelligence and cognitive processes (e.g., object permanency, symbolic play), whereas school-age assessment and beyond require more complex testing to assess problem-solving, literacy, and numeracy. There is increased recognition that Bayley II and III scores <70 predict complex cognitive and learning challenges among school-age children. However, among children with 2-year Bayley scores of 71–84 (1–2 standard deviations below the mean), they may be uniquely vulnerable to the lack of quality early childhood education and preschool experiences, especially in socially disadvantaged families (Patrianakos-Hoobler et al. 2009). Therefore, one needs to be cautious in using developmental assessments in the first 2 years of life to fully assess the spectrum of cognitive and learning disorders in all children, not only those preterm and growing up in vulnerable circumstances. The limitations in Bayley assessments are due to the dynamic processes of higher cortical functioning in childhood. Additionally, the assessment of developmental delay is intertwined with perceptual and sensory skills as well as early learning experiences and neuroplasticity. Learning, communication, and social challenges may not be apparent until there is increased complexity of tasks for academic skills and behavioral/attention regulatory capacity required by school environments.

In order to address higher-level skills at school entry, one strategy is to examine children's status at kindergarten entry. EPI cohorts born in the 1980s from Hamilton, Ontario, Melbourne, Australia, Buffalo, New York, and Chicago, Illinois, have demonstrated that 44–56% require special education resources and 21–29% have major neurodevelopmental impairments (Baek et al. 2002; Vohr and Msall 1997). These studies indicate that, in addition to planning for major developmental disabilities, resources are required to ensure success with peers in the classroom.

Gross and colleagues followed infants born very preterm and found that 41% of preterm infants were performing at grade level versus 70% of term children. These preterm children were more likely to receive special education services and three times as likely to be diagnosed with learning disabilities. In this cohort, parental marital status and educational attainment were significantly related to educational outcomes (Gross et al. 2001). Nearly three times as many preterm children achieved grade-level performance if parents were married as compared to children from single-parent homes. Thus, preterm survivors with limited family resources are further disadvantaged and vulnerable.

In Cleveland, Litt and colleagues prospectively followed 219 surviving ELBW children born between 1992 and 1995 through middle childhood and adolescence. Surviving children had a mean birth weight of 815 g, a mean GA of 26.4 weeks; and almost 1 in 5 was from multiple birth gestations. Neonatal morbidities included bronchopulmonary dysplasia in 41%, sepsis in 29%, and sonographic parenchymal brain injury in 24% (IVH3–IVH4/PVL by cranial ultrasound). Importantly, 115 term controls from the extremely preterm survivor's community classroom were assessed at 14 years. Both the extremely preterm survivors and a prospectively recruited term control group underwent a comprehensive neuropsychological battery that included reading and mathematics and neuropsychological skills of processing speed, attention, visual memory, working memory, and planning. In addition, social capital as determined by maternal education and median household income as well as gender and minority status was used as covariates when analyzing predictors of high school functioning (Litt et al. 2012).

Though major neurosensory disabilities occurred in approximately 1 in 6 of ELBW survivors (CP 15%, blindness in 0.5%, and hearing loss requiring amplification in 1.7%), a far greater number of children experienced ID and cognitive impairments. More than 1 in 6 (18%) had ID (IQ <70), a 4.5-fold greater risk than for term peers. More than 1 in 3 (37%) were cognitively impaired (IQ 71–84), a 2.3-fold greater risk than for term peers. Most importantly, almost 1 in 2 (49%) of ELBW survivors required an individualized educational plan, a fivefold higher rate than term peers. The educational resources required for managing these highly prevalent disorders would require an additional $50,000 per child during their high school years for tutoring, smaller class size, and specific curriculum modifications (Msall 2012).

Of concern were the achievement challenges of extremely preterm survivors who experienced socioeconomic adversity. These children not only demonstrated a 6.6-point lower IQ but had standard scores that were 10 points lower in reading and 8 points lower in mathematics. Importantly, both executive function and visual memory challenges were associated with academic struggles in reading and mathematics (Johnson et al. 2009, 2011; Simms et al. 2015; Wolke et al. 2015).

4.2.1 What Does This Mean?

The first lesson brings optimism: the large majority of ELBW survivors (83%) are free of neurosensory disability. Thus, unprecedented survival without major neurosensory disability can be expected. However, despite antenatal corticosteroids, surfactant replacement, improved nutrition, and infection control, the rates of CP are over 100-fold greater than for term infants. Thus, ongoing efforts in neuroprotection remain a scientific, clinical, and political priority.

The second lesson is sobering: the majority of ELBW survivors experience ongoing and serious challenges in learning, coordination, and executive function. These children benefit from quality and comprehensive interventions and special educational accommodations with continued review of how these services promote literacy, numeracy, and life skills. Litt and colleagues' outcomes suggest that evidence-based psychoeducational management strategies for executive function and specific learning disorders may be key areas for maintaining children on positive developmental trajectories (Litt et al. 2012). An important challenge in the upcoming decade is to comprehensively implement, at a population level, appropriately targeted developmental and educational optimization strategies for all preterm survivors. With more developmentally appropriate individual- and population-level supports, their neurodevelopmental risks that currently result in costly and adverse long-term physical, behavioral, educational, and social health outcomes could be dramatically reduced.

4.2.2 Behavioral/Emotional Disorders

Behavioral and emotional disorders are more prevalent among children born premature compared to their term birth peers. Meta-analysis of behavioral outcomes by Bhutta and colleagues revealed that children born preterm have a 2.6-fold risk for developing attention-deficit hyperactivity disorder (ADHD) during school age (Bhutta et al. 2002). These children are also at high risk for externalization problems such as aggression, oppositionality, and disruptive behaviors, which also are major obstacles in establishing friendships or other social relationships (e.g., lack of patience in waiting for their turn in group play) (Farooqi et al. 2007; Saigal et al. 2003). In these studies, birth weight, family function, gender, and SES predicted the behavioral adjustment of adolescents who survived ELBW status in the 1980s or the middle childhood behavioral and childhood behavioral and social adjustment of children who survived 23–25 weeks of gestation in the 1990s.

An important discovery occurred over the past decade whereby it was noted that very and extremely preterm infants were at high risk for delays in social-emotional behavioral regulation that manifested as hyperactivity, impulsivity, and difficulty with social competencies in the preschool years (Jones et al. 2013). Importantly, those children receiving appropriate quality preschool education experiences were more ready for kindergarten both cognitively and behaviorally than those who did not access these services (Arpi and Ferrari 2013; Treyvaud et al. 2013). There has also been increased recognition that late preterm survivors are at risk for regulatory and social challenges. Recent comparative investigations of toddler outcomes for LPI versus other premature infants demonstrate more externalizing, oppositional, and aggressive behaviors, suggesting a unique vulnerability for LPIs (Shah et al. 2013). Infants more prone to distress who also experienced more critical parenting styles in infancy were more likely to demonstrate externalizing behaviors at age 3, suggesting that characteristics of both infants and parents influence preterm vulnerability (Poehlmann et al. 2012).

There has also been an increased awareness of the vulnerability of adolescent and adult survivors of very and extremely preterm birth to increased rates of behavior and mental health disorders (Gardner et al. 2004). This is highlighted in Table 4. An important review by Johnson and Marlow emphasized a life course health development framework and highlighted the increased risk of attention, socio-communicative (including autism spectrum disorder), and emotional difficulties among extremely preterm survivors (Johnson et al. 2011). Importantly they highlighted rates of autism spectrum disorder (ASD) as high as 1 in 12 EPI survivors as they enter adolescence (Johnson et al. 2011). A New Jersey cohort found a rate of 1 in 20 for ASD in moderate LBW at school exit (Pinto-Martin et al. 2011). Most recently, in a large US cohort of 889 EPI survivors born in 2002–2004, Joseph and colleagues found a rate of ASD in males at age 10 of 9% and in females of 5%. Rates of ASD were 15% at 23–24 weeks of gestation, 6.5% at 25–26 weeks of gestation, and 3.4% at 27 weeks of gestation (Joseph et al. 2016).

Table 4 Adolescent and adult behavioral health outcomes

Authors	Cohort	Age at assessment	Developmental outcome
Botting et al. (1997)	1980–1983 Liverpool, England 138 VLBW and 108 matched controls	12 years	1. Any psychiatric disorder: 28% VLBW vs. 9% controls had any psychiatric disorder 2. ADHD: 23% VLBW vs. 6% controls
Dahl et al. (2006)	1978–1989 Norway 99 VLBW	13–18 years	1. VLBW adolescents report less externalizing behaviors than NBW adolescents 2. Parents of VLBW adolescents report more externalizing behaviors and emotional problems than NBW adolescents.
Grunau et al. (2004)	1981–1986 British Columbia 79 <800 g vs. 31 term	17 years	1. No differences for focus and attention 2. Significantly more parental reported internalizing, externalizing, and problem behaviors
Jong et al. (2012)	Meta-analysis of moderate and late preterm (32–36 weeks) 28 papers reviewed	Not reported (meta-analysis)	30% higher psychiatric disorders
Kunugi et al. (2001)	Meta-analysis of LBW and schizophrenia prevalence; 750 with schizophrenia and 29,000 control subjects	Not reported (meta-analysis)	LBW prevalence: 9.5% of schizophrenics and 3.9% of controls
Levy-Shiff et al. (1994)	Israel 90 VLBW and 90 NBW	13–14 years	Significantly increased hyperactive behavior among VLBW. However paternal involvement was as predictive as birth weight for hyperactivity in childhood
Saigal et al. (2006)	1977–1982 Ontario, Canada 166 ELBW and 145 NBW	22–25 years	1.3% of ELBW had autism vs. 0% controls
Saigal et al. (2007)	Ontario, Canada 149 ELBW and 133 NBW	23 years	14.1% ELBW vs. 6% on antidepressants

4.2.3 What Does This Mean?

The current understanding of the vulnerabilities of the preterm infant brain to challenges in coordination, learning, attention, and social skills offers opportunities for understanding cumulative risk and protective strategies linked to biomarkers and neurometrics. The goal of understanding what supports are needed to protect the vulnerable preterm infant brain for learning regulatory, attention, executive function, and social competencies will require increased attention to how active health and developmental experiences shape these developmental processes and what proactive informed interventions support success academically, behaviorally, and socially. Revolutionary strategies in developmental neuroscience will help inform an evidence-based approach to early identification and intervention so that children stay on track in development. In many ways, children with prematurity can help inform a shift from categorizing children's delays as leading to low learning expectations. We can examine how attention, regulatory, and social skills can be modified and lead to pathways of resilience in academic achievement and social-emotional behavioral competencies.

5 Chronic and Acute Stress

Recent studies have produced a large body of evidence that stress is significantly correlated with the occurrence of adverse birth outcomes, including prematurity and low birth weight (Graignic-Philippe et al. 2014). Prenatal stressors can include physical and psychological stress, infections, nutritional deficiencies, and drug exposures (Bock et al. 2015). In a prospective study, Killingworth-Rein et al. combined three variables into a single stress indicator comprised of state anxiety, perceived chronic stress, and life event distress. Higher scores on this aggregated factor predicted a shortened gestation and lower birth weight (Rini et al. 1999). Torche and Kleinhaus (2012) found that females who were exposed to earthquakes in early pregnancy had higher rates of preterm delivery (Torche and Kleinhaus 2012). In a study in the southern Israeli town of Sderot (4 km away from the Gaza Strip), Wainstock et al. hypothesized that the frequent exposure to rocket attacks in this community would be associated with adverse birth outcomes when compared to Kiryat Gat, a similar town without constant rocket attack exposure. Researchers found that women living in Sderot gave birth to more babies born preterm and at low birth weight, confirming the hypothesis that stress in pregnancy increases adverse birth outcomes (Wainstock et al. 2014).

A number of other studies have demonstrated an association between prenatal stress and adverse pregnancy and birth outcomes, including effects on birth weight, gestational age, and preterm birth (Bock et al. 2015). Chronic stress and acute stress may exert different effects on fetal development and perinatal outcomes. Several authors have reported lower birth weight and shortened gestation in children born to mothers exposed to chronic stress compared to acute stress (Chrousos and Gold 1992; Rini et al. 1999; Sable and Wilkinson 2000; Wadhwa et al. 1996).

Likewise, there is increasing evidence that exposure to forms of toxic stress in early life alters stress responses in adulthood. A case-controlled longitudinal study of preterm and term infants with and without medical complications demonstrated dysregulation of the hypothalamic-pituitary-adrenal axis in adult survivors of prematurity, particularly survivors also exposed to socioeconomic disadvantage (Winchester et al. 2016).

There is also a strong association between specific early pregnancy events, such as complications in the first trimester, and increased risk of preterm delivery and very preterm delivery (van Oppenraaij et al. 2009). An increased risk of low birth weight and very low birth weight was associated with first-trimester bleeding in a large prospective study (M. A. Williams et al. 1991). These adverse infant outcomes were associated with threatened miscarriage in the first trimester in another large retrospective study (Wijesiriwardana et al. 2006).

6 Epigenetic Mechanisms

Although the mechanisms of prenatal stress are not precisely known, it has been proposed that the hypothalamic-pituitary-adrenal (HPA) axis and sympathetic nervous system stress responses could lead to complications in pregnant women during pregnancy and delivery (Graignic-Philippe et al. 2014). In particular, McLean et al. (1995) suggest that high levels of neurohormones in the HPA axis as well as placental neurohormones could induce prematurity. A growing body of evidence suggests that epigenetic mechanisms induce transient and permanent alterations in gene function, resulting in altered developmental processes in the brain that result in long-term changes in emotional and cognitive behaviors (Bock et al. 2015).

The main function of the epigenome is to regulate gene transcription and compaction of DNA into the cell nucleus through mechanisms such as DNA methylation and hydroxymethylation, histone modifications, ATP-dependent chromatin remodeling, and noncoding RNAs (Provencal and Binder 2015). Prenatal stress has been shown to reduce the expression and activity of the enzyme 11-β-hydroxysteroid dehydrogenase type 2, an enzyme that converts glucocorticoids into inactive metabolites (Bock et al. 2015). An alteration in placental permeability may lead to excess exposure to maternal stress hormones, thereby promoting developmental dysregulation. Maternal intake of steroid hormones (Marciniak et al. 2011), maternal depression (O'Connor et al. 2014), and maternal anxiety (Kane et al. 2014) have been shown to alter maternal glucocorticoid levels, with a high correlation between maternal and fetal plasma glucocorticoids (Provencal and Binder 2015). In addition to affecting birth outcomes, stressful experiences in utero or during early life may also increase the risk of neurodevelopmental and behavioral disorders later in life due to alterations in epigenetic regulation (Babenko et al. 2015).

Pregnant mothers who have anxiety disorders, post-traumatic stress disorder (PTSD), depressive disorders, or major psychoses are at higher risk of adverse birth outcomes including preterm birth, low birth weight, and small-for-gestational-age infants. Mothers with bipolar disorder are at twice the risk for these adverse outcomes (MacCabe et al. 2007). Importantly, pregnant mothers with both PTSD and major depressive episode have four times the risk of having a preterm birth (Yonkers et al. 2014).

These risks occur because the brain and placenta are closely linked by a number of peptides and proteins, including oxytocin, somatostatin, neurotensin, encephalin, cortisol, insulin-like growth factor 1, vascular endothelial growth factor, and cyclic AMP response element binding factor. Individuals with mental illness often have a tendency toward coagulation and low activity of tissue plasminogen activator, potentially contributing to placental insufficiency that may lead to increased exposure of the fetus to maternal hormones. Hyperemesis gravidarum, a condition more common in women with eating disorders and anxiety than in controls, is another risk factor for pregnancy complications which may increase the risk of miscarriage, low birth weight infants, and preterm infants (Hoirisch-Clapauch et al. 2015).

7 Prenatal Stress Reduction Strategies

Intervention programs aimed at reducing stress should be considered to potentially lower the rates of unfavorable pregnancy outcomes (Wainstock et al. 2014). Feinberg et al. examined the effects of family foundation (FF), a transition to parenthood program, through a randomized control study of 148 expectant mothers. Researchers showed that the intervention significantly reduced the negative impact of maternal cortisol on birth weight, gestational age, and days in hospital in infants, thereby decreasing the risk for adverse birth outcomes (Feinberg et al. 2015). Follow-up at age 5–7 years demonstrated improved outcomes in behavior regulation and children's school adjustment (Feinberg et al. 2014). It is important to recognize the extent to which a child is affected by a mother's stress, and mental health heavily depends on moderating factors that include quality of parenting, social support, and the length and severity of the parental disorder (Howard et al. 2014). In this respect, early identification and interventions are essential (Stein et al. 2014). A recent report estimated that the long-term economic costs of perinatal mental disorders for each annual cohort exceed 8 billion euros in the UK alone (Bauer et al. 2014). Early interventions for perinatal mental disorders could produce great economic benefits and improve maternal and child physical and mental health (Howard et al. 2014) via impacting on child's regulatory behaviors and learning opportunities.

8 The Impact of Fetal Environment and Prematurity on Adult Health Outcomes

Exposure to an unfavorable environment in early life is closely associated with an increased tendency to develop adult disease. In 1992, David Barker hypothesized that the period of pregnancy and the intrauterine environment have a profound impact on risk of developing diseases like hypertension; diabetes; cardiac, pulmonary, and renal diseases; and mental illness (Capra et al. 2013). Intrauterine environment and early postnatal life are now generally accepted as important factors that may lead to increased risk for disease in adulthood (Hofman et al. 2004). In particular, low birth weight, a marker of poor fetal growth, is linked to vascular disease, hypertension, obesity, and insulin resistance (Calkins and Devaskar 2011).

Although several studies have reported an association between low birth weight and poor adult health outcomes, it remains unclear whether this association exists for children with poor fetal growth born small for gestational age as well as premature babies whose weight is appropriate for gestational age. In a retrospective study, Kaijser et al. identified subjects born preterm or with a low birth weight at four major delivery units in Sweden from 1925 to 1945. Researchers found that future risk for ischemic heart disease was most closely mediated by fetal growth restriction instead of preterm birth without growth restriction. Of note, these results came from a 1925 to 1949 birth cohort, a period when infants did not benefit from modern neonatal care. During more recent decades, infant survival has improved substantially for children born very preterm. It may not be appropriate, therefore, to generalize these results to preterm and growth-restricted infants being born today (Kaijser et al. 2008).

Babies born prematurely, whether or not they have intrauterine growth restriction (IUGR), are also at risk as adults for poor cardiovascular health outcomes (Irving et al. 2000). In a study of mothers of 72 LBW and 54 NBW infants born in Edinburgh between November 1973 and February 1975, LBW premature babies had higher adult blood pressure and fasting plasma glucose than NBW controls born at term. Babies born prematurely also had trends for an adverse metabolic profile and were at risk for hypertension and hyperglycemia as adults. Infants with IUGR were not measurably more disadvantaged than preterm infants with birth weight appropriate for gestational age (Irving et al. 2000).

A prospective follow-up study of 458 adults at age 30 in New Zealand also aimed to distinguish the relative contributions of gestation length and fetal growth to cardiovascular risk factors in adulthood. Preterm birth, rather than poor fetal growth, was shown to be the major determinant of the association between early environment and adult health outcomes; adults born preterm had increased systolic blood pressure and insulin resistance at age 30. Birth weight, independent of gestational age, was not associated with increased adult systolic blood pressure and insulin resistance, suggesting that length of gestation may be the major contribution to cardiovascular risk in adulthood (Dalziel et al. 2007).

Adult-onset insulin resistance, an early marker for type 2 diabetes, is also associated with premature birth (Hofman et al. 2004). Exposure to an adverse environment may be responsible for this reduction to insulin sensitivity, whether during intrauterine life in infants small for gestational age or a primarily adverse postnatal environment in premature infants (Hofman et al. 2004).

For the most part, mechanisms to explain the associations between intrauterine and postnatal environments and adult health outcomes are unknown. It is hypothesized that alterations to the HPA axis may explain the link between low birth weight and later increased blood pressure (Dalziel et al. 2007). Furthermore, it is theorized that earlier maturation of organ system exposure to nutritional, metabolic, hormonal, sensory, and respiratory environments at earlier time points in premature babies may also lead to abnormal development of organ systems involved in cardiovascular health (Curhan et al. 1996). Preterm infants and small-for-gestational-age infants often experience a period of "catchup growth" in the postnatal period, which may influence changes in their metabolism that are related to increased risk for these diseases (Smith and Ryckman 2015).

Increasing preterm infant survival has critical implications on the burden of adult diseases such as diabetes and cardiovascular disease. In fact, the historic trends in preterm survival and birth may be playing a critical, yet underappreciated, role in the population trend toward increasing prevalence of diabetes and cardiovascular disease (Dalziel et al. 2007).

9 Postnatal and Social Risk

Despite knowledge that supports that intervention in early childhood can positively impact disability trajectories, large gaps in services exist and disproportionally impact disadvantaged families. A 1997–2000 study looked at access to early intervention services among a population of infants aged birth to 3 years. Even in the highest risk neonates, access to community and early intervention supports was problematic and fragmented at best (>40% not enrolled in early intervention). Those toddlers with higher rates of disability were more likely to receive more services, yet a significant unmet need for services was documented among milder cases (Hintz et al. 2008).

Second, a Chicago-based cohort was followed after NICU discharge and demonstrated that less than 60% of VLBW infants living in extreme poverty (<50% federal poverty level) were receiving early intervention (EI) services despite having access to a medical home and legal advocacy. Of the 415 infants deemed not automatically eligible by EI, 95% had child and family impairments (e.g., gastrostomy, feeding delays, income <$10 K per year, parental mental or developmental disorder) that met EI inclusion criteria. This data confirms that a substantial number of infants with multiple medical and social risks do not receive ongoing developmental surveillance or early intervention services (Weiss et al. 2007).

Third, in a recent analysis of the Early Childhood Longitudinal Survey-Birth Cohort, it was found that eligibility for Part C varied widely between states (2–78%), yet the proportion of children receiving services remained consistently low (1.5–7%). There is significant state-by-state variability between eligibility criteria, yet there is also a clear national trend of insufficient enrollment for children with qualifying delays (Rosenberg et al. 2008). Given that in elementary school years 10–20% of children nationally have Individual Educational Plans, early intervention rates less than 5% reflect significant missed opportunities for secondary and tertiary prevention.

Among both VLBW and ELBW survivors, disproportionate numbers live in communities with high rates of school dropouts and poorly performing schools. This will result in barriers to accessing quality early and middle childhood educational experiences. The combination of developmental vulnerability due to LBW and preterm birth with social and family distress has shown to have cumulative impacts (Hille et al. 1994). In an 8–10-year follow-up study of infants who were the sickest and tiniest and had the most medical complications in the newborn period, Msall and colleagues found that not only were favorable vision and functional motor status at kindergarten entry associated with significantly lower rates of special education and below-grade-level educational achievement, but higher SES was also associated with positive academic and developmental outcomes. Factors strongly associated with increased risk for special education services included minority status, poverty, lack of access to a car, and Supplemental Social Security Income because of disability and poverty (Msall et al. 2004).

9.1 Adolescent and Adult Outcomes

Clinical research to date on the outcomes for preterm infants during adolescence and adulthood reveals a spectrum of strengths and challenges in physical and behavioral health, educational achievement and supports, and community participation. However, the social, educational/vocational, and independent adaptive life skills required for adulthood are inherently more quantitatively and qualitatively complex than basic developmental milestones in an infant or school achievement in middle childhood. A few crude measures of adult success have been used to examine adolescent and adult outcomes, but much work remains to unveil more meaningful multidimensional measures of adult physical and behavioral health, daily functioning, social participation, family formation, and economic well-being.

Educational attainment is a frequently examined adult outcome in the literature. The studies highlighted in Table 5 demonstrate lower rates of academic achievement, high school completion, and postsecondary education among preterm survivors. Premature survivors show high rates of

Table 5 Cognitive, executive function and academic achievement in adolescence and adulthood

Authors	Cohort	Assessment age	Developmental outcome
Botting et al. (1998)	1980–1983 Liverpool, England 138 VLBW 108 matched controls	12 years	1. VLBW lower IQ 2. Lower math and reading comprehension
Saigal et al. (2000)	1977–1982 Ontario, Canada 141 ELBW 124 matched controls	12–16 years	1. 28% reported neurosensory impairments 2. 25% of ELBW vs. 6% repeated a grade 3. 49% of ELBW vs. 10% required special education services 4. 22% ELBW required full-time educational assistance (vs. 0%) 5. Lower mean WISC-R DQ 6. Lower mean WRAT-R
Rushe et al. (2001)	1979–1980 London, England <33 weeks; 75 premature and 53 FT	14–15 years	1. No differences for tests of executive function, verbal memory, attention 2. Preterm group had impaired verbal fluency
Lefebvre et al. (2005)	1976–1981 Montreal, Canada 57 ELBW and 44 NBW	18 years	1. 56.1% ELBW vs. 84.6% controls completed HS 2. 33% vs. 9% required special education 3. Significant differences in low IQ (<85)
Hack et al. (2002)	1977–1979 Cleveland, Ohio 242 VLBW and 233 controls	20 years	1. 74% VLBW graduated HS vs. 83% NBW 2. 30% pursued secondary education vs. 53% NBW 3. 40% repeated grade vs. 27% NBW 4. Scored 1/3 SD lower on WAIS-R
Lindstrom et al. (2009)	1973–1979 Sweden 24–28 weeks vs. FT	1987–2002 national registry	71% vs. 78.6% completed 12 or more years of school
Moster et al. (2008)	1976–1983 Norway 325 preterm (23–27 weeks) vs. 828,227 FT	20–36 years	1. 67.7 preterm vs. 75.4% completed HS 2. 4.4% preterm vs. 0.1% fullterm with ID
Nomura et al. (2009) Johns Hopkins Collaborative Perinatal Study	1960–1965 Baltimore 226 near-term and 1393 FT	27–33 years	1. Near-term birth associated with lower adult educational attainment only for those living below poverty line 2. SGA had no association with educational attainment
Saigal et al. (2006)	1977–1982 Ontario, Canada 166 ELBW and 145 controls	22–25 years	No significant difference in: 1. % graduation from high school 2. Pursuit of postsecondary education

HS high school, *SD* standard deviation, *WAIS-R* Wechsler Adult Intelligence Scale-Revised, *WISC-R* Wechsler Intelligence Scale for Children-Revised, *DQ* deviation quotient, *WRAT-R* Wide Range Achievement Test-Revised, *FT* full term

need for special education supports, both in general special education services and with individual assistants, and have higher rates of grade repetition than their normal birth weight peers (Saigal et al. 2003). Furthermore, preterm survivors are less likely to graduate high school and pursue secondary education (Hack et al. 2002; Moster et al. 2008).

However, this outcome is also influenced by contextual factors. When high school graduation rates are adjusted for parental SES, there is evidence of mitigation of the difference in educational attainment. In a study by Nomura et al., it was found that in near-term survivors, only those living at incomes close to poverty line differed from full-term peers on educational attainment. The relationship between cognitive testing in adulthood and gestational age has also been significantly mitigated by socioeconomic factors (Ekeus et al. 2010). There is compelling evidence that the same risk factors disproportionately distributing premature birth to poorer, less educated mothers are also at play with the long-term outcomes of low birth weight progeny, compounding the disadvantage of the disadvantaged.

IQ outcomes have been repeatedly tested and show consistently lower scores for ELBW adults compared to matched peers. However, many studies are unable to match for socioeconomic status or parental IQ which are highly influential mediating factors. Maternal education and income have been shown consistently to predict IQ within these cohorts, indeed often with stronger correlation coefficients than LBW status (Drillien 1961; Drillien et al. 1980). There is evidence that IQ in middle childhood is strongly predictive of IQ at adolescence, suggesting that, on this measure, there is neither increasing gap nor improved catch-up to normal birth weight peers. Alternatively, one study highlighted a widening IQ gap in later childhood (Botting et al. 1998), which may be due to the complexity of the involved intellectual task in testing at older ages or the additional components of social/emotional intelligence, which are not entirely captured by younger measures of IQ. Furthermore, studies that evaluate both educational and professional attainment do not consistently demonstrate strong correlation; 50% of preterm adults in the 1983 Dutch cohort who reported poor educational attainment during the school years held full-time employment as young adults (Hille et al. 2007). How this translates to US cohorts in the ongoing economic crisis for those without college degrees is yet unknown. Other educational outcomes, such as reading and math achievement, have shown significant gaps in core educational outcomes between VLBW and age-matched peers. However given that many term children in low-income urban or rural communities in the United States also are struggling with reading, mathematics, science, and social studies performance, it is difficult to make international comparisons.

Additional evidence demonstrates the power of socioeconomic status in modifying the effect of prematurity; Lefebvre et al. assessed the cognitive and academic achievement outcomes in early adulthood of a cohort of 82 ELBW subjects in Montreal (Lefebvre et al. 2005). There were significant differences between ELBW and NBW groups in full-scale IQ (94 versus 108), verbal IQ (93 versus 106), and performance IQ (97 versus 109). However, father's low socioeconomic status contributed significantly to the prevalence of IQ <85 (19% versus 2%, $p = 0.012$), schooling in mainstream education with a regular curriculum for age (36% versus 68%), requirement for special classes or schools (33% versus 9%), and high school graduation for those 18 years or older (56% versus 85%).

Adolescent/adult self-perceptions of health, quality of life, and overall functioning are important outcomes, which may guide our clinical understanding and facilitate improved anticipatory guidance to families of premature neonates. A socioeconomically diverse cohort of adolescents born in 1983–1984 at <801 g (Brown et al. 2003) reported themselves and was reported by their parents as having lower functional status than normal birth weight peers; however, overall these health concerns did not significantly interfere with tasks of daily living. On rating scales of externalizing and internalizing problems, however, (The Behavioral Assessment System for Children- BASC), there were no differences between preterm and comparison groups. Additionally, using a self-perception profile, which included domains of scholastic competence, social acceptance, athletic competence, and global self-worth, responses did not significantly differ. In a similar cohort of adults (born at weight <1250 g in Zurich), preterm and term controls did not differ on overall physical health

Table 6 Adult outcomes after very preterm birth

Authors	Cohort	Age at assessment	Developmental outcome
Baumgardt et al. (2012)	1983–1985 Zurich, Switzerland 52 preterm (<1250 g) 75 controls	23 years	No difference in overall self-reported quality of life
Hack et al. (2007)	1977–1979 Cleveland, Ohio 241 VLBW 232 NBW	20 years	1. No difference on self-reported health satisfaction 2. No difference on self-reported comfort (physical or emotional) 3. Decreased self-reported resiliency 4. Increased self-reported risk avoidance
Hille et al. (2008)	1983 Netherlands 959 adult survivors of prematurity (<32 weeks or VLBW)	19 years	1. 11.4% had moderate/severe problem with profession 2. ½ of individuals with moderate/severe problems in education had full-time employment
Moster et al. (2008)	1976–1983; Norway 325- 23–27 weeks 1608- 28–30 weeks 6363- 31–33 weeks 31,169- 34–36 weeks 828,227- full term	20–36 years	1. 10.6% vs. 1.7% receiving disability pension 2. Lower gestation less likely to have found life partner 3. Lower gestation less likely to have children
Saigal et al. (2006)	1977–1982 Ontario, Canada 166 ELBW and 145 controls	22–25 years	No significant difference in rates of 1. Employment 2. Independent living 3. Married/cohabitation 4. Parenthood

VLBW very low birth weight (<1500 g), *ELBW* extremely low birth weight (<1000 g), *NBW* normal birth weight (>2500 g), *CPT* Conners' continuous performance task

or mental health scores on the Short Form 36 Health Survey (Baumgardt et al. 2012) (Table 6).

Adult males who survived prematurity rated themselves significantly lower than male term adults on the "physical functioning domain," but females did not differ from matched controls in any subset. Patterns of high risk and protective health habits varied: the use of marijuana was significantly lower among adults who survived prematurity, yet significantly more control adults practiced sports and more males exercised. The overall trend appears that adolescents and adult survivors of prematurity, by and large, consider themselves similar to normal term survivors on self-ratings of physiologic and psychological functioning. Some studies suggest that females may be more similar to full-term peers than males, suggesting that males may be somewhat more vulnerable to the long-term effects of prematurity and LBW. It deserves mentioning that the discrepancy between self-reported health and external measures of health has been reported in other health conditions; overall persons with a health condition rate the impact of that condition more positively than health professionals may surmise (Groot 2000).

Research on long-term consequences of low birth weight has focused on adolescent and early adult life – especially the negative impact of low birth weight on academic achievement, high school graduation and years of school completion, and college attendance. Low birth weight has been linked to these outcomes through the effects of low birth weight on kindergarten preparedness and weak performance in the first few years of schooling. Poor educational performance in subsequent years is negatively linked to both poor school readiness and accomplishment on subsequent school performance and the lingering health effects of low birth weight. The latter often includes not only growth and respiratory sequelae but increased vulnerability to a spectrum of neurobehavioral disorders that impact attention and mood. Importantly, buffers for these disorders include attention to caregiver mental health and child behavior health in the context of increasing school and community successes. While longer-term effects of low birth weight, mediated by poor educational performance and continued weak health, are hypothesized, little research has examined the midlife consequences of low birth weight and what factors contribute to thriving.

An additional complexity of measuring adolescent and adult outcomes is the shift of health status reporting from the parent of a premature survivor to the adolescent or adult himself/herself. In an adolescent follow-up of 99 very low birth weight babies born in Norway, there was found to be a significant discrepancy between adolescent and parental reporters, with the overall trend being parents reporting significantly more emotional and behavior problems than the adolescents reported in themselves (Dahl et al. 2006). In these later stages of follow-up, investigators must consider the inherent bias in asking parents vs. adolescents to report on health and behavior.

This research limitation can be remedied through analysis of data from two population datasets that include information on weight at birth and current health and well-being – the Wisconsin Longitudinal Study (WLS) and the Midlife in the United States: A National Study of Health and Well-Being (MIDUS). Additionally, utilizing these cohorts from the United States may help remedy the current data gap between well-tracked international cohorts and the dearth of longitudinal US data. International cohorts, which have lower rates of single parenthood and more homogenous racial ethnic and socioeconomic composition as compared to the United States, dominate the current knowledge base of long-term outcomes for premature babies. Extrapolating from their long-term outcomes likely vastly underestimates the need for social support throughout the life course in the United States. Additionally, international countries with single-payer systems tend to diagnose and provide more consistent social support for persons with disabilities when compared to the fragmented nature of health care in the United States.

The Wisconsin Longitudinal Study (WLS) is a long-term study of a random sample of 10,317 men and women who graduated from Wisconsin high school in 1957. The WLS provides an opportunity to study the life course, intergenerational transfers and relationships, family functioning, physical and mental health and well-being, and morbidity and mortality from late adolescence (in 1957) through early geriatric (in 2008). WLS data also cover social background, youthful aspirations, schooling, military service, labor market experiences, family characteristics and events, social participation, psychological characteristics, and retirement. Survey data were collected from the original respondents or their parents in 1957, 1964, 1975, 1992, and 2004 (when they were approximately at age 64 or 65). The WLS includes end-of-life data for members of the cohort who have died. Sibling and twin data for the original respondents, as well as gene-environment interactions from late adolescent to the retirement years, will permit models that separate the effects of family origins from the impact of low birth weight at retirement age.

The first national representative survey of Midlife Development in the United States (MIDUS) was conducted in 1995–1996. MIDUS is a 1994 national sample survey of 7189 randomly chosen adults ages 25–74 years, as well as 1914 respondents to a separate nationally representative sample of twin pairs. The wide age range of the sample was intended to permit comparisons on persons in their early adult life to those in midlife and old age. The survey permits the assessment of many psychological factors such as personality traits, sense of control, and goal commitments and their linkages to marital status, family structure, socioeconomic standing, social participation, social support, employment status, health status, and health-care utilization. MIDUS respondent follow-ups were conducted from 2002 to 2006, and there were a third round of interviews from 2006 to 2011. This dataset, including sibling data, will permit models that separate the effects of family origins and early life experiences from the impact of low birth weight at retirement age and beyond.

10 Conclusion

The interdependent challenges of prematurity and socioeconomic risk create numerous hurdles for achieving optimal physical, developmental, and emotional health. With over 50,000 surviving extremely preterm and very preterm infants per year in the United States, we have the equivalent of an ongoing annual polio crisis in the pre-vaccination era. Not only are many of these children growing up in families that are strapped for material resources, services and time, but our current early intervention and preschool systems are not delivering child health, developmental, and behavioral supports on a population basis. Therefore, there is decreased likelihood that the 325,000 late preterm survivors who annually enter kindergarten will be healthy and ready to learn. Nor will they stay on track during the first three grades, achieving adequate levels of literacy, numeracy, information handling, and social participation; they will need to succeed in school and life. As their development lags and their academic performance falters, there is too often a response of educational systems, especially during the middle school years, to divert children by using grade repetition, expulsions, and nonevidence-based remediation that only increase the likelihood that the child will leave school or be classified with behavioral problems. Importantly, unlike their middle-class and affluent counterparts, low-income children with a spectrum of neurodevelopmental dysfunction will have less access to high-quality medical care, appropriately targeted and responsive parent-child interactions, quality educational accommodations and explicit strategies for promoting basic competencies, and extracurricular activities.

Although potentially detrimental to a child's future, his/her gestational age and birth weight are rarely the major determining factors when long-term educational, social, and behavioral outcomes are considered. In this chapter we have examined several research studies that emphasized the importance of family, social, and economic environmental factors, which can either aggravate or moderate neonatal risks caused by premature birth. Much is to be gained by attention to how adversity impacts allostatic load, and through epigenetic mechanisms and complex protective buffers of parenting, health promotion, and social supports, leads to long-term outcomes of thriving across physical, behavioral, and social health outcomes. With so much to lose while living under suboptimal conditions, it is of critical importance that both health and educational professionals create systems for enhancing access to early childhood learning experiences, parenting supports, quality preschool education services, and biopsychosocial strategies in middle childhood to help children achieve basic educational, behavioral, and social competencies and adolescent supports of mentoring, preparation for independent living, and proactive behavioral health strategies for stress, time management, mood disorders, and self-efficacy. We need more research about how to spread and scale successful biopsychosocial health development strategies at a community level to insure that VLBW and ELBW survivors do not miss out on the critical experiences, which have potential to compensate for birth disadvantage, and are critical for long-term adult success. A summary of the gaps and recommendations for increasing research in life course health development after prematurity follows.

Research in life course health development for children who survive prematurity has made the following advances:

1. *Medical advances in pregnancy*: Over the past decades, there has been improved management of high-risk pregnancy disorders such as hypertension, diabetes, multiple gestation, intrauterine growth restriction, prenatal infections, and fetal malformations. There has been growing awareness that women's health involving the use of tobacco, alcohol, illicit drugs, anticonvulsants, and antidepressants has subtle neurobehavioral consequences on child development. Additionally, society has

had greater recognition that poverty, social adversity involving basic resources as well as lack of partner/family supports, previous preterm birth, minority status, limited education, and low health literacy increase the risk of low birth weight, prematurity, and early childhood health and developmental impairments.

2. *Medical advances in the neonatal period*: Over the last decades, there has been remarkable improvement in the management of premature labor and delivery. In particular, the widespread screening for and treatment of Group B *Streptococcus* colonization and the use of maternal corticosteroids when preterm labor presents have had marked improvements in premature survival and sequelae of neonatal infections. We have had improved resuscitation and neonatal transport to tertiary care centers. Throughout the vulnerable neonatal course, improved respiratory support (the use of positive pressure and noninvasive ventilator techniques after surfactant), evidence-based nutritional interventions, and infection control management have improved neonatal survival.

Although there is increased recognition that very and extremely preterm survivors experience a variety of health (e.g., growth, pulmonary), neurological (e.g., sensory impairments, seizures), neurodevelopmental (e.g., CP, ID, ASD), and learning and behavior impairment, the population-level risks have not been systematically measured. In order to improve life course health development, we propose seven theme research agenda.

11 Recommendations for an After Prematurity Life Course Health Disparities Research Agenda

1. Establish national registries.

   It is imperative to create national registries for children from birth to 5 years old who are at highest risk of CP and neurodevelopmental disabilities such as intellectual disability, neurosensory disability, and autism spectrum disorders. These registries would not only include preterm infants but also include term infants with history of critical illness from cardiac, pulmonary, infectious, neurological, or genetic disorders. Such registries would allow for the investigation of diverse interventions and link health, early intervention, special education, and rehabilitation services to long-term outcomes across the life course. Most importantly attention must be paid to maternal health, adversity, and mental health. Registries ought to include placental samples as well as cord blood and newborn screening blood spots, in order to allow for the evaluation of early biomarkers of toxic stress during early childhood.

2. Build population-based datasets.

   To understand health across the life course, it is imperative to create population-based datasets which originate at delivery and during newborn primary care visits. We must be able to link information on birth certificates with early childhood health, developmental, and educational outcomes through collaborative arrangements between public health, regional neonatal follow-up, early intervention, and district-wide educational testing. We should use these population databases to engage in ongoing health and developmental surveillance of all children with all degrees of prematurity requiring neonatal intensive care, especially those with seizures, neonatal encephalopathy, congenital heart disease, malformation requiring surgery, and abnormalities in newborn genetic and hearing screening. We should model our US efforts on the Longitudinal Study of Australian Children to understand diverse trajectories of health, development, and behavior for those with and without special health-care needs.

   Preterm infants need the establishment of longitudinal data collection registries that can collect information that is similar to the National Survey of Children's Health and NHIS disability follow-up studies. We must determine the risk factors for trajectories of positive and negative outcomes across cohorts of middle childhood, adolescence, and adulthood for sequential preterm survivors who were <28 weeks of gestation, 29–31 weeks of gestation, 32–36 weeks of gestation, and term gestation. Only with informed, collaborative, and comprehensive life course health development registries will we determine ways to support resiliency among preterm offspring of high-risk mothers with respect to health, developmental, educational, and social outcomes over the life course.

3. Expansion and evaluation of comprehensive health and developmental surveillance interventions on a population level.

   We need to improve population surveillance for children exposed to high-risk maternal conditions such as hypertension, diabetes, obesity, asthma, seizure disorders, depression, ADHD, anxiety, and maternal use of tobacco, alcohol, and illegal substances. In the setting of these risk factors, we must evaluate what factors promote maternal and child resiliency and promote positive newborn and developmental outcomes. We must understand which factors mitigate the negative effect of these exposures on growth, obesity, developmental delays, and regulatory disorders. We should seek to determine the impact of positive parenting, quality early child education (early intervention, head start preschool programming), and pediatric medical homes especially using neonatal and epigenetic biomarkers.

   Surveillance should extend beyond the neonatal period into preschool (ages 2–4 years) to identify young children who lack the basic numeracy, literacy, and social and emotional maturity needed to enter kindergarten ready to learn. Kindergarten is also a key transition for measuring health and developmental status, yet there are no systematic screening modalities in place at kindergarten entry across diverse biomedical and social risks.

4. Integration of twenty-first-century technologies to improve care coordination and integrated health and engage families in time-efficient interventions.

   Diagnostic tools such as fidgety movements are shown to have high reliability in detection of future motor delays; texting has been shown to improve parental engagement with early childhood development; and telemedicine has enabled the delivery of highly specialized care to remote or mobility-challenged populations. These growing technologies, increasingly available across socioeconomic populations, must be fully embraced and leveraged for population surveillance and therapeutic interventions.

5. Shift research methodology from antiquated methods studying individuals and parent-child dyads to novel techniques examining clusters of families and communities.

   Increasingly we need to better understand the power of parent-child interactions on determining developmental trajectories in conjunction with genetic and epigenetic biomarkers. Furthermore, siblings certainly impact health and development of one another, yet most research fails to consider the contribution of sibling factors. We must seek to develop and improve our research modalities, which look beyond a single child as the unit of measure and examine interrelatedness among family and community factors.

6. Research on impacting parent-child interventions.

   A critical need is to formally evaluate the caregiving environment of premature infants and determine how cumulative parent-child interactions impact the child's developmental capacities and parental health and well-being. Examine developmental activities as a part of everyday childcare tasks to promote early parent involvement and positive health and regulatory trajectories.

7. Determine what types of interventions effectively impact maternal mental health in the setting of adversities.

It is incompletely known how maternal mental health stressors (depression, anxiety, isolation, and violence) increase vulnerability of children when they do not receive quality early childhood social learning and behavioral supports. Strategies for integrating maternal and child physical and behavioral health have the potential to increase resilience for high-risk populations.

By combining themes from this research agenda to populations involving life course health development and the ICF model for promoting health, functioning, and participation, we have the opportunities to improve thriving after prematurity and measure our impact on long-term health, education, and community costs.

Acknowledgments This work was supported in part by NIH NINR03095 (Sullivan, Msall). Dr. Msall was also supported in part by NIH/NICHD Grant P30 HD0544275 JP Kennedy Intellectual and Developmental Disabilities Research Center and HRSA-DHHS T73 MC 11047 Leadership Education in Neurodevelopmental and Related Disorders Training Program (LEND).

References

Allen, M. C., Cristofalo, E. A., & Kim, C. (2011). Outcomes of preterm infants: Morbidity replaces mortality. *Clinics in Perinatology, 38*(3), 441–454. doi:10.1016/j.clp.2011.06.011.

Aron, L., & Loprest, P. (2012). Disability and the education system. *The Future of Children, 22*(1), 97–122.

Arpi, E., & Ferrari, F. (2013). Preterm birth and behaviour problems in infants and preschool-age children: A review of the recent literature. *Developmental Medicine and Child Neurology, 55*(9), 788–796. doi:10.1111/dmcn.12142.

Babenko, O., Kovalchuk, I., & Metz, G. A. (2015). Stress-induced perinatal and transgenerational epigenetic programming of brain development and mental health. *Neuroscience and Biobehavioral Reviews, 48*, 70–91. doi:10.1016/j.neubiorev.2014.11.013.

Baek, Y., Vohr, B. R., Alksninis, B., Cashore, W. J., Hogan, D. P., & Msall, M. E. (2002). Kindergarten readiness in very low birth weight (VLBW) children. *Pediatric Research, 51*(4), 293A.

Bauer, A., Parsonage, M., Knapp, M., Iemmi, V., & Adelaja, B. (2014). *The costs of perinatal mental health problems*. London: Cemtre for Mental Health and London School of Economics.

Baumgardt, M., Bucher, H. U., Mieth, R. A., & Fauchere, J. C. (2012). Health-related quality of life of former very preterm infants in adulthood. *Acta Paediatrica, 101*(2), e59–e63. doi:10.1111/j.1651-2227.2011.02422.x.

Bhutta, A. T., Cleves, M. A., Casey, P. H., Cradock, M. M., & Anand, K. J. (2002). Cognitive and behavioral outcomes of school-aged children who were born preterm: A meta-analysis. *JAMA, 288*(6), 728–737.

Bock, J., Wainstock, T., Braun, K., & Segal, M. (2015). Stress in utero: Prenatal programming of brain plasticity and cognition. *Biological Psychiatry*. doi:10.1016/j.biopsych.2015.02.036.

Botting, N., Powls, A., Cooke, R. W., & Marlow, N. (1998). Cognitive and educational outcome of very-low-birthweight children in early adolescence. *Developmental Medicine and Child Neurology, 40*(10), 652–660.

Brown, K. J., Kilbride, H. W., Turnbull, W., & Lemanek, K. (2003). Functional outcome at adolescence for infants less than 801 g birth weight: Perceptions of children and parents. *Journal of Perinatology, 23*(1), 41–47. doi:10.1038/sj.jp.7210850.

Calkins, K., & Devaskar, S. U. (2011). Fetal origins of adult disease. *Current Problems in Pediatric and Adolescent Health Care, 41*(6), 158–176. doi:10.1016/j.cppeds.2011.01.001.

Capra, L., Tezza, G., Mazzei, F., & Boner, A. L. (2013). The origins of health and disease: The influence of maternal diseases and lifestyle during gestation. *Italian Journal of Pediatrics, 39*, 7. doi:10.1186/1824-7288-39-7.

Chrousos, G. P., & Gold, P. W. (1992). The concepts of stress and stress system disorders. Overview of physical and behavioral homeostasis. *JAMA, 267*(9), 1244–1252.

Crouter, A. C., & Booth, A. (Eds). (2014). *Work-family challenges for low-income parents and their children*. Routledge. Abingdon, UK.

Curhan, G. C., Willett, W. C., Rimm, E. B., Spiegelman, D., Ascherio, A. L., & Stampfer, M. J. (1996). Birth weight and adult hypertension, diabetes mellitus, and obesity in US men. *Circulation, 94*(12), 3246–3250.

Dahl, L. B., Kaaresen, P. I., Tunby, J., Handegard, B. H., Kvernmo, S., & Ronning, J. A. (2006). Emotional, behavioral, social, and academic outcomes in adolescents born with very low birth weight. *Pediatrics, 118*(2), e449–e459. doi:10.1542/peds.2005-3024.

Dalziel, S. R., Parag, V., Rodgers, A., & Harding, J. E. (2007). Cardiovascular risk factors at age 30 following pre-term birth. *International Journal of Epidemiology, 36*(4), 907–915. doi:10.1093/ije/dym067.

Diagnostic and Statistical Manual of Mental Disorders: DSM-5. (2013). (5th ed.). Washington, DC: American Psychiatric Association.

Dmowska, A., Andrews, B., Schreiber, M., & Msall, M. E. (2016). Preterm survivors: Community support to lessen health disparities. In J. Merrick & L. Rubin (Eds.), *Environmental health disparities: Costs and benefits of breaking the cycle*. Hauppauge, NY: Nova Publishers.

Drillien, C. M. (1961). A longitudinal study of the growth and development of prematurely and maturely born children. VIII. Morbidity in the age period 2-5 years. *Archives of Disease in Childhood, 36*, 515–525.

Drillien, C. M., Thomson, A. J., & Burgoyne, K. (1980). Low-birthweight children at early school-age: A longitudinal study. *Developmental Medicine and Child Neurology, 22*(1), 26–47.

Ekeus, C., Lindstrom, K., Lindblad, F., Rasmussen, F., & Hjern, A. (2010). Preterm birth, social disadvantage, and cognitive competence in Swedish 18- to 19-year-old men. *Pediatrics, 125*(1), e67–e73. doi:10.1542/peds.2008-3329.

Farooqi, A., Hagglof, B., Sedin, G., Gothefors, L., & Serenius, F. (2007). Mental health and social competencies of 10- to 12-year-old children born at 23 to 25 weeks of gestation in the 1990s: A Swedish national prospective follow-up study. *Pediatrics, 120*(1), 118–133. doi:10.1542/peds.2006-2988.

Feinberg, M. E., Jones, D. E., Roettger, M. E., Solmeyer, A., & Hostetler, M. L. (2014). Long-term follow-up of a randomized trial of family foundations: Effects on children's emotional, behavioral, and school adjustment. *Journal of Family Psychology, 28*(6), 821–831. doi:10.1037/fam0000037.

Feinberg, M. E., Roettger, M. E., Jones, D. E., Paul, I. M., & Kan, M. L. (2015). Effects of a psychosocial couple-based prevention program on adverse birth outcomes. *Maternal and Child Health Journal, 19*(1), 102–111. doi:10.1007/s10995-014-1500-5.

Gardner, F., Johnson, A., Yudkin, P., Bowler, U., Hockley, C., Mutch, L., et al. (2004). Behavioral and emotional adjustment of teenagers in mainstream school who were born before 29 weeks' gestation. *Pediatrics, 114*(3), 676–682. doi:10.1542/peds.2003-0763-L.

Graignic-Philippe, R., Dayan, J., Chokron, S., Jacquet, A. Y., & Tordjman, S. (2014). Effects of prenatal stress on fetal and child development: A critical literature review. *Neuroscience and Biobehavioral Reviews, 43*, 137–162. doi:10.1016/j.neubiorev.2014.03.022.

Groot, W. (2000). Adaptation and scale of reference bias in self-assessments of quality of life. *Journal of Health Economics, 19*(3), 403–420.

Gross, S. J., Mettelman, B. B., Dye, T. D., & Slagle, T. A. (2001). Impact of family structure and stability on academic outcome in preterm children at 10 years of age. *The Journal of Pediatrics, 138*(2), 169–175. doi:10.1067/mpd.2001.111945.

Hack, M., Flannery, D. J., Schluchter, M., Cartar, L., Borawski, E., & Klein, N. (2002). Outcomes in young adulthood for very-low-birth-weight infants. *The New England Journal of Medicine, 346*(3), 149–157. doi:10.1056/NEJMoa010856.

Hamilton, B. E., Martin, J. A., Osterman, M. J., Curtin, S. C., & Matthews, T. J. (2015). Births: Final data for 2014. *National Vital Statistics Reports, 64*(12), 1–64. Retrieved from http://www.ncbi.nlm.nih.gov/pubmed/26727629.

Hille, E. T., den Ouden, A. L., Bauer, L., van den Oudenrijn, C., Brand, R., & Verloove-Vanhorick, S. P. (1994). School performance at nine years of age in very premature and very low birth weight infants: Perinatal risk factors and predictors at five years of age. Collaborative project on preterm and small for gestational age (POPS) infants in The Netherlands. *The Journal of Pediatrics, 125*(3), 426–434.

Hille, E. T., Weisglas-Kuperus, N., van Goudoever, J. B., Jacobusse, G. W., Ens-Dokkum, M. H., de Groot, L., et al. (2007). Functional outcomes and participation in young adulthood for very preterm and very low birth weight infants: The Dutch project on preterm and small for gestational age infants at 19 years of age. *Pediatrics, 120*(3), e587–e595. doi:10.1542/peds.2006-2407.

Himmelmann, K., & Uvebrant, P. (2014). The panorama of cerebral palsy in Sweden. XI. Changing patterns in the birth-year period 2003-2006. *Acta Paediatrica, 103*(6), 618–624. doi:10.1111/apa.12614.

Hintz, S. R., Kendrick, D. E., Vohr, B. R., Poole, W. K., & Higgins, R. D. (2008). Community supports after surviving extremely low-birth-weight, extremely preterm birth: Special outpatient services in early childhood. *Archives of Pediatrics & Adolescent Medicine, 162*(8), 748–755. doi:10.1001/archpedi.162.8.748.

Hofman, P. L., Regan, F., Jackson, W. E., Jefferies, C., Knight, D. B., Robinson, E. M., et al. (2004). Premature birth and later insulin resistance. *The New England Journal of Medicine, 351*(21), 2179–2186. doi:10.1056/NEJMoa042275.

Hoirisch-Clapauch, S., Brenner, B., & Nardi, A. E. (2015). Adverse obstetric and neonatal outcomes in women with mental disorders. *Thrombosis Research, 135*(Suppl 1), S60–S63. doi:10.1016/s0049-3848(15)50446-5.

Holzmann, R., & Jørgensen, S. (2001). Social risk management: A new conceptual framework for social protection, and beyond. *International Tax and Public Finance, 8*(4), 529–556. doi:10.1023/A:1011247814590.

Howard, L. M., Piot, P., & Stein, A. (2014). No health without perinatal mental health. *The Lancet, 384*(9956), 1723–1724. doi:10.1016/S0140-6736(14)62040-7.

Huston, A. C. (1991). *Children in poverty : Child development and public policy*. Cambridge, NY: Cambridge University Press.

Income, Poverty, and Health Insurance Coverage in the United States: 2005 (2006). In U. S. C. Bureau (Ed.).

Irving, R. J., Belton, N. R., Elton, R. A., & Walker, B. R. (2000). Adult cardiovascular risk factors in premature babies. *Lancet, 355*(9221), 2135–2136. doi:10.1016/s0140-6736(00)02384-9.

Jiang Y. E. M., & Skinner C. (2015). Basic facts about low-income children: Children under 3 Years, 2013 (trans: D. o. H. P. Management). Columbia University: National Center for Children in Poverty.

Johnson, S., Hennessy, E., Smith, R., Trikic, R., Wolke, D., & Marlow, N. (2009). Academic attainment and special educational needs in extremely preterm children at 11 years of age: The EPICure study. *Archives of Disease in Childhood. Fetal and Neonatal Edition, 94*(4), F283–F289. doi:10.1136/adc.2008.152793.

Johnson, S., Wolke, D., Hennessy, E., & Marlow, N. (2011). Educational outcomes in extremely preterm children: Neuropsychological correlates and predictors of attainment. *Developmental Neuropsychology, 36*(1), 74–95. doi:10.1080/87565641.2011.540541.

Jones, K. M., Champion, P. R., & Woodward, L. J. (2013). Social competence of preschool children born very preterm. *Early Human Development, 89*(10), 795–802. doi:10.1016/j.earlhumdev.2013.06.008.

Joseph, R. M., O'Shea, T. M., Allred, E. N., Heeren, T., Hirtz, D., Paneth, N., Leviton, A., & Kuban, K. C. (2016). Prevalence and associated features of autism spectrum disorder in extremely low gestational age newborns at age 10 years. *Autism Research, 10*(2), 224–232. doi:10.1002/aur.1644.

Kaijser, M., Bonamy, A. K., Akre, O., Cnattingius, S., Granath, F., Norman, M., et al. (2008). Perinatal risk factors for ischemic heart disease: Disentangling the roles of birth weight and preterm birth. *Circulation, 117*(3), 405–410. doi:10.1161/circulationaha.107.710715.

Kane, H. S., Dunkel Schetter, C., Glynn, L. M., Hobel, C. J., & Sandman, C. A. (2014). Pregnancy anxiety and prenatal cortisol trajectories. *Biological Psychology, 100*, 13–19. doi:10.1016/j.biopsycho.2014.04.003.

Lang, C. T., & Iams, J. D. (2009). Goals and strategies for prevention of preterm birth: An obstetric perspective. *Pediatric Clinics of North America, 56*(3), 537–563.

Lefebvre, F., Mazurier, E., & Tessier, R. (2005). Cognitive and educational outcomes in early adulthood for infants weighing 1000 grams or less at birth. *Acta Paediatrica, 94*(6), 733–740. doi:10.1080/08035250510025987.

Litt, J. S., Gerry Taylor, H., Margevicius, S., Schluchter, M., Andreias, L., & Hack, M. (2012). Academic achievement of adolescents born with extremely low birth weight. *Acta Paediatrica, 101*(12), 1240–1245. doi:10.1111/j.1651-2227.2012.02790.x.

MacCabe, J. H., Martinsson, L., Lichtenstein, P., Nilsson, E., Cnattingius, S., Murray, R. M., et al. (2007). Adverse pregnancy outcomes in mothers with affective psychosis. *Bipolar Disorders, 9*(3), 305–309. doi:10.1111/j.1399-5618.2007.00382.x.

Marciniak, B., Patro-Malysza, J., Poniedzialek-Czajkowska, E., Kimber-Trojnar, Z., Leszczynska-Gorzelak, B., & Oleszczuk, J. (2011). Glucocorticoids in pregnancy. *Current Pharmaceutical Biotechnology, 12*(5), 750–757.

McLean, M., Bisits, A., Davies, J., Woods, R., Lowry, P., & Smith, R. (1995). A placental clock controlling the length of human pregnancy. *Nature Medicine, 1*(5), 460–463.

Morse, S. B., Zheng, H., Tang, Y., & Roth, J. (2009). Early school-age outcomes of late preterm infants. *Pediatrics, 123*(4), e622–e629. doi:10.1542/peds.2008-1405.

Moster, D., Lie, R. T., & Markestad, T. (2008). Long-term medical and social consequences of preterm birth. *The New England Journal of Medicine, 359*(3), 262–273. doi:10.1056/NEJMoa0706475.

Msall, M. E. (2012). Academic achievement after extreme prematurity: Optimizing outcomes for vulnerable children in times of uncertainty. *Acta Paediatrica, 101*(12), 1196–1197. doi:10.1111/apa.12038.

Msall, M. E., Phelps, D. L., DiGaudio, K. M., Dobson, V., Tung, B., McClead, R. E., et al. (2000). Severity of neonatal retinopathy of prematurity is predictive of neurodevelopmental functional outcome at age 5.5 years. Behalf of the Cryotherapy for retinopathy of prematurity cooperative group. *Pediatrics, 106*(5), 998–1005.

Msall, M. E., Phelps, D. L., Hardy, R. J., Dobson, V., Quinn, G. E., Summers, C. G., et al. (2004). Educational and social competencies at 8 years in children with threshold retinopathy of prematurity in the CRYO-ROP multicenter study. *Pediatrics, 113*(4), 790–799.

O'Connor, T. G., Monk, C., & Fitelson, E. M. (2014). Practitioner review: Maternal mood in pregnancy and child development--implications for child psychology and psychiatry. *Journal of Child Psychology and Psychiatry, 55*(2), 99–111. doi:10.1111/jcpp.12153.

van Oppenraaij, R. H., Jauniaux, E., Christiansen, O. B., Horcajadas, J. A., Farquharson, R. G., & Exalto, N. (2009). Predicting adverse obstetric outcome after early pregnancy events and complications: A review. *Human Reproduction Update, 15*(4), 409–421. doi:10.1093/humupd/dmp009.

Patrianakos-Hoobler, A. I., Msall, M. E., Marks, J. D., Huo, D., & Schreiber, M. D. (2009). Risk factors affecting school readiness in premature infants with respiratory distress syndrome. *Pediatrics, 124*(1), 258–267. doi:10.1542/peds.2008-1771.

Pinto-Martin, J. A., Levy, S. E., Feldman, J. F., Lorenz, J. M., Paneth, N., & Whitaker, A. H. (2011). Prevalence of autism spectrum disorder in adolescents born weighing <2000 grams. *Pediatrics, 128*(5), 883–891. doi:10.1542/peds.2010-2846.

Poehlmann, J., Hane, A., Burnson, C., Maleck, S., Hamburger, E., & Shah, P. E. (2012). Preterm infants who are prone to distress: Differential effects of parenting on 36-month behavioral and cognitive outcomes. *Journal of Child Psychology and Psychiatry, 53*(10), 1018–1025. doi:10.1111/j.1469-7610.2012.02564.x.

Preterm Birth: Causes, Consequences, and Prevention (2007). In R. E. Behrman, & A. S. Butler (Eds.). Washington, DC: Committee on Understanding Premature Birth and Assuring Healthy Outcomes, Institute of Medicine of the Academies.

Provencal, N., & Binder, E. B. (2015). The effects of early life stress on the epigenome: From the womb to adulthood and even before. *Experimental Neurology, 268*, 10–20. doi:10.1016/j.expneurol.2014.09.001.

Requejo, J., Merialdi, M., Althabe, F., Keller, M., Katz, J., & Menon, R. (2013). Born too soon: Care during pregnancy and childbirth to reduce preterm deliveries and improve health outcomes of the preterm baby. *Reproductive Health, 10*(Suppl 1), S4. doi:10.1186/1742-4755-10-s1-s4.

Rini, C. K., Dunkel-Schetter, C., Wadhwa, P. D., & Sandman, C. A. (1999). Psychological adaptation and birth outcomes: The role of personal resources, stress, and sociocultural context in pregnancy. *Health Psychology, 18*(4), 333–345.

Rosenberg, S. A., Zhang, D., & Robinson, C. C. (2008). Prevalence of developmental delays and participation in early intervention services for young children. *Pediatrics, 121*(6), e1503–e1509. doi:10.1542/peds.2007-1680.

Rubens, C. E., Sadovsky, Y., Muglia, L., Gravett, M. G., Lackritz, E., & Gravett, C. (2014). Prevention of preterm birth: Harnessing science to address the global epidemic. *Science Translational Medicine, 6*(262), 262sr265. doi:10.1126/scitranslmed.3009871.

Sable, M. R., & Wilkinson, D. S. (2000). Impact of perceived stress, major life events and pregnancy attitudes on low birth weight. *Family Planning Perspectives, 32*(6), 288–294.

Saigal, S., & Doyle, L. W. (2008). An overview of mortality and sequelae of preterm birth from infancy to adulthood. *Lancet, 371*(9608), 261–269. doi:10.1016/s0140-6736(08)60136-1.

Saigal, S., Pinelli, J., Hoult, L., Kim, M. M., & Boyle, M. (2003). Psychopathology and social competencies of adolescents who were extremely low birth weight. *Pediatrics, 111*(5 Pt 1), 969–975.

Shah, P. E., Robbins, N., Coelho, R. B., & Poehlmann, J. (2013). The paradox of prematurity: The behavioral vulnerability of late preterm infants and the cognitive susceptibility of very preterm infants at 36 months post-term. *Infant Behavior & Development, 36*(1), 50–62. doi:10.1016/j.infbeh.2012.11.003.

Simms, V., Gilmore, C., Cragg, L., Clayton, S., Marlow, N., & Johnson, S. (2015). Nature and origins of mathematics difficulties in very preterm children: A different etiology than developmental dyscalculia. *Pediatric Research, 77*(2), 389–395. doi:10.1038/pr.2014.184.

Smith, C. J., & Ryckman, K. K. (2015). Epigenetic and developmental influences on the risk of obesity, diabetes, and metabolic syndrome. *Diabetes Metab Syndr Obes, 8*, 295–302. doi:10.2147/dmso.s61296.

Stein, A., Pearson, R. M., Goodman, S. H., Rapa, E., Rahman, A., McCallum, M., et al. (2014). Effects of perinatal mental disorders on the fetus and child. *Lancet, 384*(9956), 1800–1819. doi:10.1016/s0140-6736(14)61277-0.

Stephens, B. E., & Vohr, B. R. (2009). Neurodevelopmental outcome of the premature infant. *Pediatric Clinics of North America, 56*(3), 631–646., Table of Contents. doi:10.1016/j.pcl.2009.03.005.

The March of Dimes data book for policy makers: Maternal, infant, and child health in the United States (2012). Washington, DC: March of Dimes.

Torche, F., & Kleinhaus, K. (2012). Prenatal stress, gestational age and secondary sex ratio: The sex-specific effects of exposure to a natural disaster in early pregnancy. *Human Reproduction, 27*(2), 558–567. doi:10.1093/humrep/der390.

Treyvaud, K., Ure, A., Doyle, L. W., Lee, K. J., Rogers, C. E., Kidokoro, H., et al. (2013). Psychiatric outcomes at age seven for very preterm children: Rates and predictors. *Journal of Child Psychology and Psychiatry, 54*(7), 772–779. doi:10.1111/jcpp.12040.

Vohr, B. (2013). Long-term outcomes of moderately preterm, late preterm, and early term infants. *Clinics in Perinatology, 40*(4), 739–751. doi:10.1016/j.clp.2013.07.006.

Vohr, B. R., & Msall, M. E. (1997). Neuropsychological and functional outcomes of very low birth weight infants. *Seminars in Perinatology, 21*(3), 202–220.

Wadhwa, P. D., Dunkel-Schetter, C., Chicz-DeMet, A., Porto, M., & Sandman, C. A. (1996). Prenatal psychosocial factors and the neuroendocrine axis in human pregnancy. *Psychosomatic Medicine, 58*(5), 432–446.

Wainstock, T., Anteby, E. Y., Glasser, S., Lerner-Geva, L., & Shoham-Vardi, I. (2014). Exposure to life-threatening stressful situations and the risk of preterm birth and low birth weight. *International Journal of Gynaecology and Obstetrics, 125*(1), 28–32. doi:10.1016/j.ijgo.2013.09.035.

Weiss, E. L., Msall, M.E., & Muhammad, C. (2007). Barriers to receipt of early intervention. *Passages*. doi:E-PAS2007:616311.10.

Weitzman, M., Byrd, R. S., Aligne, C. A., & Moss, M. (2002). The effects of tobacco exposure on children's behavioral and cognitive functioning: Implications for clinical and public health policy and future research. *Neurotoxicology and Teratology, 24*(3), 397–406.

Wijesiriwardana, A., Bhattacharya, S., Shetty, A., Smith, N., & Bhattacharya, S. (2006). Obstetric outcome in women with threatened miscarriage in the first trimester. *Obstetrics and Gynecology, 107*(3), 557–562. doi:10.1097/01.AOG.0000199952.82151.de.

Williams, M. A., Mittendorf, R., Lieberman, E., & Monson, R. R. (1991). Adverse infant outcomes associated with first-trimester vaginal bleeding. *Obstetrics and Gynecology, 78*(1), 14–18.

Williams, J., Lee, K. J., & Anderson, P. J. (2010). Prevalence of motor-skill impairment in preterm children who do not develop cerebral palsy: A systematic review. *Developmental Medicine and Child Neurology, 52*(3), 232–237. doi:10.1111/j.1469-8749.2009.03544.x.

Winchester, S. B., Sullivan, M. C., Roberts, M. B., & Granger, D. A. (2016). Prematurity, birth weight and socioeconomic status are linked to atypical diurnal hypothalamic-pituitary-adrenal Axis activity in young adults. *Research in Nursing & Health, 39*(1), 15–29.

Wolke, D., Strauss, V. Y., Johnson, S., Gilmore, C., Marlow, N., & Jaekel, J. (2015). Universal gestational age effects on cognitive and basic mathematic processing: 2 cohorts in 2 countries. *J Pediatr, 166*(6), 1410–1416. doi:10.1016/j.jpeds.2015.02.065.

World Health Organization. (2007). *ICF-CY, international classification of functioning, disability, and health: Children & Youth version*. Geneva: World Health Organization.

Yonkers, K. A., Smith, M. V., Forray, A., Epperson, C. N., Costello, D., Lin, H., et al. (2014). Pregnant women with posttraumatic stress disorder and risk of preterm birth. *JAMA Psychiatry, 71*(8), 897–904. doi:10.1001/jamapsychiatry.2014.558.

7

Early in the Life Course: Time for Obesity Prevention

Summer Sherburne Hawkins, Emily Oken, and Matthew W. Gillman

1 Introduction

Although the dramatic rise in obesity in the USA experienced in recent decades (Wang and Beydoun 2007) may have now stabilized (Ogden et al. 2014; Wen et al. 2012), the prevalence of obesity remains high. The most recent nationally representative data collected in 2012 showed that 17% of children ages 2–19 years were obese (Ogden et al. 2014). From 2003 through 2010, the prevalence of obesity in low-income children aged 2–4 years remained at approximately 15% (Pan et al. 2012), while one regional study suggested that from 2004 through 2008, obesity prevalence started to drop among 0 to 6-year-olds from non-low-income families (Wen et al. 2012). The reasons for this potential slowing or slight reversal of the trend among some subgroups in the USA remain unknown. However, obesity has not affected all segments of the population equally (Wang and Beydoun 2007; Wang et al. 2011), and racial/ethnic differences in obesity are already evident by the preschool years (Ogden et al. 2014).

The short- and long-term consequences of obesity include conditions involving nearly every organ system, such as asthma, type 2 diabetes, high blood pressure, cardiovascular disease, depression, and orthopedic problems, starting in childhood and escalating among adults (Han et al. 2010; Lobstein et al. 2004). Children who are obese are much more likely to be obese adults, and obesity at any age is very difficult to treat (Lobstein et al. 2004). Furthermore, the population-level effects of obesity are substantial. Nationwide, 9.1% of annual medical spending is attributable to adult obesity, representing a cost of $147 billion per year (Finkelstein et al. 2009). This combination of evidence on the epidemiology, health consequences, and public health impact of obesity suggests that prevention is essential.

2 Conceptual Framework

One of the reasons for the intractability of childhood obesity is the failure to take into account the complexity and interconnectedness of contributing factors ranging from the social, built and economic environments to behavior, physiology, and epigenetics. These factors may also interact with each other creating a self-perpetuating cycle

S.S. Hawkins (✉)
Boston College, Chestnut Hill, MA, USA
e-mail: summer.hawkins@bc.edu

E. Oken • M.W. Gillman
Harvard Medical School and Harvard Pilgrim Health Care Institute, Boston, MA, USA
e-mail: emily_oken@harvardpilgrim.org; matthew.gillman@nih.gov

of obesity, as we illustrate using gestational diabetes mellitus (Sect. 4.3; Gillman 2016). Based on the life course health development approach to chronic disease epidemiology, biological, behavioral, and psychosocial exposures that occur at particular stages in the life course may have differential and/or lasting effects on later outcomes (Ben-Shlomo and Kuh 2002; Halfon and Forrest 2017).

The effects of these exposures can be cumulative across an individual's life as well as operate across generations to influence future generation's risk for chronic disease. Factors can also interact with each other over the life course and be more or less important at particular stages. These periods of particular influence are often termed critical or sensitive (Ben-Shlomo and Kuh 2002). Throughout the chapter, we demonstrate that multiple critical and sensitive periods for obesity risk exist across the life course, although practically they may be hard to identify. Given the plasticity inherent in early human development, the pre- and perinatal periods may present the most important opportunity for critical or sensitive period effects. Added to the fact that treatment of obesity is impeded by cultural, behavioral, and physiological feedback loops, modifying environment, behaviors, and physiology early in life is likely an especially effective strategy for preventing obesity and its consequences.

Consistent with LCHD principles (see Halfon and Forrest 2017), Glass and McAtee (2006) propose that the multilevel approach shown in Fig. 1 places obesity prevention in a complex system with individual risk factors being influenced by multiple "above-water" levels (families, neighborhood, policies) as well as by the interaction with biology and "underwater" levels (genes, epigenetics, physiology) over time. This framework adds to a life course health development approach by emphasizing feedback loops and cross-level influences, such as gene-environment interactions, thus highlighting the need for methodology that takes into account these complex relationships to help identify the important and modifiable levers of change (Huang and Glass 2008).

We have organized this chapter to reflect the current thinking on periods in the life course that appear to be most important for the development of obesity. We focus primarily on the early portion of the life course, but also discuss later periods that may be key time points for intervening. These periods often represent times of active growth or turning points when the primary sources of influence change.

At each stage of the life course, we discuss specific macro-level factors if they are directly relevant to that time period. Most macro-level factors, however, either indirectly or directly influence all age groups, so we present them together after reviewing each life course stage individually. While this chapter does not represent a systematic review of the literature, we present key examples at each stage of the life course to illustrate important risk factors, mechanisms, and gaps in research. We conclude with recommendations for future work on methodology, research in emerging areas, and implications for practice and policy.

3 Measurement of Overweight and Obesity

Body mass index (BMI; weight/height^2) is the most commonly used indirect measure of adiposity, or fatness, at the population level. The US Centers for Disease Control and Prevention (CDC) recommends monitoring growth in children aged 0–2 years using the World Health Organization weight for recumbent length growth standards and defines excess weight as at or above the 97.7th percentile (Grummer-Strawn et al. 2010). The CDC defines obesity in children aged 2–19 years as a BMI at or above the 95th percentile for age and sex, with overweight between the 85th and 95th percentiles, using the CDC sex-specific BMI-for-age growth charts from 2000 (Kuczmarski et al. 2002; Ogden and Flegal 2010).

4 Prenatal Period

4.1 Birth Weight

Numerous studies have confirmed the associations of higher birth weight with risk of later obesity and type 2 diabetes mellitus; lower birth

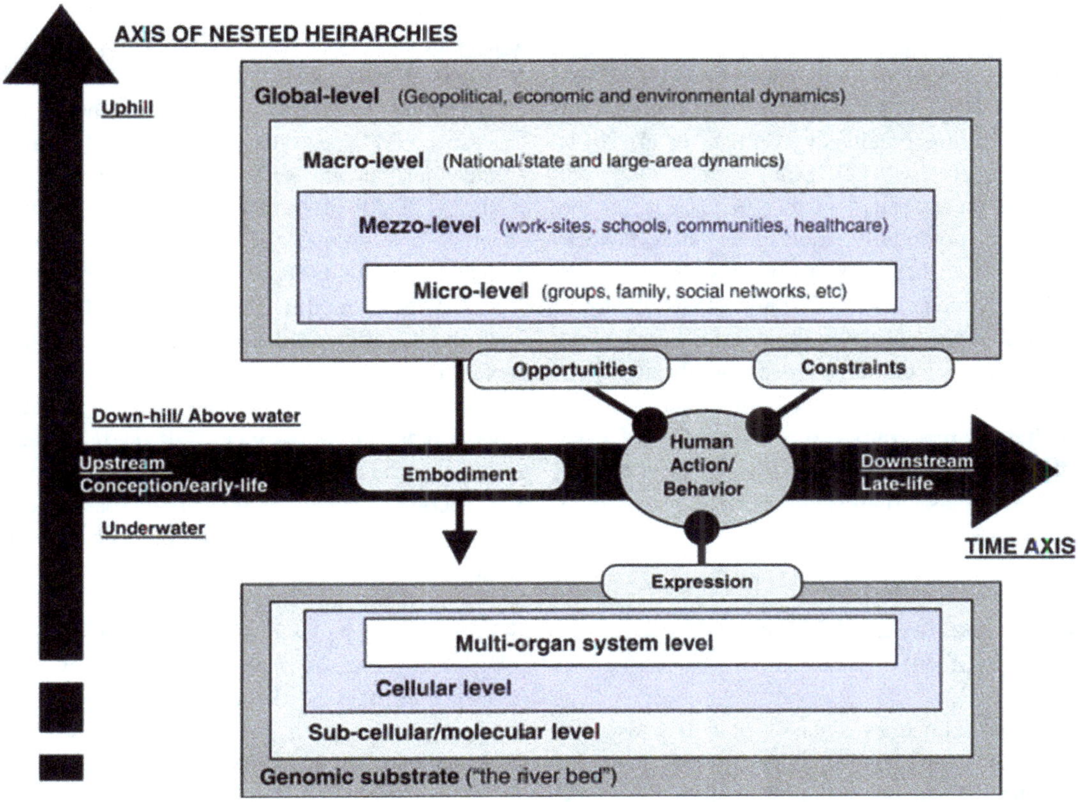

Fig. 1 Conceptual framework for etiology of childhood obesity (Reproduced from Glass and McAtee (2006))

weight is consistently associated with increased risk for central adiposity and its metabolic correlates, including type 2 diabetes mellitus and cardiovascular disease (Parsons et al. 1999; Yu et al. 2011). Birth weight, however, is not an etiologic factor in itself. Some have used birth weight as a marker of in utero programming during sensitive periods of development (Gillman 2005). However, many factors could explain the relationship between birth weight and later obesity. For example, maternal obesity, a risk factor for higher birth weight, is also highly related to childhood obesity (Perng et al. 2014). This association may be due to genomic inheritance and shared postnatal environment of eating habits and physical activity or inactivity in addition to in utero effects (Gillman and Poston 2012). However, even after controlling for maternal obesity, sociodemographic characteristics, and other risk factors, the birth weight-obesity association remains, raising the possibility of a lasting effect of fetal programming on later health (Gillman 2004; Oken and Gillman 2003).

4.2 Maternal Prepregnancy Obesity

Many women start their pregnancy already overweight or obese. In 2009, a representative survey from 20 states found that 21% of women were obese prepregnancy and an additional 25% were overweight (Fisher et al. 2013). Mothers who are overweight or obese prepregnancy are more likely to have infants with higher birth weight and an increased risk for being large-for-gestational age (LGA; >90th percentile of weight-for-gestational age) or macrosomic (birth weight > 4000 g) (Institute of Medicine 2009).

Women who are overweight or obese going into pregnancy are at higher risk for developing gestational diabetes mellitus (Torloni et al. 2009) and more likely to gain excessive amounts of weight during pregnancy (Battista et al. 2011; Dalenius et al. 2012). Studies must take into account these related factors to tease apart the roles of potentially modifiable risk factors. Furthermore, these risk factors may also be markers for shared genes and/or the postnatal environment (including lifestyle behaviors), which could also influence children's risk for obesity. This issue of interrelated factors—which may serve as mediators, moderators, or confounders of each other—is applicable not just to the prenatal period, but also to all stages of life course health development.

4.3 Gestational Diabetes Mellitus (GDM)

GDM is defined as diabetes first diagnosed in pregnancy, typically between 24 and 28 weeks gestation. Data on 59 million births from the National Hospital Discharge Survey showed that GDM increased from 1.9% to 4.2% from 1989 through 2004 (Getahun et al. 2008). Over this time period, the relative increase in GDM was 94% for white women (from 2.2% to 4.2%), but 260% for black women (from 0.6% to 2.1%) (Getahun et al. 2008).

GDM may be fueling the obesity epidemic (Battista et al. 2011; Herring and Oken 2011). Figure 2 shows the interrelationships of maternal, fetal, and child factors across the life course that may propagate the intergenerational transmission of obesity and diabetes (Gillman 2016). Both maternal prepregnancy obesity and excessive gestational weight gain (GWG) independently increase mothers' risk for developing GDM. A systematic review found that higher maternal prepregnancy BMI was associated with an increase in risk for GDM, such that overweight, moderately obese, and morbidly obese women were 2, 3, and 5.5 times more likely to develop GDM compared to women with normal BMI (Torloni et al. 2009). Excess GWG during pregnancy may also increase mothers' risk for GDM, independent of women's prepregnancy weight (Hedderson et al. 2010). Compared to women with adequate levels of weight gain, women with excessive GWG are also more likely to have greater postpartum weight retention (Nehring et al. 2011). All of these factors increase women's risk for subsequent health problems. Women with a history of GDM are more likely to develop type 2 diabetes mellitus, particularly within the first decade after delivery (Kim et al. 2002). Developing GDM in one pregnancy increases mothers' risk for the recurrence of GDM in subsequent pregnancies (Kim et al. 2007). If women do not lose the excess weight they gained before they become pregnant again, this increased adiposity reinforces the cycle in the subsequent pregnancy.

Prepregnancy obesity, excessive GWG, and GDM are associated with higher fetal growth and subsequent increases in children's adiposity and risk for obesity (Fig. 2) (Gillman 2016). Infants born to mothers with prepregnancy obesity or GDM are more likely to be of higher birth weight or be macrosomic (Battista et al. 2011; Institute of Medicine 2009), and trials of GDM treatment show reductions in macrosomia (Crowther et al. 2005; Gillman et al. 2010; Landon et al. 2009). A study found that children born to mothers with GDM had higher levels of adiposity and insulin secretion at age 5–10 years, independent of current BMI (Chandler-Laney et al. 2012). Boney et al. (2005) found that children who were LGA at birth and exposed to either GDM or maternal obesity in utero were at an increased risk for developing metabolic syndrome. The cycle continues when girls who are obese mature and have children of their own.

Plausible developmental mechanisms exist for the influence of GDM on childhood obesity. Pancreatic β-cells normally increase their insulin secretion to compensate for the insulin resistance during pregnancy. Glucose intolerance results when the β-cells are not able to respond to this increasing demand (Battista et al. 2011). Since glucose crosses the placenta but insulin does not, the fetus is exposed to greater levels of glucose (Freinkel 1980). The developing fetal pancreas

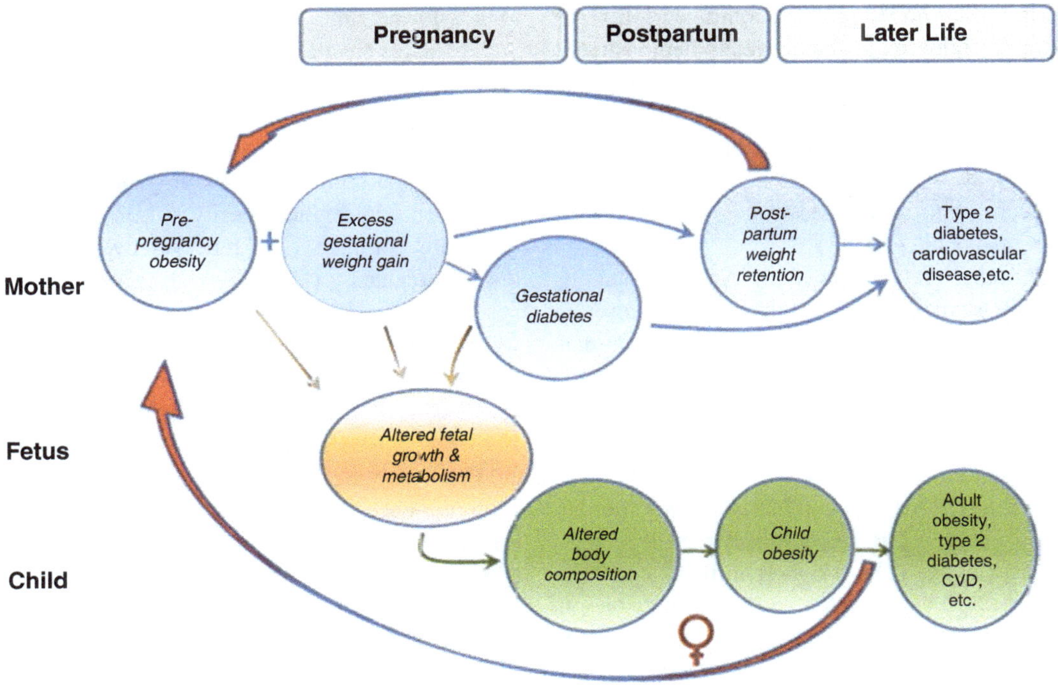

Fig. 2 Intergenerational transmission of obesity and gestational diabetes mellitus (Reproduced from Gillman (2016))

responds to the additional glucose by producing insulin, which can increase fetal adiposity (Freinkel 1980). Current research on the mechanisms of GDM is focusing on the areas of genetics, glucose, amino acid, lipid transport, and adipokines (Harlev and Wiznitzer 2010).

Methodological challenges abound in studying the association between GDM and later obesity. Kim et al. (2011) have argued that many studies combine pregestational diabetes mellitus and GDM into one category, examine only exposed or high-risk infants without an appropriate control group, and fail to control for potential confounding factors, most notably BMI. Their systematic review identified 12 studies of children exposed prenatally to GDM (excluding pregestational diabetes), with resulting crude odds ratios of 0.7–6.3 for offspring obesity. However, in many studies, it is not possible to distinguish women with GDM with true onset during pregnancy from undiagnosed pregestational diabetes (Herring and Oken 2011; Kim et al. 2011). In the two studies that adjusted for maternal prepregnancy BMI, results attenuated and were no longer significant after the covariate was included (Kim et al. 2011), which suggests that GDM may be a marker for preexisting maternal factors.

Randomized controlled trials (RCTs) of risk factor manipulation in pregnancy with childhood follow-up are especially valuable because they minimize the effect of confounding and thus are the most direct assessment of in utero programming in humans. In a US-based RCT of the treatment for mild GDM on pregnancy-related outcomes, Landon et al. (2009) found reduction in LGA and macrosomia; however, no childhood follow-up has been done. Gillman et al. (2010) followed up a subset of children who participated in an Australian-based multicenter RCT of treatment for mild GDM. Although the parent trial showed halving of macrosomia at birth, there were no differences in child BMI at age 4–5 years. One possible explanation for the null result is that offspring of mothers with GDM appear to lose their excess fat in the first year of life and do not again begin to diverge from their unexposed peers until school age; thus, continued follow-up of these children may be needed to demonstrate a longer-lasting effect of prenatal GDM treatment. Furthermore, as this study included women with mild GDM only, a more dramatic benefit of treatment may be experienced among offspring of women with more extreme hyperglycemia (Gillman et al. 2010).

Another method for minimizing confounding is sibling-pair designs, which partially control for differences in the pre- and postnatal environment (Brion 2010). This method relies on discrepant in utero exposure between siblings, such that the mother experienced GDM during her pregnancy with one sibling but not the other. Lawlor and colleagues (2011b) conducted a sibling-pair study of over 280,000 Swedish men through a record linkage study of their military conscription medical examination with birth information. They found that BMI at age 18 was higher in men whose mothers had GDM during pregnancy than those who did not; these differences were still evident in the within-sibling analyses and independent of maternal BMI. The authors concluded that GDM may influence later obesity risk through intrauterine mechanisms (Lawlor et al. 2011b).

4.4 Gestational Weight Gain (GWG)

In 1990, the Institute of Medicine (IOM) (1990) issued guidelines for the appropriate amount of weight women should gain during pregnancy. However, over the last two decades, excessive GWG has been common and increasing. In 2010, based on the Pregnancy Nutrition Surveillance System (PNSS) from 29 states and the District of Columbia, approximately 48% of low-income women gained more weight than recommended (Dalenius et al. 2012). Excessive weight gain is associated with adverse infant outcomes, including macrosomia and LGA infants, as well as postpartum weight retention in mothers (Siega-Riz et al. 2009). In 2009, the IOM published new guidelines, which for the first time include a weight gain range for obese women that recommends lower gains than for women with lower weight status (Institute of Medicine 2009).

GWG may also have a lasting effect on body size across the life course through in utero conditioning. Although some evidence suggests that extreme undernutrition during pregnancy may be associated with higher obesity risk in offspring, the more common occurrence is overnutrition during pregnancy (Herring et al. 2012). Recent systematic reviews found that excessive GWG was associated with an increased risk for offspring obesity compared to adequate GWG (Lau et al. 2014; Mamun Mamun et al. 2014; Nehring et al. 2013), with an overall pooled odds ratio of 1.4 (Mamun et al. 2014; Nehring et al. 2013). For example, Perng et al. (2014) found that every 5 kilograms of GWG was associated with greater adiposity (measured total fat and trunk fat) and higher leptin in children at ages 6–10 years, independent of maternal prepregnancy BMI.

GWG may influence childhood obesity through several potential developmental pathways. Mothers who are more prone to gain weight through genetic risk, poor diet, or other behavioral factors may have children who are also themselves exposed to these same risks. However, associations still remain after adjustment for maternal and paternal BMI, reducing some influence of shared genes and the postnatal environment. An alternative explanation may be through fetal conditioning (Gillman 2005), similar to that proposed for GDM. In animal models, overnutrition during pregnancy has resulted in insulin resistance, increased adiposity, and hypertension in offspring (Alfaradhi and Ozanne 2011).

One methodology to test causality is through an intervention aimed at influencing maternal weight gain during pregnancy through positive lifestyle changes. Three recent meta-analyses summarized the evidence on RCTs for prenatal dietary, physical activity, and behavioral or lifestyle interventions on maternal weight gain and infant outcomes (Agha et al. 2014; Oteng-Ntim et al. 2012; Thangaratinam et al. 2012). The reviews found that dietary and lifestyle interventions resulted in a small reduction in GWG (1.42–2.21 kg), but together the interventions did not appear to influence birth weight or LGA (Agha et al. 2014; Oteng-Ntim et al. 2012; Thangaratinam et al. 2012). However, none of the trials to date have looked at longer-term outcomes of child adiposity. Several ongoing RCTs targeted at changing GWG will follow offspring for development of obesity and its consequences (Dodd et al. 2011; Moholdt et al. 2011; Vesco et al. 2012). Vesco et al. (2014) found that obese women randomized to a dietary intervention gained less weight during pregnancy and had a lower proportion of babies born LGA, with further follow-up planned.

Two separate sibling-pair analyses have examined GWG and offspring obesity. Lawlor and colleagues (2011a) examined the association of maternal weight gain during pregnancy with obesity in men at age 18 years. They found that among mothers with a normal BMI, there was no relationship between GWG and later obesity. However, among mothers who were already overweight or obese, GWG was associated with an increased risk for later obesity, even in the within-sibling analyses, suggesting an influence of the intrauterine environment (Lawlor et al. 2011a). Although Branum et al. (2011) found that women with higher prepregnancy BMI and gestational weight gain had children with a higher BMI at age 4, differences were no longer significant in the sibling fixed-effects analysis. The interaction between maternal prepregnancy BMI and GWG on childhood obesity risk is an area of active investigation (Institute of Medicine 2009).

4.5 Maternal Smoking During Pregnancy

In 2010, approximately 9% of US women smoked during pregnancy, with white mothers and mothers with lower education more likely to smoke during pregnancy (Hawkins and Baum 2014). Many short- and long-term health effects of smoking during pregnancy on mothers and infants are well known, including lower fetal growth (U.S. Department of Health and Human Services 2004). It may seem paradoxical then that numerous studies, as summarized in recent meta-analyses, have shown that prenatal smoking exposure is associated with an increased risk for later obesity, even in studies that adjusted for potential confounding factors (Oken et al. 2008; Weng et al. 2012). Although mechanisms for the relationship between maternal smoking during pregnancy and childhood obesity are not fully understood, animal studies have shown an association between prenatal nicotine exposure and increased adiposity in offspring (Gao et al. 2005).

However, the extent to which this association, seen mainly in observational studies, is causal remains uncertain, especially since smoking is so strongly socially patterned. Several approaches have been used to minimize confounding, including accounting for paternal smoking, a proxy for sociodemographic risk that is likely to provide little direct exposure to the fetus. One study with information on both maternal smoking during pregnancy and paternal smoking status postpartum found that the association remained after adjustment for sociodemographic characteristics and paternal smoking (von Kries et al. 2008), while in another study the association was no longer evident after adjustment (Fleten et al. 2012).

Others have used alternative study designs to test whether the association may be causal. Although RCTs have demonstrated that smoking cessation during pregnancy reduces rates of low birth weight and preterm birth (Lumley et al. 2009), none have examined later child obesity risk. Two studies have used sibling-pair designs to examine smoking during pregnancy (Gilman et al. 2008; Iliadou et al. 2010). Although both found a relationship between smoking and later obesity, the association was no longer evident after including the sibling fixed-effect. These results raise the possibility that the association may be confounded by unmeasured factors that are shared within families rather than being causal.

4.6 Hormonal Influences: Leptin

In 1973, Douglas L. Coleman published his seminal work in two papers, discussing an unknown circulating factor responsible for the obese/diabetic state in the *ob/ob* mouse, later called leptin (Grayson and Seeley 2012). Leptin is a hormone primarily produced by adipose tissue known to be responsible for the regulation of appetite, energy expenditure, and neuroendocrine function (Hauguel-de Mouzon et al. 2006). It is sometimes called the satiety hormone because of its effects on inducing a sense of fullness.

The developmental role of leptin in the perinatal period may differ from that later in the life course. The placenta releases leptin into maternal and fetal circulation, which may influence appetite and weight regulation. Maternal plasma leptin concentrations during gestation are two times higher than during non-gravid periods (Hauguel-de Mouzon et al. 2006). Fetuses born to obese mothers and mothers with GDM have higher cord leptin levels than fetuses of lean mothers or mothers without GDM, respectively (Catalano et al. 2009; Okereke et al. 2002). Umbilical cord leptin levels are positively associated with fetal fat mass, percent body fat, and birth weight (Okereke et al. 2002).

Sensitive period(s) may exist for the role of leptin in later obesity risk. A series of studies from Project Viva, a US pre-birth cohort, has examined relationships of leptin with early growth. Lower cord blood leptin levels were associated with smaller size at birth, but higher weight gain from birth to 6 months and higher BMI at age 3 years (Mantzoros et al. 2009; Parker et al. 2011). In a follow-up study, Boeke et al. (2013) found that lower leptin levels during pregnancy and in cord blood were associated with more adiposity at age 3 years; however, higher leptin levels at age 3 were associated with greater weight gain and higher adiposity through age 7. These findings were independent of maternal BMI and birth weight. The authors concluded there may be a sensitive period of leptin influence during the prenatal period followed by accumulation of leptin tolerance during early childhood, with different effects of leptin exposure by timing (Boeke et al. 2013). These observations are consistent with animal studies showing conditioning impact of heightened leptin sensitivity on later obesity, with differences evident across the life course (Bouret et al. 2004). There is great interest in identifying the correct sensitive period(s) for leptin to influence fetal development and reduce later obesity risk. To date, however, little is known about modifiable factors influencing fetal leptin regulation in humans (Boeke et al. 2013).

5 Infancy

5.1 Rapid Weight Gain

Infants grow in both length and weight, and weight changes include growth in both fat-free mass and fat mass. Many studies have used change in weight as a proxy for gain in adiposity, which may or may not be a valid assumption. There are many different definitions of rapid growth, which are often based on country- or population-specific references (Monteiro and Victora 2005).

Several meta-analyses have demonstrated that infants who gain weight more quickly than average during the first 2 years of life are at higher risk for later obesity (Baird et al. 2005; Monteiro and Victora 2005; Weng et al. 2012). Taveras and colleagues (2011c) examined the number of major weight-for-length percentiles crossed on the CDC 2000 growth chart during each of the 6-month periods from birth to 2 years with outcomes of obesity at ages 5 and 10 years. They found that crossing upward 2 or more percentiles in the first 2 years was associated with an increased risk for obesity at both ages. The highest prevalence of later obesity was seen in children with the crossing upward of 2 or more weight-for-length percentiles within the first 6 months of life (Taveras et al. 2011c).

Debate continues as to the exact time frame that rapid weight gain matters the most for later obesity risk. A major limitation of current research is the lack of repeated measurements at small intervals during infancy. Studies with repeat detailed measurements often include small, homogeneous samples of children, and thus their generalizability is limited. An important area of future research is to more precisely define the critical window for rapid gain in adiposity (or length) as well as modifiable determinants of rapid weight gain.

Although based on the research we summarize here a potential conclusion might be to limit rapid weight gain in infants to prevent later obesity, an important consideration is the potential detrimental effects of restricting weight gain for other organ systems. For infants born preterm, more rapid postnatal weight gain has an important benefit for neurodevelopment and attained size (Ehrenkranz et al. 2006) Although no association was seen between slower infant weight gain and poorer neurodevelopmental outcomes in a study of healthy, term infants (Belfort et al. 2008), this area requires more study to help determine optimal length and BMI patterns to promote healthy neurodevelopment as well as reduce childhood obesity.

One important modifiable determinant of the rate of infant weight gain is infant feeding, both the type and the approach. Although exclusively breastfed infants gain weight more rapidly in the early postnatal period, infants who are formula fed or fed a combination of breast milk and formula gain BMI more rapidly during the latter half of the first year of life (Kramer et al. 2004). In an Australian RCT promoting positive feeding practices, Mihrshahi et al. (2011) found that formula feeding and feeding on a schedule were independently associated with rapid weight gain between birth and age 4–7 months. Although the association between breastfeeding and childhood obesity is discussed in the next section, infant gain in length or adiposity and nutrition are closely linked and, in fact, may be challenging to tease apart.

5.2 Breastfeeding

Despite the numerous demonstrated health benefits of breastfeeding (Section on Breastfeeding 2012), according to the CDC's 2014 Breastfeeding Report Card, only 79% of US mothers initiated breastfeeding and only 49% breastfed for at least 6 months (Centers for Disease Control and Prevention 2014). Moreover, racial/ethnic disparities in breastfeeding are substantial. Using national data from 2004 to 2008, there was a 20% point differential between black and white mothers for both breastfeeding initiation (54% versus 74%) and breastfeeding for at least 6 months (27% versus 43%) (Centers for Disease Control and Prevention 2010).

Systematic reviews and meta-analyses of observational studies have demonstrated an inverse association of breastfeeding initiation or duration with later obesity (Arenz et al. 2004; Harder et al. 2005; Owen et al. 2005b). Two reviews found that an inverse relationship still remained after adjusting for confounding factors, such as parental obesity or social class (Arenz et al. 2004; Owen et al. 2005b). However, a third showed attenuation of the association with BMI to null after such adjustment (Owen et al. 2005a). There was also evidence for a dose-response relationship, such that a longer duration of breastfeeding conferred a greater reduction in obesity risk (Harder et al. 2005; Owen et al. 2005b). As the majority of study samples were often homogeneous with children of mostly white European descent, there is debate about the extent to which these relationships apply to all racial/ethnic groups (Gillman 2011; Harder et al. 2005).

Plausible mechanisms abound for the relationship between breastfeeding and childhood obesity (Bartok and Ventura 2009). Breastfed infants may be better at self-regulation than bottle-fed infants because they come off the breast when they are full, which may help them learn to regulate energy intake (Li et al. 2010). Breast milk contains hormones, such as leptin, involved in regulating growth and development during infancy (Savino and Liguori 2008). After the first 3 months of life, breastfed infants have slower weight gain for the remainder of the year than formula-fed infants (Savino and Liguori 2008).

Nevertheless, evidence is mounting to question the extent to which this relationship is causal (Gillman 2011). The majority of research has been based on observational studies, and associations may still be due to unmeasured factors. The few studies using a sibling-pair design showed that breastfeeding duration reduced risk for later obesity, but because mothers often breastfeed similarly across siblings, there are a limited number of discordant pairs to detect effects (Gillman et al. 2006; Metzger and McDade 2010; Nelson et al.

2005; O'Tierney et al. 2009). Furthermore, these designs may not eliminate the role of infant growth and behavior as a predictor—rather than result—of breastfeeding intensity and duration.

Another methodological design to infer causality is to examine the association in a context with different social gradients for both the exposure and outcome measures (Brion 2010; Gillman 2011). Brion et al. (2011) compared the association between breastfeeding duration and BMI from two cohorts—in England where breastfeeding is associated with more advantaged social circumstances and in Brazil where there is little social patterning. There was an inverse association between breastfeeding duration and obesity risk for children in England, but no such association for children in Brazil, from which the authors concluded the effects are likely due to residual confounding (Brion et al. 2011). Similarly, a study in Hong Kong also found no association between breastfeeding and childhood obesity, where breastfeeding and obesity follow different social patterns (Kwok et al. 2010).

The Promotion of Breastfeeding Intervention Trial (PROBIT) in Belarus is a cluster-randomized trial of breastfeeding promotion (Kramer et al. 2001). Mothers who started breastfeeding were randomly assigned to an intervention group that provided additional breastfeeding support or a standard care control group. Although mothers in the breastfeeding promotion group showed increases in duration and exclusivity of breastfeeding, there was no evidence for a protective effect of breastfeeding on skinfold thickness or obesity in children at age 6.5 or 11 years (Kramer et al. 2007; Martin et al. 2013). Based on the existing evidence, breastfeeding may only confer modest protection against obesity rather than being a major determinant (Gillman 2011).

5.3 Disparities in Obesity Partially Explained by Early-Life Factors

Beyond breastfeeding, many other early-life obesogenic exposures may be socially patterned (Dixon et al. 2012). Several investigators have attempted to investigate whether observed racial/ethnic disparities in obesity rates (Ogden et al. 2014) are related to early-life factors. Taveras and colleagues (2010) have shown that compared to white children, black and Hispanic children were more likely to have risk factors for childhood obesity including excessive weight gain during infancy and early introduction of solid foods, while after 2 years, they were more likely to have a television in their bedrooms, shorter sleep duration, and higher intake of sugar-sweetened beverages and fast food (Taveras et al. 2010). In contrast, they were less likely to be exposed to factors associated with protection against obesity, including exclusive breastfeeding (Taveras et al. 2010). The same investigators more recently examined whether racial/ethnic differences in childhood obesity at age 7 were explained by these early risk factors (Taveras et al. 2013). Although black and Hispanic children had higher BMI z-scores than white children, there were no longer differences in BMI after adjustment for infancy- and childhood-related risk factors. The authors conclude that racial/ethnic disparities in obesity may be determined by modifiable factors in early life (Taveras et al. 2013).

6 Early to Mid-childhood

6.1 Family

Although family members have similar levels of adiposity, meaning that children are more likely to have a high BMI if their parents have a high BMI (Patel et al. 2011), the influence of parents on child adiposity almost certainly extends beyond shared genes. Parents (including caregivers) also share a similar family, neighborhood, and social environment. During the early years, parents are the primary influence on children's dietary and physical activity/inactivity choices. Parents not only physically provide children with food and opportunities for physical activity, but they also influence children's preferences through modeling or other experiences (Birch and Davison 2001; Van Der Horst et al. 2007). In the next two sections on early childhood to mid-childhood and adolescence, we focus on "above-water" macro-level factors where there is potential for population-level interventions and public health impact.

6.2 Diet, Physical Activity, and Inactivity

In the simplest terms, excessive weight gain occurs when there is more "energy in" than "energy out." The dietary and physical activity patterns of children and adolescents in the USA have changed substantially over the last few decades. Total energy intake and portion sizes from energy-dense, nutrient-poor foods have increased, and more meals are being eaten away from home (Duffey and Popkin 2013; Piernas and Popkin 2011). Among school-aged children, daily calories from sugar-sweetened beverages have increased from 130 to 212 kcal/day over the last 20 years (Lasater et al. 2011). Although children and adolescents are recommended to participate in 60 min or more of physical activity daily (U.S. Department of Health and Human Services 2008), many children are not achieving this goal. In 2013, nationwide, 15% of students did not engage in at least 60 min of physical activity on any of the prior 7 days (Kann et al. 2014). As children transition from childhood through adolescence, physical activity levels decrease (Kahn et al. 2008), and media exposure and sedentary behaviors increase (Kann et al. 2014; Rideout and Hamel 2006). In recent decades, screen time and media use have increased. Currently, 41% of students play video or computer games 3 or more hours per day, and an additional 33% watch television 3 or more hours per day (Kann et al. 2014). Even by age 1, children are using approximately 50 min of screen media daily, which increases to nearly 2 hours by age 4–6 years (Rideout and Hamel 2006).

As media use has increased, so has children's exposure to advertisements and food marketing. Food advertising has been linked to influencing children's food preferences, purchasing requests, and consumption patterns (McGinnis et al. 2006), suggesting a potential mechanism by which television and media use may increase children's risk for obesity. US guidelines for the responsible advertising to children are voluntary self-regulatory initiatives, and the Rudd Center for Food Policy and Obesity (2013) suggested that loopholes in industry pledges may provide for more public relations benefits than health benefits.

6.3 Food Insecurity

In 2013, 14% of US households with children were food insecure at least once during the year, meaning they were unable to provide adequate food for one or more household members due to insufficient means (Coleman-Jensen et al. 2014). Black and Hispanic households, low-income households, and single-parent households with children had rates of food insecurity higher than the national average (Coleman-Jensen et al. 2014). Since children from lower-income families are at higher risk for obesity, the challenge for many families is to dependably provide nutritious and high-quality food rather than obtaining enough food (Ludwig et al. 2012). The Supplemental Nutrition Assistance Program (SNAP) has no regulations on the quality of foods purchased (US Department of Agriculture, 2013b), and families may be spending their limited food budget on foods that are high in calories but with low nutrient quality such as sugar-sweetened beverages.

Three systematic reviews found that although food insecurity was associated with an increased risk for obesity in adults, particularly women, the evidence was mixed for children (Dinour et al. 2007; Eisenmann et al. 2011; Franklin et al. 2012). A challenge for studies is identifying whether the measure of food insecurity is at the family or child level as parents may protect children from being food insecure. Echoing the conclusion from a review by Eisenmann et al. (2011), even if the association is not causal, both food insecurity and obesity exist in low-income households. It is essential, therefore, to learn more about purchasing patterns, diet, and physical activity in these families to learn why food insecurity and obesity coexist and identify areas for intervention.

6.4 Child Care and School

Policies and programs in child care and school can influence children's dietary intake, physical activity patterns, and risk for obesity. Approximately 30% of children are in center-based programs by age 2 and 40% of children by age 3, spending nearly 30 hours in nonparental care each week (National Center for Education Statistics 2005). Thus, child care is a setting in which obesogenic behaviors can be allowed or prevented (Larson et al. 2011a). A review by Larson and colleagues (2011b) identified 18 obesity prevention interventions that take place in child care centers/preschools and 2 of the 5 interventions that used weight status as an outcome found evidence for reduced weight.

In 2007, Benjamin et al. (2008) reviewed state child care regulations for policies related to nutrition and physical activity that may contribute to childhood obesity. They found that 80% of states had regulations to ensure that water is freely available in child care centers, 33% regulated screen time, 18% had regulations for the provision of breast milk, 14% restricted sugar-sweetened beverages, and only three states required a specified number of minutes of physical activity. Four states had no policies related to obesogenic practices in child care. The proportion of states with these regulations for family child care homes—as opposed to centers—was either the same or less. As of 2013, up to one quarter of states did not comply with any of the five recommendations from the IOM to promote physical activity among infants in child care centers or family child care homes (Slining et al. 2014). Benjamin et al. (2009) showed that infants who attended home-based child care early in life had an increased weight for length at 1 year and BMI at 3 years, suggesting that more research is needed into the food and physical activity policies of family child care homes. Additional studies in Denmark (Neelon et al. 2015) and Finland (Lehto et al. 2015) have demonstrated an association between starting child care before age 1 and an increased risk for later obesity. In 2011, the White House Task Force on Childhood Obesity supported the development of new national standards for healthy eating, encouraging breastfeeding, promoting physical activity, and limiting screen time in early-care settings (American Academy of Pediatrics, American Public Health Association, and National Resource Center for Health and Safety in Child Care and Early Education 2012).

Since children spend most of their time in school and may eat two daily meals there, the school environment can play an important role in shaping health behaviors (Institute of Medicine 2007; Story et al. 2009). A systematic review and meta-analysis by Waters et al. (2011) identified 55 interventions for preventing obesity in children aged 0–18 years, with 5 of the 6 most promising strategies related to the school environment: school curricula that include healthy eating and physical activity, increases in opportunities for physical activity throughout the school week, improvements in the nutritional quality of the food served in schools, environments and cultural practices that support children eating healthier foods and being active throughout the day, and support for teachers and staff to implement health promotion strategies and activities. They also concluded that interventions did not increase disparities. There have been a number of reviews that examined the impact of school-based interventions overall or school food and physical activity, separately, on obesity risk (Gonzalez-Suarez et al. 2009; Katz et al. 2008; Kropski et al. 2008).

Food and beverages available in schools are either part of the federal school lunch and breakfast programs or are competitive foods sold outside the federal programs. Meals served in the National School Lunch Program and School Breakfast Program must adhere to federally defined nutrition standards in order for schools to be eligible for federal subsidies (Institute of Medicine 2007). In 2013, the US Department of Agriculture issued the new "Smart Snacks in Schools" nutrition standards for competitive foods and beverages, which limit calories, fat, sugar, and sodium (U.S. Department of Agriculture 2013a). A study by Masse et al. (2013) found that between 2003 and 2008, states significantly strengthened their school nutrition-related laws, particularly those related to the sale of competitive foods. Overall, laws for competitive food policies were stronger for elementary schools than for middle and high schools. As of 2008, 7 states had no school nutrition laws across the 16 categories they examined (Masse et al. 2013).

The National Association for Sport and Physical Education (NASPE) sets standards for physical education, including time allotment, curriculum, and staffing (National Association for Sport and Physical Education 2004). Perna et al. (2012) found that public schools in states with specific and stringent physical education laws reported more weekly time for physical education: specifically, elementary schools reported 40 more minutes and middle schools reported 60 more minutes than schools within states with no laws. There were no differences between high schools. However, overall, only 8.5% of schools fully met the NASPE guidelines for physical education time (Perna et al. 2012). Without federal legislation for physical education, policies vary widely by state and even by schools themselves.

7 Adolescence

7.1 Social Influences

Adolescence is a developmental period characterized by hormonal changes and a period of rapid growth both physically and psychologically (Viner et al. 2012). As children become more independent, their sphere of influence moves from parents to peers with increasing autonomy in making choices. Although influences of dietary and physical activity habits on obesity risk are similar to those described during the early- to mid-childhood periods, these habits are often influenced by peer norms. Strong peer relationships are an important developmental change during adolescence, and peer groups can influence health behaviors both positively and negatively (Viner et al. 2012).

Using social network theory and analysis, Christakis and colleagues (2007) found that weight gain in one person spread through social ties and influenced risk of obesity in a friend, sibling, or spouse among adults in the Framingham Study. Trogdon et al. (2008) used the National Longitudinal Study of Adolescent Health (Add Health) to examine the influence of peer effects on adolescents' own BMI by constructing a detailed definition of peer groups based on nominated friendship relationships. They found that mean peer BMI was associated with adolescent BMI, females were more sensitive to peer BMI and overweight status than males, and peer weight was more influential among adolescents with the highest BMI (Trogdon et al. 2008).

Ali et al. (2011) also used data from the Add Health study to understand potential mechanisms of peer effects on obesity-related health behaviors. They found evidence for the influence of peers on adolescents pursuing an active sport, regular exercise, and eating in fast-food restaurants, but no consistent relationships with television viewing, short sleep duration, or other dietary factors (Ali et al. 2011). Although additional research is needed to confirm these findings, the potential implications are that obesity prevention programs aimed at adolescents will need to consider the influence of peer groups.

8 Macro-level Factors

Although we have touched upon policies and social issues that have their strongest influence in particular age groups, this section presents macro-level factors that either indirectly or directly influence obesity risk across all stages in life course health development.

8.1 Environment

The term "obesogenic environment" often refers to features of the built and natural environments that limit healthful behaviors related to eating, sleeping, screen time, and physical activity. The definition used to study the built environment varies widely across studies (Dunton et al. 2009; Lovasi et al. 2009; Papas et al. 2007). The most common measures of access to food are distances to the nearest fast-food restaurants or grocery stores or density of food outlets within a defined area. The most common measures of access to physical activity resources are measured distance to facilities for physical activity such as parks, density of such facilities, walkability, or aspects of community design. Related measures included assessments of aesthetics or neighborhood safety. Papas et al. (2007) found that 17 of the 20 studies identified found a significant association between some aspect of the built environment and risk for obesity across the life course, with the majority of studies looking at features of the environment related to physical activity. Dunton et al. (2009) examined aspects of the built environment related to physical activity and childhood obesity. While they found few consistent findings in children, in adolescents obesity was associated with access to equipment and facilities, neighborhood type (urban/rural), and urban sprawl. Lovasi et al. (2009) examined how the built environment may be contributing to disparities in obesity and its risk factors. They focused on studies that included individuals who were poor or of low socioeconomic status, black, or Hispanic. The authors found that lack of access to supermarkets, exercise facilities or places to be active, and safety because of crime or traffic was all associated with BMI or related behaviors, and they concluded that prevention strategies should focus on these areas (Lovasi et al. 2009).

There are many methodological challenges to understanding the effects of the neighborhood environment on children because of the diversity of populations, measures, and outcomes across studies (Dunton et al. 2009; Lovasi et al. 2009; Papas et al. 2007). A further limitation is that nearly all of the studies have been cross-sectional, so the temporality of associations is not clear. Effects of the built environment on health vary across the life course because exposure to and interaction with the environment change by age. For example, distance to playgrounds matters more for children than adolescents, whereas walkability may have less impact on young children. While subjective measures of the built environment are often from parents or children themselves, more studies are using objective measures of the environment, such as geographic information system (GIS) mapping or even personal devices to determine time, place, and activity simultaneously. The most important aspect is the definition of the built environment. Studies that examine the same construct, such as walkability, may be using different definitions and measurements, which limit the ability to synthesize the evidence. As Dunton et al. (2009) conclude, it is imperative to identify "modifiable and specific" features of the built environment to inform the development of interventions.

Neighborhoods vary in many ways, most of which are unmeasured but likely interrelated; observed associations that remain after adjustment are still subject to residual confounding. RCTs, which balance both measured and unmeasured confounders, are uncommon in this area primarily due to the feasibility of manipulating aspects of the built environment. The Department of Housing and Urban Development conducted a unique social experiment from 1994 through 1998 to better understand the effects of neighborhood characteristics on health and social outcomes (Sanbonmatsu et al. 2011). Women with children living in public housing in high-poverty areas were randomly assigned to one of three groups: experimental housing vouchers redeemable only if they moved to a low-poverty area, unrestricted traditional vouchers, and a control group that offered neither opportunity (Ludwig et al. 2011). Ludwig et al. (2011) followed up the participants from 2008 to 2010 and found that women assigned to the experimental group had lower levels of extreme obesity and diabetes than women in the control group, although there were no baseline measures of these outcomes. However, among youth, there were no differences in physical health outcomes, including obesity (Sanbonmatsu et al. 2011). The authors concluded that although the mechanisms for these reductions were unknown, the intervention provides some causal evidence for the impact of the neighborhood environment on health (Ludwig et al. 2011).

A methodology for future research in this area is quasi-experimental designs that evaluate a clearly defined change—often a wide-ranging policy—that are referred to as natural experiments. Taking measurements of residents before and after this change, or using secondary measures such as data from electronic medical records, especially in comparison with an unexposed control group, can help assess the impact of neighborhood factors on obesity itself or related health behaviors. Such alternative study designs are needed to identify important levers of change to help inform the development of interventions conducted at the neighborhood or community levels.

8.2 Local and State

In recent years, city and state governments have taken bold actions to change the environment and encourage healthy choices. New York City (NYC) has been a pioneer in this effort by using a multiagency approach to tackle obesity and its risk factors (Mello 2009). In 2006, NYC passed the first regulation in the USA banning trans fat use in restaurants. An evaluation comparing food purchase data before and after the ban found a significant decrease in the trans fat content of purchases from fast-food chains after the law, with benefits for patrons from both high- and low-poverty neighborhoods (Angell et al. 2012). In 2008, NYC required chain restaurants to post calorie information prominently on menu boards and menus. Although children and adolescents' reported they noticed the posted information, there were no differences in calories purchased after versus before the introduction of calorie postings (Elbel et al. 2011). NYC initiatives have also extended to schools and the built environment (Office of the Mayor 2012). NYC established nutritional standards for every city agency that purchases or serves meals to clients, including the 1.1 million students that attend city schools, as well as standards for city vending machines. The most controversial proposal was to limit the size of sugar-sweetened beverages sold in food service establishments to 16 ounces, which caused much debate both for and against this measure and was ultimately blocked (Grynbaum 2012).

Although these policies in NYC provide assessable natural experiments to allow for evaluation of specific environmental factors that might promote weight gain (or loss), a challenge is learning what may be the critical lever(s) for change. When policies and programs are implemented simultaneously or within short time periods, it may not be possible to tease apart the individual effects of each policy. Furthermore, these efforts may not be generalizable; budgets are often limited, and other cities or states may not have the resources to implement the whole suite of policies that have been enacted in NYC. Nevertheless, these efforts provide valuable data to clinicians and policy makers to help elucidate what policies or programs will have the biggest effect on obesity levels.

A relatively new area is using legislation to financially penalize the purchase and consumption of obesogenic foods and beverages. One approach draws from the lessons of tobacco control and the success of cigarette taxes. Taxes on sugar-sweetened beverages are a prime example, although taxes have also been proposed to reduce the consumption of fast food (Powell et al. 2013). The consumption of sugar-sweetened beverages is strongly related to increased body weight (Te Morenga et al. 2012). As of January 2014, 34 states and DC had a sales tax on regular soda sold in food stores, with a mean tax rate of 5.2% (Chriqui et al. 2014). A systematic review by Powell et al. (2013) found that soda taxes had little impact on weight outcomes, but the authors argued that they were based on state-level sales taxes that were relatively low and therefore unlikely to effect substantial change in behavior.

Brownell et al. (2009) have proposed a national excise tax on sugar-sweetened beverages as a public health strategy to address the obesity epidemic. They recommended implementing an excise tax of 1 cent per ounce for beverages that have any added caloric sweetener, which would increase the cost of a 20-ounce soda by 15–20% (Brownell et al. 2009). This type of tax, which is similar to cigarette excise taxes, is preferable to a sales tax because it provides an incentive to reduce the amount of sugar per ounce of sugar-sweetened beverage (Brownell et al. 2009). Since the cost would be passed onto retailers, they would likely increase the retail price, and consumers would be aware of the cost when they are deciding to purchase the product. Andreyeva et al. (2011) estimated that a 1 cent per ounce tax on sugar-sweetened beverages could reduce consumption by 24% and daily per capita caloric intake from sugar-sweetened beverages from current levels of 190–200 calories to 145–150 calories. Brownell et al. (2009) suggest that the public health impact could be greater for groups at higher risk for obesity, such as children and low-income groups, who consume greater amounts of sugar-sweetened beverages.

An alternative approach to promoting a healthful diet is a subsidy to reduce price and encourage the consumption of healthful foods. Unfortunately, in recent decades, just the opposite situation has occurred. The real inflation-adjusted price of fruits and vegetables has increased, while soda prices have declined and fast-food prices have remained stable (Powell et al. 2013). In the USA, subsidies on food have been designed to alleviate food insecurity for low-income families rather than increasing consumption of healthful foods by everyone. Powell et al. (2013) found that lower fruit and vegetable prices were associated with lower body weight among low-income populations; however, cohort studies are mixed when it comes to the effects of fruits and vegetables on weight gain (Casazza et al. 2013). Based on the long history of tobacco control, the area of taxes and subsidies related to obesity is still in its infancy.

8.3 National

Reducing and preventing obesity is a federal priority. At a national level, the White House Task Force on Childhood Obesity and the accompanying *Let's Move!* campaign aim to reduce childhood obesity and raise a healthier generation through an intra-agency collaboration (White House Task Force on Childhood Obesity 2010). The 70 recommendations were summarized into five themes: getting children a healthy start on life; empowering parents and caregivers; providing healthy foods in schools; improving access to healthy, affordable food; and getting children more physically active. The strategy emphasized that changes are needed at many macro levels to promote healthy behaviors, including improvements to schools and the built environment. The White House Task Force reported some progress on many of these areas after just 1 year (White House Task Force on Childhood Obesity 2011). The IOM's Standing Committee on Childhood Obesity Prevention (Institute of Medicine 2011) and the US Department of Health and Human Services' National Prevention Strategy (National Prevention Council 2011) echo these priorities.

9 Recommendations

9.1 Major Themes

A multilevel approach for obesity prevention is needed, which takes into account individual risk factors that operate at multiple levels ("above-water" and "underwater" influences) and recognizes that these factors also interact across the life course (Fig. 1). We reviewed phases of life course health development, prenatal through adolescence, that appear to be most important for the development of obesity. We also presented alternative methodological approaches to observational studies that can help disentangle causal associations. The following sections outline research priorities and data/methods development priorities, and conclude with recommendations for practice and policy.

9.2 Research Priorities

Of the many emerging risk factors for obesity, we briefly highlight sleep duration, endocrine-disrupting chemicals, epigenetic markers, and microbial colonization.

- Sleep duration and quality: Disruption of sleep may have adverse health consequences, including childhood obesity. Biologically plausible mechanisms exist for why short sleep duration could increase children's risk for obesity: tiredness and fatigue lead to reduced physical activity; hormone changes associated with insufficient sleep, particularly lower leptin levels and higher ghrelin levels, result in increased hunger and eating; and with less sleep, there is more awake time to eat (Taheri 2006). Although most of the studies in this area have been cross-sectional, prospective cohort studies do provide some evidence for causality. Chen et al. (2008) identified 17 studies from 1980 to 2007 on sleep duration and adiposity in children, of which 3 were prospective cohort studies. Nielsen et al. (2011) reviewed the literature from 2007 to 2009 and identified an additional 13 studies in children. Of the eight prospective cohort studies, all found a significant inverse relationship between duration of sleep and adiposity (Nielsen et al. 2011). Recent studies from Project Viva have shown that chronic sleep curtailment from infancy was associated with an increase in adiposity and metabolic risk at age 7 (Cespedes et al. 2014; Taveras et al. 2014).

- Early relational environment: Two aspects of children's early relational environment—the quality of parental relationships and children's exposure to adverse experiences—have been identified as potential risk factors for child and adolescent obesity. The psychological and physiological consequences of insecure attachments and trauma are well established, including poor emotional regulation and heightened stress responses, which may directly lead to obesity through biological changes (Glaser and Kiecolt-Glaser 2005) or indirectly through emotional eating (Michopoulos et al. 2015; Torres and Nowson 2007) and sleep disturbances (Vgontzas et al. 2008). Studies in children and adolescents have found that those with poor-quality maternal-child relationships (Anderson et al. 2012) or insecure attachment (Anderson and Whitaker 2011) in early childhood were more likely to be obese compared to those with higher-quality relationships. Danese and Tan (2014) conducted a meta-analysis of 41 studies and found that childhood maltreatment was associated with an increased risk of obesity across the life course with an overall pooled odds ratio of 1.36 and associations remained after adjustment for socioeconomic status and health behaviors. An additional meta-analysis of 23 cohort studies found that adults who reported physical, emotional, sexual, or general abuse during childhood were more likely to be obese (pooled odds ratios of 1.28–1.45) and four studies reported dose-response relationships (Hemmingsson et al. 2014). While this evidence suggests a role of children's early relational environment in the development of obesity, further research is needed to better understand the mechanisms to help inform interventions.
- Endocrine-disrupting chemicals (EDCs): EDCs are compounds that mimic or interfere with the normal actions of endocrine hormones, including estrogens, androgens, and thyroid and pituitary hormones (Newbold et al. 2007). Although some EDCs are naturally occurring, man-made organic compounds pose greater risks to human health and include flame retardants, bisphenol A (BPA), pesticides, and polychlorinated biphenyls (PCBs). EDCs that are lipophilic, resistant to metabolism, and/or able to bioconcentrate up the food chain become stored in body fats and are of particular concern (Elobeid and Allison 2008). Thus, in utero exposure to environmental chemicals, including EDCs, during critical periods may play a role in the development of obesity through fetal programming (Newbold et al. 2007). Only recently has evidence been synthesized from animal models and epidemiologic studies in humans to suggest a possible link between EDCs and later obesity (Elobeid and Allison 2008). Trasande et al. (2012) found that urinary BPA concentrations were associated with obesity in children and adolescents, although alternative explanations cannot be ruled out because the study was cross-sectional.
- Epigenetics: The notion that early environmental influences, such as maternal diet, or toxic substances, like air pollution, alter offspring outcomes through epigenetic changes that influence gene regulation could unite several strands of human and animal observations about the origins of obesity. Proof of principle emanates from agouti mice (Waterland and Jirtle 2004). The epigenetic mechanism associated with dif-

ferences in body fat and cardiometabolic disease risk of the offspring involves switching off the agouti gene by methyl groups from a dietary supplement (Waterland and Jirtle 2004). These and similar findings show, in principle, how genetically identical individuals raised in similar postnatal environments can nonetheless develop widely differing phenotypes.

- Gut microbiota: Infants get their first priming dose of microbes in utero via the placenta, followed by a more thorough colonization as they pass through the birth canal and are exposed to the mother's skin, so that by the time they are a few days or weeks old, their gastrointestinal tracts are colonized by a population of microbes notable not only for their abundance but also variety. Gut microbiota are likely to affect many organs and systems, including the regulation of energy balance and weight gain. Although research on animal models suggests a role of gut microbiota in the development of obesity, studies in humans are limited (DiBaise et al. 2008). One model system for evaluating the role of gut microbiota is the route of delivery. Microbes from the mother and the environment colonize the infant's intestinal tract during delivery (Neu and Rushing 2011). During cesarean delivery, the direct contact with maternal vaginal and intestinal flora is absent. The intestinal microbial composition of infants via cesarean delivery resembles that of the mother's skin, whereas the intestinal flora of infants born vaginally resembles the mother's vaginal flora and intestinal tract (Dominguez-Bello et al. 2010). A systematic review by Li et al. (2013) found that delivery by cesarean section was associated with an increased risk for overweight/obesity across the life course compared to vaginal delivery, with an overall pooled odds ratio of 1.33.

9.3 Data/Methods Development Priorities

There are a number of major challenges to understanding causal influences on obesity risk throughout the life course. Here, we discuss some of these challenges as well as approaches to overcoming or minimizing them.

- One recurrent issue is the extent to which associations described in observational studies are causal. One notable example is breastfeeding (Gillman 2011). Mothers who choose to breastfeed often have substantially different social and economic circumstances from mothers who do not breastfeed their infants. Furthermore, factors that predict successful initiation and long-term maintenance of breastfeeding, such as maternal obesity and cesarean delivery, are themselves putative causes of child obesity. Also, it is possible that infant characteristics themselves predict breastfeeding duration, since mothers may be more likely to supplement faster growing infants, who appear hungrier.
- In cross-sectional studies, both confounding and reverse causation are important considerations. Longitudinal cohort studies with adjustment for multiple measured characteristics can go part of the way in minimizing confounding, but other approaches such as sibling-pair design, maternal versus paternal effects, cohorts with different confounding structures, and RCTs can help control for unmeasured confounding. Others have applied Mendelian randomization, a method that takes advantage of variation in genes of known function to examine the causal effect of a modifiable exposure on disease in nonexperimental studies (Smith and Ebrahim 2003). The genotype must affect the disease status only via its effect on the exposure of interest and should be randomly distributed with respect to other covariates (Ding and Hu 2008). This approach can produce unbiased estimates of the effects of a putative causal variable without a traditional RCT. One example is the study of the maternal and offspring FTO genotype and offspring obesity risk, which suggests that maternal obesity affects childhood obesity only through pathways other than the intrauterine environment (Lawlor et al. 2008). However, many times these approaches are not feasible. For example, data may not be readily available on

large numbers of siblings with discordant exposures; RCTs are costly and may not be ethical; and the few common genes that influence obesity risk do not have strong associations and also may influence multiple metabolic pathways.

- Another challenge is that of appropriate exposure assessment, which is relevant for multiple factors of great interest including diet, physical activity, and the toxic, built, and social environments. Multiple factors may interact among each other. For example, breastfeeding may particularly affect childhood obesity risk only in the presence of an obesogenic environment, whereas two important null studies of breastfeeding and obesity (Brion et al. 2011; Kramer et al. 2007; Martin et al. 2013) were both conducted in middle-income countries with relatively low population obesity rates (Belarus and Brazil).
- Current statistical techniques typically cannot take into account the multitude of factors both hierarchically and across the life course that impact obesity. Traditional longitudinal analyses, even those that account for multiple levels of influence, are often not powerful enough to account for the complexity and interconnectedness of obesity. Systems science approaches such as agent-based and system dynamics modeling can include not only longitudinal and multiple levels but also more complex features of relationships like nonlinearity, path dependence, loops, and tipping (Hammond 2009; Huang et al. 2009). These approaches have just recently been imported into public health from disciplines such as engineering (Mani et al. 2010) and evolutionary biology (Kitano 2002) and may very well contribute to understanding and ultimately solving childhood obesity.

9.4 Translational Priorities

The key to reducing childhood obesity is finding the right level and time in the life course to intervene for the maximal effectiveness and efficiency. Many intervention studies early in the life course are getting underway or are ongoing, and will be invaluable in informing not only what factors to change but how to change them. Such interventions may be complex and costly, but ultimately may be what is required to reverse the tide of obesity.

- Interventions to modify determinants of obesity through life course health development may invoke multiple settings, e.g., medical care, homes, child care, and school (Foster et al. 2010; Taveras et al. 2011a, b, 2012); involve multiple components, e.g., system redesign and individual behavior change strategies including e-technology (Lubans et al. 2010; Taveras et al. 2012); and target single or multiple factors (Dodd et al. 2011; Taveras et al. 2011b; Vesco et al. 2012). Interventions within medical care may be especially valuable during pregnancy and infancy, when individuals see their providers more often than any other time during the life course.
- Some recommendations are already clear. For prenatal factors, smoking avoidance has been a priority for decades (U.S. Department of Health and Human Services 2004). Guidelines exist for appropriate GWG (Institute of Medicine 2009). For mild-moderate GDM, treatment with lifestyle and insulin reduces neonatal complications (Crowther et al. 2005; Landon et al. 2009); the protocol and criteria for diagnosing GDM are undergoing new scrutiny.
- Among early childhood factors, "feeding up" small-for-gestational age infants should be abandoned for most because such infants who gain weight rapidly in infancy are at higher risk of chronic disease and derive no neuro-cognitive benefits (Belfort and Gillman 2011). The World Health Organization recommends exclusive breastfeeding for 6 months, but in the developed world, recommendations are moving toward 4–6 months (Section on Breastfeeding 2012); that interval appears to be appropriate for introducing solid foods for obesity prevention (Huh et al. 2011; Pearce et al. 2013).
- Among dietary factors, evidence is strongest for intake of sugary beverages at many ages. Avoiding introducing these into infant diets may be especially valuable, given most

humans'—especially children's—inherent "sweet tooth" (Ventura and Mennella 2011).

- The American Academy of Pediatrics recommends zero screen time under age 2 years and no more than 2 hours/day of screen time for child age 2 years and older (Strasburger 2011). Avoiding from the outset having a TV in the room where a child sleeps appears to be key to reducing screen time (Schmidt et al. 2012).
- Among the newer risk factors, improving sleep duration and quality may be an especially effective maneuver—and preliminary studies suggest it is feasible (Taveras et al. 2011a)—because all parents want more sleep!

Funding Funded by grants from NIH R00 HD068506 to Dr. Hawkins, K24 HD069408 and P30 DK092924 to Dr. Oken, and K24 HL060841 to Dr. Gillman. The content is solely the responsibility of the authors and does not necessarily represent the official views of the National Institutes of Health.

References

Agha, M., Agha, R. A., & Sandell, J. (2014). Interventions to reduce and prevent obesity in pre-conceptual and pregnant women: A systematic review and meta-analysis. *PloS One, 9*(5), e95132.

Alfaradhi, M. Z., & Ozanne, S. E. (2011). Developmental programming in response to maternal overnutrition. *Frontiers in Genetics, 2*, 27.

Ali, M. M., Amialchuk, A., & Heiland, F. W. (2011). Weight-related behavior among adolescents: The role of peer effects. *PloS One, 6*(6), e21179.

American Academy of Pediatrics, American Public Health Association, and National Resource Center for Health and Safety in Child Care and Early Education. (2012). *Preventing childhood obesity in early care and education: Selected standards from caring for our children; National health and safety performance standards; Guidelines for early care and education programs, 3rd edition.* http://nrckids.org/CFOC3/PDFVersion/preventing_obesity.pdf. Accessed 8 Feb 2013.

Anderson, S. E., Gooze, R. A., Lemeshow, S., & Whitaker, R. C. (2012). Quality of early maternal–child relationship and risk of adolescent obesity. *Pediatrics, 129*(1), 132–140.

Anderson, S. E., & Whitaker, R. C. (2011). Attachment security and obesity in US preschool-aged children. *Archives of Pediatrics & Adolescent Medicine, 165*(3), 235–242.

Andreyeva, T., Chaloupka, F. J., & Brownell, K. D. (2011). Estimating the potential of taxes on sugar-sweetened beverages to reduce consumption and generate revenue. *Preventive Medicine, 52*(6), 413–416.

Angell, S. Y., Cobb, L. K., Curtis, C. J., Konty, K. J., & Silver, L. D. (2012). Change in trans fatty acid content of fast-food purchases associated with New York City's restaurant regulation: A pre-post study. *Annals of Internal Medicine, 157*(2), 81–86.

Arenz, S., Ruckerl, R., Koletzko, B., & von Kries, R. (2004). Breast-feeding and childhood obesity–a systematic review. *International Journal of Obesity and Related Metabolic Disorders, 28*(10), 1247–1256.

Baird, J., Fisher, D., Lucas, P., Kleijnen, J., Roberts, H., & Law, C. (2005). Being big or growing fast: Systematic review of size and growth in infancy and later obesity. *BMJ, 331*(7522), 929.

Bartok, C. J., & Ventura, A. K. (2009). Mechanisms underlying the association between breastfeeding and obesity. *International Journal of Pediatric Obesity, 4*(4), 196–204.

Battista, M. C., Hivert, M. F., Duval, K., & Baillargeon, J. P. (2011). Intergenerational cycle of obesity and diabetes: How can we reduce the burdens of these conditions on the health of future generations? *Experimental Diabetes Research, 2011*, 596060.

Belfort, M. B., & Gillman, M. W. (2011). Healthy infant growth: What are the trade-offs in the developed world? In M. W. Gillman, P. D. Gluckman, & R. G. Rosenfeld (eds): *Recent Advances in Growth Research: Nutritional, Molecular and Endocrine Perspectives*. Nestlé Nutr Inst Workshop Ser, vol 71, pp 171–184

Belfort, M. B., Rifas-Shiman, S. L., Rich-Edwards, J. W., Kleinman, K. P., Oken, E., & Gillman, M. W. (2008). Infant growth and child cognition at 3 years of age. *Pediatrics, 122*(3), e689–e695.

Ben-Shlomo, Y., & Kuh, D. (2002). A life course approach to chronic disease epidemiology: Conceptual models, empirical challenges and interdisciplinary perspectives. *International Journal of Epidemiology, 31*(2), 285–293.

Benjamin, S. E., Cradock, A., Walker, E. M., Slining, M., & Gillman, M. W. (2008). Obesity prevention in child care: A review of U.S. state regulations. *BMC Public Health, 8*, 188.

Benjamin, S. E., Rifas-Shiman, S. L., Taveras, E. M., Haines, J., Finkelstein, J., Kleinman, K., & Gillman, M. W. (2009). Early child care and adiposity at ages 1 and 3 years. *Pediatrics, 124*(2), 555–562.

Birch, L. L., & Davison, K. K. (2001). Family environmental factors influencing the developing behavioral controls of food intake and childhood overweight. *Pediatric Clinics of North America, 48*(4), 893–907.

Boeke, C. E., Mantzoros, C. S., Hughes, M. D., L Rifas-Shiman, S., Villamor, E., Zera, C. A., & Gillman, M. W. (2013). Differential associations of leptin with adiposity across early childhood. *Obesity, 21*(7), 1430–1437.

Boney, C. M., Verma, A., Tucker, R., & Vohr, B. R. (2005). Metabolic syndrome in childhood: Association with birth weight, maternal obesity, and gestational diabetes mellitus. *Pediatrics, 115*(3), e290–e296.

Bouret, S. G., Draper, S. J., & Simerly, R. B. (2004). Trophic action of leptin on hypothalamic neurons that regulate feeding. *Science, 304*(5667), 108–110.

Branum, A. M., Parker, J. D., Keim, S. A., & Schempf, A. H. (2011). Prepregnancy body mass index and gestational weight gain in relation to child body mass index among siblings. *American Journal of Epidemiology, 174*(10), 1159–1165.

Brion, M. J. (2010). Commentary: Assessing the impact of breastfeeding on child health: Where conventional methods alone fall short for reliably establishing causal inference. *International Journal of Epidemiology, 39*(1), 306–307.

Brion, M. J., Lawlor, D. A., Matijasevich, A., Horta, B., Anselmi, L., Araujo, C. L., Menezes, A. M., Victora, C. G., & Smith, G. D. (2011). What are the causal effects of breastfeeding on IQ, obesity and blood pressure? Evidence from comparing high-income with middle-income cohorts. *International Journal of Epidemiology, 40*(3), 670–680.

Brownell, K. D., Farley, T., Willett, W. C., Popkin, B. M., Chaloupka, F. J., Thompson, J. W., & Ludwig, D. S. (2009). The public health and economic benefits of taxing sugar-sweetened beverages. *The New England Journal of Medicine, 361*(16), 1599–1605.

Casazza, K., Fontaine, K. R., Astrup, A., Birch, L. L., Brown, A. W., Bohan Brown, M. M., Durant, N., Dutton, G., Foster, E. M., Heymsfield, S. B., McIver, K., Mehta, T., Menachemi, N., Newby, P. K., Pate, R., Rolls, B. J., Sen, B., Smith, D. L., Jr., Thomas, D. M., & Allison, D. B. (2013). Myths, presumptions, and facts about obesity. *The New England Journal of Medicine, 368*(5), 446–454.

Catalano, P. M., Presley, L., Minium, J., & Hauguel-de Mouzon, S. (2009). Fetuses of obese mothers develop insulin resistance in utero. *Diabetes Care, 32*(6), 1076–1080.

Centers for Disease Control and Prevention. (2010). Racial and ethnic differences in breastfeeding initiation and duration, by state – National Immunization Survey, United States, 2004–2008. *MMWR. Morbidity and Mortality Weekly Report, 59*(11), 327–334.

Centers for Disease Control and Prevention. (2014). Breastfeeding report card: United States, 2014. http://www.cdc.gov/breastfeeding/pdf/2014breastfeedingreportcard.pdf. Accessed 2 Dec 2014.

Cespedes, E. M., Rifas-Shiman, S. L., Redline, S., Gillman, M. W., Pena, M. M., & Taveras, E. M. (2014). Longitudinal associations of sleep curtailment with metabolic risk in mid-childhood. *Obesity, 22*(12), 2586–2592.

Chandler-Laney, P. C., Bush, N. C., Granger, W. M., Rouse, D. J., Mancuso, M. S., & Gower, B. A. (2012). Overweight status and intrauterine exposure to gestational diabetes are associated with children's metabolic health. *Pediatr Obes, 7*(1), 44–52.

Chen, X., Beydoun, M. A., & Wang, Y. (2008). Is sleep duration associated with childhood obesity? A systematic review and meta-analysis. *Obesity, 16*(2), 265–274.

Chriqui, J. F., Eidson, S. S., & Chaloupka, F. J. (2014). State sales taxes on regular soda (as of January 2014) – BTG Fact Sheet. http://www.bridgingthegapresearch.org/_asset/s2b5pb/BTG_soda_tax_fact_sheet_April2014.pdf. Accessed 3 Dec 2014.

Christakis, N. A., & Fowler, J. H. (2007). The spread of obesity in a large social network over 32 years. *The New England Journal of Medicine, 357*(4), 370–379.

Coleman-Jensen, A., Gregory, C., & Singh, A. (September 2014). *Household food security in the United States in 2013, ERR-173*. Washington, DC: U.S. Department of Agriculture, Economic Research Service.

Crowther, C. A., Hiller, J. E., Moss, J. R., McPhee, A. J., Jeffries, W. S., & Robinson, J. S. (2005). Effect of treatment of gestational diabetes mellitus on pregnancy outcomes. *The New England Journal of Medicine, 352*(24), 2477–2486.

Dalenius, K., Brindley, P., Smith, B. L., Reinold, C. M., & Grummer-Strawn, L. (2012). *Pregnancy nutrition surveillance 2010 report*. Atlanta, GA: US Department of health and human services; Centers for Disease Control and Prevention.

Danese, A., & Tan, M. (2014). Childhood maltreatment and obesity: Systematic review and meta-analysis. *Molecular Psychiatry, 19*(5), 544–554.

DiBaise, J. K., Zhang, H., Crowell, M. D., Krajmalnik-Brown, R., Decker, G. A., & Rittmann, B. E. (2008). Gut microbiota and its possible relationship with obesity. *Mayo Clinic Proceedings, 83*(4), 460–469.

Ding, E. L., & Hu, F. B. (2008). Determining origins and causes of childhood obesity via Mendelian randomization analysis. *PLoS Medicine, 5*(3), e65.

Dinour, L. M., Bergen, D., & Yeh, M. C. (2007). The food insecurity-obesity paradox: A review of the literature and the role food stamps may play. *Journal of the American Dietetic Association, 107*(11), 1952–1961.

Dixon, B., Pena, M. M., & Taveras, E. M. (2012). Lifecourse approach to racial/ethnic disparities in childhood obesity. *Advances in Nutrition, 3*(1), 73–82.

Dodd, J. M., Turnbull, D. A., McPhee, A. J., Wittert, G., Crowther, C. A., & Robinson, J. S. (2011). Limiting weight gain in overweight and obese women during pregnancy to improve health outcomes: The LIMIT randomised controlled trial. *BMC Pregnancy and Childbirth, 11*, 79.

Dominguez-Bello, M. G., Costello, E. K., Contreras, M., Magris, M., Hidalgo, G., Fierer, N., & Knight, R. (2010). Delivery mode shapes the acquisition and structure of the initial microbiota across multiple body habitats in newborns. *Proceedings of the National Academy of Sciences of the United States of America, 107*(26), 11971–11975.

Duffey, K. J., & Popkin, B. M. (2013). Causes of increased energy intake among children in the U.S., 1977–2010.

American Journal of Preventive Medicine, 44(2), e1–e8.

Dunton, G. F., Kaplan, J., Wolch, J., Jerrett, M., & Reynolds, K. D. (2009). Physical environmental correlates of childhood obesity: A systematic review. *Obesity Reviews, 10*(4), 393–402.

Ehrenkranz, R. A., Dusick, A. M., Vohr, B. R., Wright, L. L., Wrage, L. A., & Poole, W. K. (2006). Growth in the neonatal intensive care unit influences neurodevelopmental and growth outcomes of extremely low birth weight infants. *Pediatrics, 117*(4), 1253–1261.

Eisenmann, J. C., Gundersen, C., Lohman, B. J., Garasky, S., & Stewart, S. D. (2011). Is food insecurity related to overweight and obesity in children and adolescents? A summary of studies, 1995–2009. *Obesity Reviews, 12*(5), e73–e83.

Elbel, B., Gyamfi, J., & Kersh, R. (2011). Child and adolescent fast-food choice and the influence of calorie labeling: A natural experiment. *International Journal of Obesity, 35*(4), 493–500.

Elobeid, M. A., & Allison, D. B. (2008). Putative environmental-endocrine disruptors and obesity: A review. *Current Opinion in Endocrinology, Diabetes, and Obesity, 15*(5), 403–408.

Finkelstein, E. A., Trogdon, J. G., Cohen, J. W., & Dietz, W. (2009). Annual medical spending attributable to obesity: Payer-and service-specific estimates. *Health Affairs, 28*(5), 822–831.

Fisher, S. C., Kim, S. Y., Sharma, A. J., Rochat, R., & Morrow, B. (2013). Is obesity still increasing among pregnant women? Prepregnancy obesity trends in 20 states, 2003–2009. *Preventive Medicine, 56*(6), 372–378.

Fleten, C., Nystad, W., Stigum, H., Skjaerven, R., Lawlor, D. A., Davey Smith, G., & Naess, O. (2012). Parent-offspring body mass index associations in the Norwegian Mother and Child Cohort Study: A family-based approach to studying the role of the intrauterine environment in childhood adiposity. *American Journal of Epidemiology, 176*(2), 83–92.

Foster, G. D., Linder, B., Baranowski, T., Cooper, D. M., Goldberg, L., Harrell, J. S., Kaufman, F., Marcus, M. D., Treviño, R. P., & Hirst, K. (2010). A school-based intervention for diabetes risk reduction. *The New England Journal of Medicine, 363*(5), 443–453.

Franklin, B., Jones, A., Love, D., Puckett, S., Macklin, J., & White-Means, S. (2012). Exploring mediators of food insecurity and obesity: A review of recent literature. *Journal of Community Health, 37*(1), 253–264.

Freinkel, N. (1980). Banting lecture 1980. Of pregnancy and progeny. *Diabetes, 29*(12), 1023–1035.

Gao, Y. J., Holloway, A. C., Zeng, Z. H., Lim, G. E., Petrik, J. J., Foster, W. G., & Lee, R. M. (2005). Prenatal exposure to nicotine causes postnatal obesity and altered perivascular adipose tissue function. *Obesity Research, 13*(4), 687–692.

Getahun, D., Nath, C., Ananth, C. V., Chavez, M. R., & Smulian, J. C. (2008). Gestational diabetes in the United States: Temporal trends 1989 through 2004. *American Journal of Obstetrics and Gynecology, 198*(5), e521–e525.

Gillman, M. W. (2004). A life course approach to obesity. In D. Kuh (Ed.), *A life course approach to chronic disease epidemiology*. Oxford: Oxford University Press.

Gillman, M. W. (2005). Developmental origins of health and disease. *The New England Journal of Medicine, 353*(17), 1848–1850.

Gillman, M. W. (2011). Commentary: Breastfeeding and obesity–the 2011 Scorecard. *International Journal of Epidemiology, 40*(3), 681–684.

Gillman, M. W. (2016). Interrupting intergenerational cycles of maternal obesity. In M. S. Fewtrell, F. Haschke, & S. L. Prescott (eds): Preventive Aspects of Early Nutrition. Nestlé Nutr Inst Workshop Ser, vol 85, pp 59–69.

Gillman, M. W., Oakey, H., Baghurst, P. A., Volkmer, R. E., Robinson, J. S., & Crowther, C. A. (2010). Effect of treatment of gestational diabetes mellitus on obesity in the next generation. *Diabetes Care, 33*(5), 964–968.

Gillman, M. W., & Poston, L. (2012). *Maternal obesity*. Cambridge, UK: Cambridge University Press.

Gillman, M. W., Rifas-Shiman, S. L., Berkey, C. S., Frazier, A. L., Rockett, H. R., Camargo, C. A., Jr., Field, A. E., & Colditz, G. A. (2006). Breast-feeding and overweight in adolescence: Within-family analysis [corrected]. *Epidemiology, 17*(1), 112–114.

Gilman, S. E., Gardener, H., & Buka, S. L. (2008). Maternal smoking during pregnancy and children's cognitive and physical development: A causal risk factor? *American Journal of Epidemiology, 168*(5), 522–531.

Glaser, R., & Kiecolt-Glaser, J. K. (2005). Stress-induced immune dysfunction: Implications for health. *Nature Reviews Immunology, 5*(3), 243–251.

Glass, T. A., & McAtee, M. J. (2006). Behavioral science at the crossroads in public health: Extending horizons, envisioning the future. *Social Science & Medicine, 62*(7), 1650–1671.

Gonzalez-Suarez, C., Worley, A., Grimmer-Somers, K., & Dones, V. (2009). School-based interventions on childhood obesity: A meta-analysis. *American Journal of Preventive Medicine, 37*(5), 418–427.

Grayson, B. E., & Seeley, R. J. (2012). Deconstructing obesity: The face of fatness before and after the discovery of leptin. *Diabetologia, 55*(1), 3–6.

Grummer-Strawn, L. M., Reinold, C., & Krebs, N. F. (2010). Use of World Health Organization and CDC growth charts for children aged 0–59 months in the United States. *MMWR – Recommendations and Reports, 59*(RR-9), 1–15.

Grynbaum, M. M. (2012). Will soda restrictions help New York win the war on obesity? *BMJ, 345*, e6768.

Halfon, N., & Forrest, C. B. (2017). The emerging theoretical framework of life course health development. In N. Halfon, C. B. Forrest, R. M. Lerner, & E. Faustman (Eds.), *Handbook of life course health-development science*. Cham: Springer.

Hammond, R. A. (2009). Complex systems modeling for obesity research. *Preventing Chronic Disease, 6*(3), A97.

Han, J. C., Lawlor, D. A., & Kimm, S. Y. (2010). Childhood obesity. *Lancet, 375*(9727), 1737–1748.

Harder, T., Bergmann, R., Kallischnigg, G., & Plagemann, A. (2005). Duration of breastfeeding and risk of overweight: A meta-analysis. *American Journal of Epidemiology, 162*(5), 397–403.

Harlev, A., & Wiznitzer, A. (2010). New insights on glucose pathophysiology in gestational diabetes and insulin resistance. *Current Diabetes Reports, 10*(3), 242–247.

Hauguel-de Mouzon, S., Lepercq, J., & Catalano, P. (2006). The known and unknown of leptin in pregnancy. *American Journal of Obstetrics and Gynecology, 194*(6), 1537–1545.

Hawkins, S. S., & Baum, C. F. (2014). Impact of state cigarette taxes on disparities in maternal smoking during pregnancy. *American Journal of Public Health, 104*(8), 1464–1470.

Hedderson, M. M., Gunderson, E. P., & Ferrara, A. (2010). Gestational weight gain and risk of gestational diabetes mellitus. *Obstetrics and Gynecology, 115*(3), 597–604.

Hemmingsson, E., Johansson, K., & Reynisdottir, S. (2014). Effects of childhood abuse on adult obesity: A systematic review and meta-analysis. *Obesity Reviews, 15*(11), 882–893.

Herring, S. J., & Oken, E. (2011). Obesity and diabetes in mothers and their children: Can we stop the intergenerational cycle? *Current Diabetes Reports, 11*(1), 20–27.

Herring, S. J., Rose, M. Z., Skouteris, H., & Oken, E. (2012). Optimizing weight gain in pregnancy to prevent obesity in women and children. *Diabetes, Obesity & Metabolism, 14*(3), 195–203.

Huang, T. T., Drewnosksi, A., Kumanyika, S., & Glass, T. A. (2009). A systems-oriented multilevel framework for addressing obesity in the 21st century. *Preventing Chronic Disease, 6*(3), A82.

Huang, T. T., & Glass, T. A. (2008). Transforming research strategies for understanding and preventing obesity. *JAMA, 300*(15), 1811–1813.

Huh, S. Y., Rifas-Shiman, S. L., Taveras, E. M , Oken, E., & Gillman, M. W. (2011). Timing of solid food introduction and risk of obesity in preschool-aged children. *Pediatrics, 127*(3), e544–e551.

Iliadou, A. N., Koupil, I., Villamor, E., Altman, D., Hultman, C., Langstrom, N., & Cnattingius, S. (2010). Familial factors confound the association between maternal smoking during pregnancy and young adult offspring overweight. *International Journal of Epidemiology, 39*(5), 1193–1202.

Institute of Medicine. (1990). *Nutrition during pregnancy. Part I, weight gain*. Washington, DC: National Academies Press.

Institute of Medicine. (2007). *Nutrition standards for foods in schools: Leading the way toward healtheir youth*. Washington, DC: National Academies Press.

Institute of Medicine. (2009). *Weight gain during pregnancy: Reexamining the guidelines*. Washington, DC: National Academies Press.

Institute of Medicine. (2011). *Early childhood obesity prevention policies*. Washington DC: National Academies Press.

Kahn, J. A., Huang, B., Gillman, M. W., Field, A. E., Austin, S. B., Colditz, G. A., & Frazier, A. L. (2008). Patterns and determinants of physical activity in U.S. adolescents. *The Journal of Adolescent Health, 42*(4), 369–377.

Kann, L., Kinchen, S., Shanklin, S. L., Flint, K. H., Kawkins, J., Harris, W. A., Lowry, R., Olsen, E. O., McManus, T., Chyen, D., Whittle, L., Taylor, E., Demissie, Z., Brener, N., Thornton, J., Moore, J., Zaza, S., & Centers for Disease Control and Prevention (CDC). (2014). Youth risk behavior surveillance–United States, 2013. *MMWR Surveillance Summaries, 63*(4), 1–168.

Katz, D. L., O'Connell, M., Njike, V. Y., Yeh, M. C., & Nawaz, H. (2008). Strategies for the prevention and control of obesity in the school setting: Systematic review and meta-analysis. *International Journal of Obesity, 32*(12), 1780–1789.

Kim, C., Berger, D. K., & Chamany, S. (2007). Recurrence of gestational diabetes mellitus: A systematic review. *Diabetes Care, 30*(5), 1314–1319.

Kim, C., Newton, K. M., & Knopp, R. H. (2002). Gestational diabetes and the incidence of type 2 diabetes: A systematic review. *Diabetes Care, 25*(10), 1862–1868.

Kim, S. Y., England, J. L., Sharma, J. A., & Njoroge, T. (2011). Gestational diabetes mellitus and risk of childhood overweight and obesity in offspring: A systematic review. *Experimental Diabetes Research, 2011*, 541308.

Kitano, H. (2002). Systems biology: A brief overview. *Science, 295*(5560), 1662–1664.

Kramer, M. S., Chalmers, B., Hodnett, E. D., Sevkovskaya, Z., Dzikovich, I., Shapiro, S., Collet, J. P., Vanilovich, I., Mezen, I., Ducruet, T., Shishko, G., Zubovich, V., Mknuik, D., Gluchanina, E., Dombrovsky, V., Ustinovitch, A., Ko, T., Bogdanovich, N., Ovchinikova, L., & Helsing, E. (2001). Promotion of Breastfeeding Intervention Trial (PROBIT): A randomized trial in the Republic of Belarus. *JAMA, 285*(4), 413–420.

Kramer, M. S., Guo, T., Platt, R. W., Vanilovich, I., Sevkovskaya, Z., Dzikovich, I., Michaelsen, K. F., Dewey, K., & Promotion of Breastfeeding Intervention Trials Study Group. (2004). Feeding effects on growth during infancy. *The Journal of Pediatrics, 145*(5), 600–605.

Kramer, M. S., Matush, L., Vanilovich, I., Platt, R. W., Bogdanovich, N., Sevkovskaya, Z., Dzikovich, I., Shishko, G., Collet, J. P., Martin, R. M., Davey Smith, G., Gillman, M. W., Chalmers, B., Hodnett, E., Shapiro, S., & PROBIT Study Group. (2007). Effects of prolonged and exclusive breastfeeding on child height, weight, adiposity, and blood pressure at age 6.5 y: Evidence from a large randomized trial. *The American Journal of Clinical Nutrition, 86*(6), 1717–1721.

Kropski, J. A., Keckley, P. H., & Jensen, G. L. (2008). School-based obesity prevention programs: An evidence-based review. *Obesity, 16*(5), 1009–1018.

Kuczmarski, R. J., Ogden, C. L., Guo, S. S., Grummer-Strawn, L. M., Flegal, K. M., Mei, Z., Curtin, L. R., Roche, A. F., & Johnson, C. L. (2002). 2000 CDC growth charts for the United States: Methods and development. *Vital and Health Statistics, 11*(246), 1–190.

Kwok, M. K., Schooling, C. M., Lam, T. H., & Leung, G. M. (2010). Does breastfeeding protect against childhood overweight? Hong Kong's 'Children of 1997' birth cohort. *International Journal of Epidemiology, 39*(1), 297–305.

Landon, M. B., Spong, C. Y., Thom, E., Carpenter, M. W., Ramin, S. M., Casey, B., Wapner, R. J., Varner, M. W., Rouse, D. J., Thorp, J. M., Jr., Sciscione, A., Catalano, P., Harper, M., Saade, G., Lain, K. Y., Sorokin, Y., Peaceman, A. M., Tolosa, J. E., Anderson, G. B., & Eunice Kennedy Shriver National Institute of Child Health and Human Development Maternal-Fetal Medicine Units Network. (2009). A multicenter, randomized trial of treatment for mild gestational diabetes. *The New England Journal of Medicine, 361*(14), 1339–1348.

Larson, N., Ward, D., Neelon, S. B., & Story, M. (2011a). *Preventing obesity among preschool children: How can child-care settings promote healthy eating and physical activity? Research synthesis*. Princeton, NJ: Robert Wood Johnson Foundation.

Larson, N., Ward, D. S., Neelon, S. B., & Story, M. (2011b). What role can child-care settings play in obesity prevention? A review of the evidence and call for research efforts. *Journal of the American Dietetic Association, 111*(9), 1343–1362.

Lasater, G., Piernas, C., & Popkin, B. M. (2011). Beverage patterns and trends among school-aged children in the US, 1989–2008. *Nutrition Journal, 10*, 103.

Lau, E. Y., Liu, J., Archer, E., McDonald, S. M., & Liu, J. (2014). Maternal weight gain in pregnancy and risk of obesity among offspring: A systematic review. *Journal of Obesity, 2014*, 524939.

Lawlor, D. A., Lichtenstein, P., Fraser, A., & Langstrom, N. (2011a). Does maternal weight gain in pregnancy have long-term effects on offspring adiposity? A sibling study in a prospective cohort of 146,894 men from 136,050 families. *The American Journal of Clinical Nutrition, 94*(1), 142–148.

Lawlor, D. A., Lichtenstein, P., & Langstrom, N. (2011b). Association of maternal diabetes mellitus in pregnancy with offspring adiposity into early adulthood: Sibling study in a prospective cohort of 280,866 men from 248,293 families. *Circulation, 123*(3), 258–265.

Lawlor, D. A., Timpson, N. J., Harbord, R. M., Leary, S., Ness, A., McCarthy, M. I., Frayling, T. M., Hattersley, A. T., & Smith, G. D. (2008). Exploring the developmental overnutrition hypothesis using parental-offspring associations and FTO as an instrumental variable. *PLoS Medicine, 5*(3), e33.

Lehto, R., Mäki, P., Ray, C., Laatikainen, T., & Roos, E. (2015). Childcare use and overweight in Finland: Cross-sectional and retrospective associations among 3- and 5-year-old children. *Pediatric Obesity, 11*(2), 136–143. doi:10.1111/ijpo.12036.

Li, H. T., Zhou, Y. B., & Liu, J. M. (2013). The impact of cesarean section on offspring overweight and obesity: A systematic review and meta-analysis. *International Journal of Obesity, 37*(7), 893–899.

Li, R., Fein, S. B., & Grummer-Strawn, L. M. (2010). Do infants fed from bottles lack self-regulation of milk intake compared with directly breastfed infants? *Pediatrics, 125*(6), e1386–e1393.

Lobstein, T., Baur, L., & Uauy, R. (2004). Obesity in children and young people: A crisis in public health. *Obesity Reviews, 5*(1), 4–104.

Lovasi, G. S., Hutson, M. A., Guerra, M., & Neckerman, K. M. (2009). Built environments and obesity in disadvantaged populations. *Epidemiologic Reviews, 31*, 7–20.

Lubans, D. R., Morgan, P. J., Dewar, D., Collins, C. E., Plotnikoff, R. C., Okely, A. D., Batterham, M. J., Finn, T., & Callister, R. (2010). The Nutrition and Enjoyable Activity for Teen Girls (NEAT girls) randomized controlled trial for adolescent girls from disadvantaged secondary schools: Rationale, study protocol, and baseline results. *BMC Public Health, 10*, 652.

Ludwig, D. S., Blumenthal, S. J., & Willett, W. C. (2012). Opportunities to reduce childhood hunger and obesity: Restructuring the supplemental nutrition assistance program (the food stamp program). *JAMA, 308*(24), 2567–2568.

Ludwig, J., Sanbonmatsu, L., Gennetian, L., Adam, E., Duncan, G. J., Katz, L. F., Kessler, R. C., Kling, J. R., Lindau, S. T., Whitaker, R. C., & McDade, T. W. (2011). Neighborhoods, obesity, and diabetes–a randomized social experiment. *The New England Journal of Medicine, 365*(16), 1509–1519.

Lumley, J., Chamberlain, C., Dowswell, T., Oliver, S., Oakley, L., & Watson, L. (2009). Interventions for promoting smoking cessation during pregnancy. *Cochrane Database of Systematic Reviews, 3*, CD001055.

Mamun, A. A., Mannan, M., & Doi, S. A. (2014). Gestational weight gain in relation to offspring obesity over the life course: A systematic review and bias-adjusted meta-analysis. *Obesity Reviews, 15*(4), 338–347.

Mani, M., Mandre, S. B., & M. (2010). Events before droplet splashing on a solid surface. *Journal of Fluid Mechanics, 647*, 163.

Mantzoros, C. S., Rifas-Shiman, S. L., Williams, C. J., Fargnoli, J. L., Kelesidis, T., & Gillman, M. W. (2009). Cord blood leptin and adiponectin as predictors of adiposity in children at 3 years of age: A prospective cohort study. *Pediatrics, 123*(2), 682–689.

Martin, R. M., Patel, R., Kramer, M. S., Guthrie, L., Vilchuck, K., Bogdanovich, N., Sergeichick, N., Gusina, N., Foo, Y., Palmer, T., Rifas-Shiman, S. L., Gillman, M. W., Smith, G. D., & Oken, E. (2013). Effects of promoting longer-term and exclusive breastfeeding on adiposity and insulin-like growth factor-I at age 11.5 years: A randomized trial. *JAMA, 309*(10), 1005–1013.

Masse, L. C., Perna, F., Agurs-Collins, T., & Chriqui, J. F. (2013). Change in school nutrition-related laws from 2003 to 2008: Evidence from the school nutrition-environment state policy classification system. *American Journal of Public Health, 103*(9), 1597–1603.

McGinnis, J. M., Gootman, J. A., & Kraak, V. I. (2006). *Food marketing to children and youth: Threat or opportunity?* Washington, DC: National Academies Press.

Mello, M. M. (2009). New York City's war on fat. *The New England Journal of Medicine, 360*(19), 2015–2020.

Metzger, M. W., & McDade, T. W. (2010). Breastfeeding as obesity prevention in the United States: A sibling difference model. *American Journal of Human Biology, 22*(3), 291–296.

Michopoulos, V., Powers, A., Moore, C., Villarreal, S., Ressler, K. J., & Bradley, B. (2015). The mediating role of emotion dysregulation and depression on the relationship between childhood trauma exposure and emotional eating. *Appetite, 91*, 129–136.

Mihrshahi, S., Battistutta, D., Magarey, A., & Daniels, L. A. (2011). Determinants of rapid weight gain during infancy: Baseline results from the NOURISH randomised controlled trial. *BMC Pediatrics, 11*, 99.

Moholdt, T. T., Salvesen, K., Ingul, C. B., Vik, T., Oken, E., & Morkved, S. (2011). Exercise Training in Pregnancy for obese women (ETIP): Study protocol for a randomised controlled trial. *Trials, 12*, 154.

Monteiro, P. O., & Victora, C. G. (2005). Rapid growth in infancy and childhood and obesity in later life–a systematic review. *Obesity Reviews, 6*(2), 143–154.

National Association for Sport and Physical Education. (2004). *Moving into the future: National standards for physical education* (2nd ed.). Reston, VA: McGraw-Hill.

National Prevention Council. (2011). *National prevention strategy*. Washington, DC: U.S. Department of Health and Human Services, Office of the Surgeon General.

Neelon, S. B., Andersen, C. S., Morgen, C. S., Kamper-Jørgensen, M., Oken, E., Gillman, M. W., & Sørensen, T. I. A. (2015). Early child care and obesity at 12 months of age in the Danish National Birth Cohort. *International Journal of Obesity, 39*(1), 33–38.

Nehring, I., Lehmann, S., & von Kries, R. (2013). Gestational weight gain in accordance to the IOM/NRC criteria and the risk for childhood overweight: A meta-analysis. *Pediatric Obesity, 8*(3), 218–224.

Nehring, I., Schmoll, S., Beyerlein, A., Hauner, H., & von Kries, R. (2011). Gestational weight gain and long-term postpartum weight retention: A meta-analysis. *The American Journal of Clinical Nutrition, 94*(5), 1225–1231.

Nelson, M. C., Gordon-Larsen, P., & Adair, L. S. (2005). Are adolescents who were breast-fed less likely to be overweight? Analyses of sibling pairs to reduce confounding. *Epidemiology, 16*(2), 247–253.

Neu, J., & Rushing, J. (2011). Cesarean versus vaginal delivery: Long-term infant outcomes and the hygiene hypothesis. *Clinics in Perinatology, 38*(2), 321–331.

Newbold, R. R., Padilla-Banks, E., Snyder, R. J., Phillips, T. M., & Jefferson, W. N. (2007). Developmental exposure to endocrine disruptors and the obesity epidemic. *Reproductive Toxicology, 23*(3), 290–296.

Nielsen, L. S., Danielsen, K. V., & Sorensen, T. I. (2011). Short sleep duration as a possible cause of obesity: Critical analysis of the epidemiological evidence. *Obesity Reviews, 12*(2), 78–92.

Office of the Mayor. (2012). Reversing the epidemic: The New York City obesity task force plan to prevent and control obesity. http://www.nyc.gov/html/om/pdf/2012/otf_report.pdf. Accessed 5 Feb 2013.

O'Tierney, P. F., Barker, D. J., Osmond, C., Kajantie, E., & Eriksson, J. G. (2009). Duration of breast-feeding and adiposity in adult life. *The Journal of Nutrition, 139*(2), 422S–425S.

Ogden, C. L., Carroll, M. D., Kit, B. K., & Flegal, K. M. (2014). Prevalence of childhood and adult obesity in the United States, 2011–2012. *JAMA, 311*(8), 806–814.

Ogden, C. L., & Flegal, K. M. (2010). Changes in terminology for childhood overweight and obesity. *National Health Statistics Reports, 25*, 1–5.

Oken, E., & Gillman, M. W. (2003). Fetal origins of obesity. *Obesity Research, 11*(4), 496–506.

Oken, E., Levitan, E. B., & Gillman, M. W. (2008). Maternal smoking during pregnancy and child overweight: Systematic review and meta-analysis. *International Journal of Obesity, 32*(2), 201–210.

Okereke, N. C., Uvena-Celebrezze, J., Hutson-Presley, L., Amini, S. B., & Catalano, P. M. (2002). The effect of gender and gestational diabetes mellitus on cord leptin concentration. *American Journal of Obstetrics and Gynecology, 187*(3), 798–803.

Oteng-Ntim, E., Varma, R., Croker, H., Poston, L., & Doyle, P. (2012). Lifestyle interventions for overweight and obese pregnant women to improve pregnancy outcome: Systematic review and meta-analysis. *BMC Medicine, 10*, 47.

Owen, C. G., Martin, R. M., Whincup, P. H., Davey-Smith, G., Gillman, M. W., & Cook, D. G. (2005a). The effect of breastfeeding on mean body mass index throughout life: A quantitative review of published and unpublished observational evidence. *The American Journal of Clinical Nutrition, 82*(6), 1298–1307.

Owen, C. G., Martin, R. M., Whincup, P. H., Smith, G. D., & Cook, D. G. (2005b). Effect of infant feeding on the risk of obesity across the life course: A quantitative review of published evidence. *Pediatrics, 115*(5), 1367–1377.

Pan, L., Blanck, H. M., Sherry, B., Dalenius, K., & Grummer-Strawn, L. M. (2012). Trends in the prevalence of extreme obesity among US preschool-aged children living in low-income families, 1998–2010. *JAMA, 308*(24), 2563–2565.

Papas, M. A., Alberg, A. J., Ewing, R., Helzlsouer, K. J., Gary, T. L., & Klassen, A. C. (2007). The built environment and obesity. *Epidemiologic Reviews, 29*, 129–143.

Parker, M., Rifas-Shiman, S. L., Belfort, M. B., Taveras, E. M., Oken, E., Mantzoros, C., & Gillman, M. W. (2011). Gestational glucose tolerance and cord blood leptin levels predict slower weight gain in early infancy. *The Journal of Pediatrics, 158*(2), 227–233.

Parsons, T. J., Power, C., Logan, S., & Summerbell, C. D. (1999). Childhood predictors of adult obesity: A systematic review. *International Journal of Obesity and Related Metabolic Disorders, 23*(8), S1–107.

Patel, R., Martin, R. M., Kramer, M. S., Oken, E., Bogdanovich, N., Matush, L., Smith, G. D., & Lawlor, D. A. (2011). Familial associations of adiposity: Findings from a cross-sectional study of 12,181 parental-offspring trios from Belarus. *PloS One, 6*(1), e14607.

Pearce, J., Taylor, M. A., & Langley-Evans, S. C. (2013). Timing of the introduction of complementary feeding and risk of childhood obesity: A systematic review. *International Journal of Obesity, 37*(10), 1295–1306.

Perna, F. M., Oh, A., Chriqui, J. F., Masse, L. C., Atienza, A. A., Nebeling, L., Agurs-Collins, T., Moser, R. P., & Dodd, K. W. (2012). The association of state law to physical education time allocation in US public schools. *American Journal of Public Health, 102*(8), 1594–1599.

Perng, W., Gillman, M. W., Mantzoros, C. S., & Oken, E. (2014). A prospective study of maternal prenatal weight and offspring cardiometabolic health in midchildhood. *Annals of Epidemiology, 24*(11), 793–800 e791.

Piernas, C., & Popkin, B. M. (2011). Increased portion sizes from energy-dense foods affect total energy intake at eating occasions in US children and adolescents: Patterns and trends by age group and sociodemographic characteristics, 1977–2006. *The American Journal of Clinical Nutrition, 94*(5), 1324–1332.

Powell, L. M., Chriqui, J. F., Khan, T., Wada, R., & Chaloupka, F. J. (2013). Assessing the potential effectiveness of food and beverage taxes and subsidies for improving public health: A systematic review of prices, demand and body weight outcomes. *Obesity Reviews, 14*(2), 110–128.

Rideout, V. J., & Hamel, E. (2006). *The media family: Electronic media in the lives of infants, toddlers, preschoolers, and their parents*. Menlo Park, CA: Kaiser Family Foundation.

Rudd Center for Food Policy & Obesity. (2013). *Industry self-regulation of food marketing.*. http://www.yaleruddcenter.org/what_we_do.aspx?id=25. Accessed 5 Feb 2013.

Sanbonmatsu, L., Ludwig, J., Katz, L. F., Gennetian, L. A., Duncan, G. J., Kessler, R. C., Adam, E., TW, M. D., & Lindau, S. T. (2011). *Moving to opportunity for fair housing demonstration program – Final impacts evaluation*. Washington, DC: U.S. Department of Housing and Urban Development.

Savino, F., & Liguori, S. A. (2008). Update on breast milk hormones: Leptin, ghrelin and adiponectin. *Clinical Nutrition, 27*(1), 42–47.

Schmidt, M. E., Haines, J., O'Brien, A., McDonald, J., Price, S., Sherry, B., & Taveras, E. M. (2012). Systematic review of effective strategies for reducing screen time among young children. *Obesity, 20*(7), 1338–1354.

Section on Breastfeeding. (2012). Breastfeeding and the use of human milk. *Pediatrics, 129*(3), e827–e841.

Siega-Riz, A. M., Viswanathan, M., Moos, M. K., Deierlein, A., Mumford, S., Knaack, J., Thieda, P., Lux, L. J., & Lohr, K. N. (2009). A systematic review of outcomes of maternal weight gain according to the Institute of Medicine recommendations: Birthweight, fetal growth, and postpartum weight retention. *American Journal of Obstetrics and Gynecology, 201*(4), 339.e331–339.e314.

Slining, M. M., Benjamin Neelon, S. E., & Duffey, K. J. (2014). A review of state regulations to promote infant physical activity in child care. *International Journal of Behavioral Nutrition and Physical Activity, 11*(1), 139.

Smith, G. D., & Ebrahim, S. (2003). 'Mendelian randomization': Can genetic epidemiology contribute to understanding environmental determinants of disease? *International Journal of Epidemiology, 32*(1), 1–22.

National Center for Education Statistics. (2005). *Number of children under 6 years old and not yet enrolled in kindergarten, percentage in center-based programs, average weekly hours in nonparental care, and percentage in various types of primary care arrangements, by selected child and family characteristics: 2005*. http://nces.ed.gov/programs/digest/d09/tables/dt09_044.asp. Accessed 5 Feb 2013.

Story, M., Nanney, M. S., & Schwartz, M. B. (2009). Schools and obesity prevention: Creating school environments and policies to promote healthy eating and physical activity. *The Milbank Quarterly, 87*(1), 71–100.

Strasburger, V. C. (2011). Children, adolescents, obesity, and the media. *Pediatrics, 128*(1), 201–208.

Taheri, S. (2006). The link between short sleep duration and obesity: We should recommend more sleep to prevent obesity. *Archives of Disease in Childhood, 91*(11), 881–884.

Taveras, E. M., Blackburn, K., Gillman, M. W., Haines, J., McDonald, J., Price, S., & Oken, E. (2011a). First steps for mommy and me: A pilot intervention to improve nutrition and physical activity behaviors of postpartum mothers and their infants. *Maternal and Child Health Journal, 15*(8), 1217–1227.

Taveras, E. M., Gillman, M. W., Kleinman, K., Rich-Edwards, J. W., & Rifas-Shiman, S. L. (2010). Racial/ethnic differences in early-life risk factors for childhood obesity. *Pediatrics, 125*(4), 686–695.

Taveras, E. M., Gillman, M. W., Kleinman, K. P., Rich-Edwards, J. W., & Rifas-Shiman, S. L. (2013). Reducing racial/ethnic disparities in childhood obesity: The role of early life risk factors. *JAMA Pediatrics, 167*(8), 731–738.

Taveras, E. M., Gillman, M. W., Pena, M. M., Redline, S., & Rifas-Shiman, S. L. (2014). Chronic sleep curtailment and adiposity. *Pediatrics, 133*(6), 1013–1022.

Taveras, E. M., Gortmaker, S. L., Hohman, K. H., Horan, C. M., Kleinman, K. P., Mitchell, K., Price, S., Prosser, L. A., Rifas-Shiman, S. L., & Gillman, M. W. (2011b). Randomized controlled trial to improve primary care to prevent and manage childhood obesity: The high five for kids study. *Archives of Pediatrics & Adolescent Medicine, 165*(8), 714–722.

Taveras, E. M., McDonald, J., O'Brien, A., Haines, J., Sherry, B., Bottino, C. J., Troncoso, K., Schmidt, M. E., & Koziol, R. (2012). Healthy habits, happy homes: Methods and baseline data of a randomized controlled trial to improve household routines for obesity prevention. *Preventive Medicine, 55*(5), 418–426.

Taveras, E. M., Rifas-Shiman, S. L., Sherry, B., Oken, E., Haines, J., Kleinman, K., Rich-Edwards, J. W., & Gillman, M. W. (2011c). Crossing growth percentiles in infancy and risk of obesity in childhood. *Archives of Pediatrics & Adolescent Medicine, 165*(11), 993–998.

Te Morenga, L., Mallard, S., & Mann, J. (2012). Dietary sugars and body weight: Systematic review and meta-analyses of randomised controlled trials and cohort studies. *BMJ, 346*, e7492.

Thangaratinam, S., Rogozinska, E., Jolly, K., Glinkowski, S., Roseboom, T., Tomlinson, J. W., Kunz, R., Mol, B. W., Coomarasamy, A., & Khan, K. S. (2012). Effects of interventions in pregnancy on maternal weight and obstetric outcomes: Meta-analysis of randomised evidence. *BMJ, 344*, e2088.

Torloni, M. R., Betran, A. P., Horta, B. L., Nakamura, M. U., Atallah, A. N., Moron, A. F., & Valente, O. (2009). Prepregnancy BMI and the risk of gestational diabetes: A systematic review of the literature with meta-analysis. *Obesity Reviews, 10*(2), 194–203.

Torres, S. J., & Nowson, C. A. (2007). Relationship between stress, eating behavior, and obesity. *Nutrition, 23*(11–12), 887–894.

Trasande, L., Attina, T. M., & Blustein, J. (2012). Association between urinary bisphenol a concentration and obesity prevalence in children and adolescents. *JAMA, 308*(11), 1113–1121.

Trogdon, J. G., Nonnemaker, J., & Pais, J. (2008). Peer effects in adolescent overweight. *Journal of Health Economics, 27*(5), 1388–1399.

U.S. Department of Agriculture. (2013a). National school lunch program and school breakfast program: Nutrition standards for all foods sold in school as required by the Healthy, Hunger-Free Kids Act of 2010; Interim Final Rule. *Federal Register, 78*(125), 39067–39120.

U.S. Department of Agriculture. (2013b). *Supplemental Nutrition Assistance Program (SNAP)*. http://www.fns.usda.gov/snap. Accessed 5 Feb 2013.

U.S. Department of Health and Human Services. (2004). *The health consequences of smoking: A report of the surgeon general*. Atlanta, GA: U.S. Department of Health and Human Services; Centers for Disease Control and Prevention; National Center for Chronic Disease Prevention and Health Promotion; Office on Smoking and Health.

U.S. Department of Health and Human Services. (2008). *2008 physical activity guidelines for Americans*. Washington, DC: U.S. Department of Health and Human Services.

Van Der Horst, K., Paw, M. J., Twisk, J. W., & Van Mechelen, W. (2007). A brief review on correlates of physical activity and sedentariness in youth. *Medicine and Science in Sports and Exercise, 39*(8), 1241–1250.

Ventura, A. K., & Mennella, J. A. (2011). Innate and learned preferences for sweet taste during childhood. *Current Opinion in Clinical Nutrition and Metabolic Care, 14*(4), 379–384.

Vesco, K. K., Karanja, N., King, J. C., Gillman, M. W., Leo, M. C., Perrin, N., CT, M. E., Eckhardt, C. L., Smith, K. S., & Stevens, V. J. (2014). Efficacy of a group-based dietary intervention for limiting gestational weight gain among obese women: A randomized trial. *Obesity, 22*(9), 1989–1996.

Vesco, K. K., Karanja, N., King, J. C., Gillman, M. W., Perrin, N., McEvoy, C., Eckhardt, C., Smith, K. S., & Stevens, V. J. (2012). Healthy moms, a randomized trial to promote and evaluate weight maintenance among obese pregnant women: Study design and rationale. *Contemporary Clinical Trials, 33*(4), 777–785.

Vgontzas, A. N., Lin, H. M., Papaliaga, M., Calhoun, S., Vela-Bueno, A., Chrousos, G. P., & Bixler, E. O. (2008). Short sleep duration and obesity: The role of emotional stress and sleep disturbances. *International Journal of Obesity, 32*(5), 801–809.

Viner, R. M., Ozer, E. M., Denny, S., Marmot, M., Resnick, M., Fatusi, A., & Currie, C. (2012). Adolescence and the social determinants of health. *Lancet, 379*(9826), 1641–1652.

von Kries, R., Bolte, G., Baghi, L., & Toschke, A. M. (2008). Parental smoking and childhood obesity–is maternal smoking in pregnancy the critical exposure? *International Journal of Epidemiology, 37*(1), 210–216.

Wang, Y., & Beydoun, M. A. (2007). The obesity epidemic in the United States–gender, age, socioeconomic, racial/ethnic, and geographic characteristics: A systematic review and meta-regression analysis. *Epidemiologic Reviews, 29*, 6–28.

Wang, Y. C., Gortmaker, S. L., & Taveras, E. M. (2011). Trends and racial/ethnic disparities in severe obesity among US children and adolescents, 1976–2006. *International Journal of Pediatric Obesity, 6*(1), 12–20.

Waterland, R. A., & Jirtle, R. L. (2004). Early nutrition, epigenetic changes at transposons and imprinted genes, and enhanced susceptibility to adult chronic diseases. *Nutrition, 20*(1), 63–68.

Waters, E., de Silva-Sanigorski, A., Hall, B. J., Brown, T., Campbell, K. J., Gao, Y., Armstrong, R., Prosser, L., & Summerbell, C. D. (2011). Interventions for preventing obesity in children. *Cochrane Database of Systematic Reviews, 12*, CD001871.

Wen, X., Gillman, M. W., Rifas-Shiman, S. L., Sherry, B., Kleinman, K., & Taveras, E. M. (2012). Decreasing prevalence of obesity among young children in Massachusetts from 2004 to 2008. *Pediatrics, 129*(5), 823–831.

Weng, S. F., Redsell, S. A., Swift, J. A., Yang, M., & Glazebrook, C. P. (2012). Systematic review and meta-analyses of risk factors for childhood overweight identifiable during infancy. *Archives of Disease in Childhood, 97*(12), 1019–1026.

White House Task Force on Childhood Obesity. (2011). *One year progress report.* http://www.letsmove.gov/sites/letsmove.gov/files/Obesity_update_report.pdf. Accessed 8 Feb 2013.

White House Task Force on Childhood Obesity. (2010). *Solving the problem of childhood obesity within a generation: The White House task force on childhood obesity report to the president* http://www.letsmove.gov/sites/letsmove.gov/files/TaskForce_on_Childhood_Obesity_May2010_FullReport.pdf. Accessed 19 July 2012.

Yu, Z. B., Han, S. P., Zhu, G. Z., Zhu, C., Wang, X. J., Cao, X. G., & Guo, X. R. (2011). Birth weight and subsequent risk of obesity: A systematic review and meta-analysis. *Obesity Reviews, 12*(7), 525–542.

8

Using the Fragile Families and Child Wellbeing Study (FFCWS) in Life Course Health Development Research

Amanda Geller, Kate Jaeger, and Garrett Pace

1 Background

1.1 Policy and Scholarly Debates

Of the many potential determinants of child health development throughout the life course, one of the most contentiously debated has been the role of marriage and nonmarital childbearing. The now-famous Moynihan Report (1965), titled *The Negro Family*, highlighted family structure, along with the legacy of slavery and sustained discrimination, and inadequate employment opportunities, as key determinants of intransigent poverty among African-Americans of the time (Massey and Sampson 2009). Moynihan's primary policy recommendation was for increased federal efforts toward economic opportunity, and he was initially praised by black leaders for focusing such high-level attention on the wellbeing of black families. However, a more enduring legacy of his report, particularly in the context of the civil rights and feminist movements of the 1960s, was his reference to the "pathological" nature of mother-headed households (ibid.) and the controversy it engendered.

In the subsequent decades, scholars and policymakers debated whether nonmarital childbearing was the result of a "culture of poverty," which encouraged choices that undermined African-American children's life chances, or of structural factors such as racial discrimination, which trapped families in circumstances of intergenerational poverty and social disadvantage (Wilson 1988). The nature and causes of poverty, and the racialized discourse about social welfare programs, single-parent families, and their implications for child wellbeing, played a significant role in policy debates as well. This rhetoric was particularly notable in passage of the 1996 welfare reform law, the Personal Responsibility and Work Opportunity Reconciliation Act (Cherlin et al. 2009).

At the same time, the prevalence of nonmarital births has grown considerably, both among blacks and other racial and ethnic groups (McLanahan 2009). This growth, illustrated in Fig. 1, engendered further debate about the nature of nonmarital childbearing and whether its widespread increase should be cause for concern.

However, in the 1990s, empirical data on unmarried parents and their children was limited

A. Geller (✉)
New York University, New York, NY, USA
e-mail: amanda.geller@nyu.edu

K. Jaeger
Princeton University, Princeton, NJ, USA

G. Pace
Doctoral Student, School of Social Work, Department of Sociology, University of Michigan, Ann Arbor, MI, USA

Fig. 1 Unmarried births as a percent of US births, 1950–2013 (National Center for Health Statistics; National Vital Statistics System). Note: Hispanics can be of any race. "*Black*" data from 1950 to 1969 refers to all non-whites

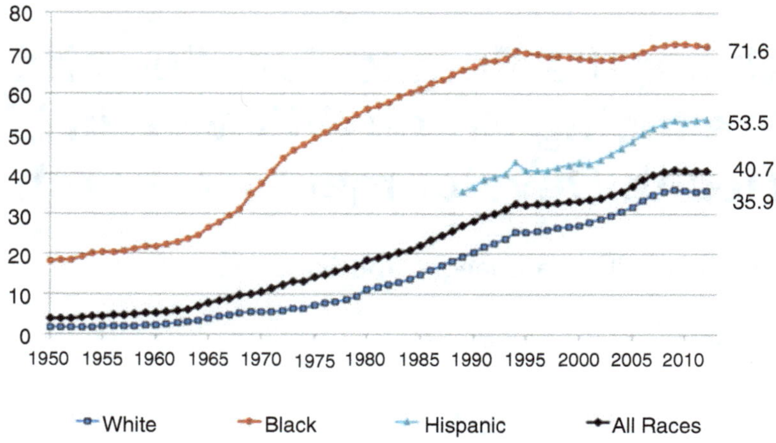

(McLanahan 2009). Scholars and analysts alternately posited that children born to unmarried parents were the result of encounters so casual that mothers might not know who the fathers were, or that nonmarital childbearing in the United States might resemble that in other Western industrialized countries in which committed, cohabiting parents raised children within the same stable unions as a married couple, "lacking only the piece of paper." Still others suggested that while unmarried parents might be committed to each other and their children, the American welfare state did not provide the support of those in other Western industrialized countries, leaving the family units at risk (McLanahan et al. 2010).

At the point when these debates were most salient, the literature on single parenthood and father absence focused predominantly on widows and divorced families (McLanahan and Sandefur 1994), who researchers suspected differed significantly from parents who never married. Some basic demographic information was available about the women who gave birth while unmarried, but very little was known about the fathers of their children or about the social and cultural environments in which their children grew up (McLanahan 2009). Still less was known about the health development outcomes of children born outside of marriage or the role of the family and social environment in their development.

1.2 Development of the Fragile Families and Child Wellbeing Study

To build a sound evidence base on the causes and consequences of nonmarital childbearing, a team of researchers at Columbia and Princeton Universities developed and implemented a large national survey, the Fragile Families and Child Wellbeing Study (FFCWS). The "Fragile Families" moniker was carefully chosen and derived from the Ford Foundation's "Strengthening Fragile Families" initiative of the 1990s (Sorensen et al. 2002). Although a variety of family transitions carried the potential for resulting instability – divorce and parental death, among others – the term "Fragile Families" referred specifically to families in which parents were not married at the time a child was born (ibid.). The word "fragile" referred to the risks that unmarried parents faced in terms of their economic and relationship stability, while the word "families" was used in recognition that unmarried partners with children represent a cohesive family unit (ibid.).[1]

The FFCWS was designed to address four key questions raised by the Moynihan Report and subsequent public discourse (Reichman et al. 2001).

[1] To avoid potential stigma associated with the term "fragile," families participating in the FFCWS were approached using more neutral terms and asked to participate in the "Survey of Parents."

1. What are the capabilities of unmarried parents (especially fathers) when their child is born? How many of the fathers hold steady jobs? How many want to be involved in raising their children?
2. What is the nature of parental relationships in fragile families at birth? How many couples are involved in stable, long-term relationships? How many expect to marry? How many experience high levels of conflict or domestic violence? How do relationships change over time?
3. What factors push new unwed parents together? What factors pull them apart? How do public policies affect parents' behaviors and living arrangements or child wellbeing? What are the long-term consequences of new welfare regulations, stronger paternity establishment, and stricter child support enforcement? What roles do childcare and healthcare policies play? How do these policies play out in different labor market environments?
4. How do parents and children fare in fragile families, and how does family structure and stability affect child wellbeing and development?

The study has since expanded to become a key source of information about family relationships and the broader social environment and their effects on child health development and wellbeing. At time of writing, the FFCWS is in the middle of its sixth wave of data collection, and the children born at the study baseline are turning 15 years old. The study is a joint effort by the Princeton University Center for Research on Child Wellbeing (CRCW) and Center for Health and Wellbeing, the Columbia Population Research Center (CPRC), and the National Center for Children and Families (NCCF) at Columbia University. The Principal Investigators of the Fragile Families Study are Sara McLanahan, Dan Notterman, Janet Currie, and Christina Paxson[2] at Princeton University and Irwin Garfinkel, Jeanne Brooks-Gunn, Ron Mincy, and Jane Waldfogel at Columbia University. The study's funding has come from the Eunice Kennedy Shriver National Institute of Child Health and Human Development, as well as a variety of other government and private funders, listed in Appendix A. More than 730 scholarly articles, theses, books, and abstracts have used the FFCWS data, which has also been used to inform testimony to policymakers at the national, state, and local levels (e.g., Sorensen et al. 2002; Geller 2011).

1.3 The FFCWS and Life Course Health Development Research

The FFCWS has several features that make it ideally suited for life course health development research on children. The Life Course Health Development (LCHD) model (see Halfon and Forrest 2017) views health as a "dynamic, emergent capacity that develops continuously over the lifespan, in a complex, nonlinear process" forming health development trajectories that are influenced by physical and social environmental as well as personal and genetic factors. Specifically, the model lays out seven principles of health development (ibid.):

1. Health is an emergent set of developmental capacities.
2. Health develops continuously over the life span.
3. Health development is a complex, nonlinear process occurring in multiple dimensions and at multiple levels and phases.
4. Health development is sensitive to the timing and social structuring of environmental exposures and experience.
5. Health development is an adaptive process that has been engendered by evolution with strategies to promote resilience and plasticity in the face of changing and often constraining environmental contexts.
6. Optimal health development promotes survival, enhances thriving, and protects against disease.
7. Health development is sensitive to the timing and synchronization of molecular, physiological, behavioral, social, and cultural function.

[2]Since the start of the FFCWS, Dr. Paxson has left Princeton University and at time of writing is the President of Brown University.

Health is a broad set of developmental capacities that are in constant and dynamic transactions with individuals' biological, physical, and social environments (National Research Council and Institute of Medicine 2004). The FFCWS measures children's environments across all of these domains: the study contains biological indicators of children's wellbeing from the time of their birth, including low birthweight (Reichman and Teitler 2006) and overweight and obesity (Kimbro et al. 2007), among others (e.g., Holt et al. 2013). In many cases the FFCWS is even able to study children's prenatal environments through their mothers' hospital records (Reichman and Nepomnyaschy 2008; Smulian et al. 2005). More recently, the study has also started to collect genetic data, to enable examination of gene-environment interactions (Mitchell et al. 2014).

The FFCWS also contains rich information on children's physical environments, examining factors with significant influence on health development throughout the life course. The study collects data on the homes and neighborhoods in which children live, exposure to lead (Boutwell et al. 2014), access to food (Corman et al. 2014), and other neighborhood conditions.

One of the richest contributions of the FFCWS is its measurement of the social environment in which children are raised. According to the theoretical principles of life course health development, health development is a multilevel construct, and the FFCWS measures children's social environments at many of the levels that influence their health development throughout the life course: the family (both biological parents and the social unit that comprises the household) (Jackson et al. 2012; Pilkauskas 2014), childcare settings (Rigby et al. 2007), schools (Razza et al. Forthcoming), neighborhoods (Suglia et al. 2013), and broader contexts such as states or local labor markets (Rigby et al. 2007; Pilkauskas et al. 2012).

In addition to the rich multilevel data contained in the FFCWS, another significant contribution the study makes to life course research is its unique sampling strategy (detailed below in Sect. 2.1). Given the study's focus on unmarried parents and nonmarital childbearing, the study systematically oversamples unmarried couples, who face disproportionate socioeconomic challenges (McLanahan 2011). The FFCWS permits the observation of these challenges on a population level, and enables the identification of factors that might exacerbate risk or promote resilience among children. By nature of the FFCWS sampling plan, the data also contain large samples of racial and ethnic minority families, who are often underrepresented in population-based surveys (Reichman et al. 2001).

Another contribution of the FFCWS is the longitudinal nature of its data collection. The study contains rich information on children's environments, health status throughout infancy, early childhood, school entry, and middle childhood, which permits the construction of health development trajectories. As important as these periods are for long-term health and wellbeing (Shonkoff and Phillips 2000; Heckman 2006), very few population-based American datasets track birth cohorts or begin in infancy or early childhood (though see Flanagan and West 2004 for information on the Early Childhood Longitudinal Study, a notable exception).

The longitudinal birth cohort structure of the FFCWS, coupled with the rich data it collects on multiple domains of health and health determinants, permits the joint analysis of children's physical and emotional health development, both of which develop continuously over the life span. Health development and environmental constructs are tracked over time, with indicators either measured repeatedly or updated to be age-appropriate, as needed. These measures are therefore able to capture the time-sensitive nature of child development. Children (and adults) experience several key transitions throughout the life course (e.g., school entry, puberty, etc.), which require new modes of adaptation to biological, psychological, or social changes (Elder 1985; Graber and Brooks-Gunn 1996). Events they experience – both positive and negative – may also serve as turning points that alter their life course trajectories (Elder 1985; Sampson and Laub 1990). The effects of turning points and other key exposures on life course trajectories may further be linked to the timing of these exposures with respect to developmental transitions (Graber and Brooks-Gunn 1996). An important strength of the FFCWS is its observation of exposures to key influences, and measurement of children's risk and resilience, throughout their health developmental trajectories.

1.4 Road Map

The rest of this chapter proceeds as follows. Section 2 lays out the sampling plan and study design of the FFCWS. Section 3 provides an inventory of the data available at time of writing. Section 4 provides greater detail on how the FFCWS data may be used for life course health development research. Section 5 lays out future plans for the FFCWS. Section 6 concludes with resources available for FFCWS data users.

2 Study Design

The FFCWS was designed to provide information on unmarried couples and their newborn children (McLanahan et al. 2010). Previous efforts to describe these "fragile families" were limited by the challenges in collecting data on unmarried fathers (Reichman et al. 2001). What little was known about men who fathered children outside of marriage suggested that they were younger and less educated than men who father children within marriage, with lower incomes and fewer attachments to the labor market (Reichman et al. 2001; Garfinkel et al. 1998). These fathers also reported more disability, more depression, and a greater prevalence of risky health behaviors such as drinking and substance use (ibid.). These factors create challenges in recruiting and retaining them in population-based surveys (Aday and Cornelius 2006). Unmarried fathers also are less likely to be their children's legal guardians and to have fewer formal ties to their families, and may be harder to locate as a result. Accordingly, it is also likely that data obtained from prior household surveys understated the disadvantage faced by families with unmarried fathers.

The FFCWS focused its study design around the objective of obtaining information about previously understudied, unmarried, and often nonresident fathers. Early pilot studies suggested that unmarried fathers were often present at the birth of their child, and that both parents were willing to be interviewed at this time (Reichman et al. 2001). Baseline data collection was designed around this "magic moment," and both mothers and fathers were initially contacted for interview while in the hospital, shortly after their child's birth. Sampling from hospitals also provided a spatial clustering of new parents that both improved response rates and kept recruitment and interview costs manageable.

2.1 Sampling Strategy

The FFCWS was based on a multistage stratified random sample: cities were sampled, then hospitals within cities, and then births within hospitals. The sampling of cities was based on all cities in the United States with populations of 200,000 or more. Some of the cities in the sampling frame had a population of over 200,000 only when outlying suburban areas were included, while some cities were considered only in terms of their inner city – the definition of each city was drawn from its vital statistics (Reichman et al. 2001). These cities were then characterized by their policy environments, as defined by three variables: the welfare generosity, the strength of the local labor market, and the strength of local child support enforcement. (See Reichman et al., at 310–311, for further details on the scoring of policy environments.)

Each city's welfare, labor market, and child support regimes were scored on a three-point scale: low, medium, or high welfare generosity and strong, medium, or weak labor markets and child support enforcement policies. Cities were then sorted into two groups: those with only extreme values (low or high) for all three dimensions (leaving 8 different "extreme cells") and cities with at least one middle value (19 remaining cells). One city was sampled from each of the 8 extreme cells, and 8 additional cities were

Table 1 Fragile Families and Child Wellbeing Study cities and sample sizes

Oakland, CA: *N = 330*[a]	Philadelphia, PA: *N = 337*	New York, NY: *N = 384*	Jacksonville, FL: *N = 100*
Austin, TX: *N = 326*	Richmond, VA: *N = 327*	San Jose, CA: *N = 326*[a]	Toledo, OH: *N = 101*
Baltimore, MD: *N = 338*	Corpus Christi, TX: *N = 331*	Boston, MA: *N = 99*	San Antonio, TX: *N = 100*
Detroit, MI: *N = 327*[a]	Indianapolis, IN: *N = 325*	Nashville, TN: *N = 102*	Pittsburgh, PA: *N = 100*
Newark, NJ: *N = 342*[a]	Milwaukee, WI: *N = 348*	Chicago, IL: *N = 155*	Norfolk, VA: *N = 99*

[a]Newark, Oakland, Detroit, and San Jose were strategically selected due to funder interest and therefore are not part of the FFCWS "national sample"

randomly sampled from the 19 remaining cities, with selection probability based on city populations. In the 8 "extreme policy" cities, the plan was to collect data on 250 nonmarital births and 75 marital births, for a total of 325. In the other 8 cities, the plan was to sample a total of 100 births. The "large sample" cities provided an ability to understand the social and policy environment and social processes within cities, as well as differences between cities. The eight "small sample" cities, selected from the cells with at least one middle value, improved the ability to observe nonlinearities in the effects of welfare, child support, and labor markets.

The 16 cities randomly selected along the systematic stratified sampling plan comprise the "national sample" of the FFCWS.[3] Four additional cities were added to the study, given their special substantive interest to funders. Table 1 lists the cities sampled in the FFCWS, whether they were selected as part of the national (i.e., random) sample and their baseline sample sizes.

The FFCWS is not only designed to be nationally representative of births in large cities but to offer detailed case studies of the included cities themselves. Hospitals were systematically sampled in order to increase coverage of nonmarital births, which led to a full sample of 75 hospitals (see Reichman et al. 2001, for the full list of included hospitals). Within each hospital, mothers of new babies were sampled from maternity ward lists. Once sampled, mothers were asked to complete a screening instrument to determine marital status and eligibility for participation in the study. Quotas were set at each hospital for the number of unmarried and married births, based on sample cities' 1996/1997 unmarried birth rates. Marital and nonmarital births were randomly sampled until preset quotas were reached for each hospital. If a mother was determined to be above the set quota for a given marital status, the case was coded "over quota," and the mother was not interviewed. In the rare cases that surveyed parents had had twins or a higher-order multiple birth, one child was designated the "focal child," the child to whom answers to the FFCWS refer.

The FFCWS oversample of nonmarital births, coupled with the significantly higher rates of nonmarital childbearing among blacks and Hispanics noted in Fig. 1, provided a study sample with a significantly higher representation of non-white families than most household surveys. Racial and ethnic classification of the mothers and fathers in the survey are provided in Table 2.

Several subgroups of parents were not included in the study: those who did not speak English or Spanish well enough to complete the interview, those who planned to place the child for adoption, those for whom the father of the baby was deceased, those whose baby died before the interview could take place, those mothers who were too ill to complete the interview (or

[3]Two cities (Baltimore and San Jose) were selected in a second round of sampling, when the research team was unable to gain access to hospitals in two of their initially sampled cities (Birmingham, AL and Santa Ana, CA).

Table 2 Racial and ethnic composition, FFCWS sample

	Mothers (%)	Fathers (%)
White, non-Hispanic	21	18
Black, non-Hispanic	47	49
Hispanic (all races)	27	28
Other races and ethnicities	4	4
Race/ethnicity unknown	<1	1
Total	100	100

Note: Mothers' race-ethnicity are based on self-reports. Fathers' race-ethnicity are based on a mix of self-reports and mother reports

whose babies were too ill for the mother to complete the interview), and, in many hospitals, parents who were under 18 and therefore prohibited by the hospital from being interviewed (Reichman et al. 2001). Because the study was designed to examine the roles of mothers and fathers in families, the study is also limited to births to heterosexual couples. As the sample is hospital-based, home births and births in other venues are also not represented. With these and other slight exceptions, the FFCWS sample is representative of the nonmarital births taking place in each city. However, the marital sample is not necessarily representative of marital births in each city because in many cities, births were purposively sampled from hospitals with the highest rates of nonmarital births. It is also important to note that the sample is representative of nonmarital births taking place in each city rather than of births to residents of each city (Reichman et al. 2001), since parents giving birth within the city may live elsewhere.

2.2 Sampling Weights

Due to the complex sampling design of the FFCWS, the data are provided with sampling weights to make the data representative of the sample cities and of urban births nationally. These weights account for the stratified random sample of cities, the sample of hospitals, and the sample of births, as well as the clustering of births by hospital, the oversample of nonmarital births, the underrepresentation of teen births, and mothers' marital status, education, race/ethnicity, and age. The survey includes six sets of weights: to make the data nationally representative and representative of sample cities, for couples and for mothers and fathers separately. These weights are provided for the five waves of data currently available, to account not only for design but for baseline nonresponse and attrition over time (Carlson 2008; CRCW 2008a, b).

2.3 Timing of Interviews

Baseline interviewing for the FFCWS took place over 3 years, between 1998 and 2000. Couples were subsequently contacted for re-interview in four additional waves, reflecting various developmental stages of the focal child's life. Interviews took place when the focal children were 1, 3, 5, and 9 years of age, and a sixth wave of the study is currently in the field (interviewing the families while the focal children are 15 years old.) Due to the short time that elapsed between the early interviews, some families were interviewed for their Year 1 (Y1) follow-up before baseline interviewing was completed for all families, for their Year 3 (Y3) follow-up before Y1 interviewing was completed, and for Year 5 (Y5) follow-up before Y3 interviewing was completed.

Because interviews were carried out over approximately 3 years in each wave, many of the early interviews provided valuable information to improve the survey while it was ongoing. Interviews took place in the first two cities (Oakland, CA and Austin, TX) approximately a full year before interviewing began in the remaining 18 cities, and the early interviews served as a form of pilot test. If questions were not well understood by the respondents, or responses did not have sufficient variation to permit meaningful analysis, these questions were revised before interviewing in the remaining 18 cities.

It also bears noting that considerable time may elapse between father and mother interviews within the same family. Of the families in which both mothers and fathers were interviewed at baseline, more than half (55%) of couples were interviewed on the same day. However, in more than 10% of families, parents were interviewed more than 1 month apart. By Year 9 (Y9), only 15% of parents who both participated were interviewed on the same day. More than 30% were interviewed more than 1 month apart from their partners, with a small number interviewed over a year apart. It is quite possible that discrepancies in mothers' and fathers' reports of family circumstance reflect differences in timing as well as differences in perspective and other traditional sources of measurement error.

2.4 Attrition and Retention

The FFCWS has been unusually successful in collecting data on its generally hard-to-reach target population. Core response rates are provided in Table 3 for mothers and fathers, by their baseline marital status. Mothers' baseline response rates are computed as the percent of mothers approached for interview who agreed to participate. Fathers' results at baseline are computed as the percent of mothers interviewed at baseline whose partners agreed to participate. Response rates in subsequent waves are computed as a percent of the couples interviewed at baseline who participated in subsequent waves. Even among the hardest-to-reach population, unmarried fathers, the majority of the sample was retained in the survey at the 9-year follow-up wave. Nearly all fathers (96% of fathers married at baseline and 87% of unmarried fathers) were interviewed at least once.

2.5 Couple Data

Another way in which the FFCWS provides unique information into its hard-to-reach target population is by the collection of couple data. Not only does the "magic moment" of the focal child's birth provide an opportunity to identify fathers who might not otherwise be located, information on these fathers is not only provided through personal interviews but also through the data collected from their partners. Mothers report not only on their own background and behavior and their personal perception of the couple relationship, but they also report detailed information on their partners' own background and behavior. This information includes the fathers' racial and ethnic background, place of residence, and educational attainment, as well as behavioral information such as labor market activity, incarceration history, parenting behavior, and other aspects of father involvement (e.g., child support payment and visitation). Likewise, fathers are asked to report on similar domains of the mothers' background and behavior.

Couple data provides value in two important ways. When both parents are interviewed, concordance or disagreement between the two parents' responses can be used to assess many domains of their relationship, subject to differences in the phrasing of some questions and the timing of each parent's interview. When only one parent is interviewed, responses about their partner provide information not directly obtainable. This is particularly important given the factors likely to influence attrition and retention. If the fathers least involved with their partners and

Table 3 Response rates, FFCWS core biological parent survey

	Mother		Father	
	Unmarried (%)	Married (%)	Unmarried (%)	Married (%)
Baseline	87	82	75	89
Year 1	90	91	71	82
Year 3	88	89	69	82
Year 5	87	86	67	78
Year 9	76	75	58	70
Ever			87	96

children are the most likely to leave the survey, analyses based only on those retained are likely to be affected by selection bias. Collecting mothers' reports of father characteristics helps to reduce this bias.

3 Current Data Availability

3.1 Data Access

As noted, five waves of FFCWS data collection have been completed as of time of writing. A sixth wave of data collection is ongoing. Baseline, Y1, Y3, Y5, and Y9 core follow-up data are available to the public through the data archive at the Office of Population Research (OPR) at Princeton University. These data, excluding Y9, are also available through the Inter-university Consortium for Political and Social Research (ICPSR). In-home data from the Y3, Y5, and Y9 waves are also available for a subset of core respondents. Additional data, described below, are available to the public via a restricted use contract.

The FFCWS restricted-use dataset (also known as the "contract data") contain more sensitive information such as geographic identifiers (i.e., the city where the focal child was born and state of respondent residence), census tract characteristics, local macroeconomic measures, genetic data, medical records data, and school characteristics. More information on these measures is provided in Appendix B. While these indicators are invaluable for researchers who are interested in children's local or school environments, gene-environment interactions, or detailed information about maternal health, it bears noting that the vast majority of FFCWS research is done using the public-use dataset.

Access to the FFCWS contract data is limited to researchers who agree to the terms and conditions contained in the Contract Data Use License. Access is limited to faculty and research personnel at institutions which have an institutional review board (IRB) or human subjects review committee registered with the US Office for Human Research Protections (OHRP) or the National Institutes of Health (NIH). Researchers must obtain IRB approval of their research and data protection plans. Students may use the FFCWS contract data for dissertation research; however, a faculty advisor must serve as the investigator and complete the application process, with the student signing a Supplemental Agreement with Research Staff form. The faculty advisor and the institution bear full responsibility for ensuring that all conditions of the license are met by the student. Further information about the data access process for both the public- and restricted-use files is available in Appendix B.

3.2 Data Modules

In every wave, participating mothers and fathers each completed a "core" survey, administered in-person for most baseline interviews and by phone in most subsequent interviews. For both mothers and fathers, each core interview included questions on household and family characteristics (including a household roster and parents' marital and coresidence status, as well as contact between nonresident parents and the focal child); sociodemographic and background characteristics; information on parenting behavior; romantic relationships (with the focal biological child's other biological parent or, where relevant, with new partners); details about each parent's health, education, employment, and income; as well as indicators of the focal child's health development and wellbeing. Many of the indicators in the core are collected using the same survey questions at each wave, enabling longitudinal analyses of family trajectories. Details on the data collected in the FFCWS core are provided in Sect. 4. In addition to the data available in the core, both the FFCWS public- and restricted-use files contain several other modules with additional information. These include in-home observations, supplemental surveys, official records, and genetic data.

3.2.1 In-Home Module (Public and Restricted Use)

In addition to the data collected by phone from both mothers and fathers in the FFCWS core data, both the public- and restricted-use files include an in-home module in the Y3, Y5, and Y9 waves. The in-home module includes several assessments of the child and his or her home environment and a survey of the child's primary caregiver (PCG), defined as person the focal child lives with at least half the time. The PCG, who can be either the biological mother or father, or a nonparental figure such as a grandparent, is interviewed in the Y3, Y5, and Y9 survey waves. Interviews include a mix of in-person and self-administered questionnaires conducted in the home and questions asked over the phone.

The PCG survey covers information about the child's home and neighborhood environment, including questions of neighborhood safety, the availability of household resources, parenting behaviors, and childcare arrangements. The PCG also provides details of the focal child's health development, which are best reported by the person the focal child spends the most time with. It is notable, however, that which questions are answered in the PCG survey and which are answered by the biological parents in the core survey vary by wave.

In addition, the in-home module in all three waves includes several systematic assessments by the interviewer, including the focal child's general health and cognitive health development, the PCG's health and cognitive abilities, and assessments of the home and neighborhood environment. These include measures of the height and weight of both the PCG and child, cognitive tests of both the PCG and child, and recorded observations of interactions between the PCG and child.

In the most recent wave (Y9), the in-home assessment also includes an interview of the focal child. In the "child survey," the focal child provides his or her perspective on the home environment, including relationships with each of their biological parents, as well as any new partners that the parents are married to or living with. The child also reports on the extent of discipline and monitoring provided by their primary caregiver and discipline provided by each of their biological parents and any new partners. The focal child also reports on relationships with his or her siblings and how and with whom he or she spends time. He or she provides self-reports of personal information that might not be accurately assessed by the parents or PCG, including health, personal safety, his or her school environment, school connectedness, bullying and bully victimization, and several aspects of behavior, including early delinquent behavior.

3.2.2 Childcare Provider and Teacher Surveys (Public and Restricted Use)

In the Y3 survey, families using nonparental childcare for at least 7 hours per week, and one consistent childcare arrangement for at least 5 hours per week, were asked if a representative of the childcare program could be interviewed. A subset of these parents and childcare providers consented to be interviewed and observed. The childcare provider survey included information on the focal child's behavior, social skills, and learning, as well as characteristics of the program. In many cases the interviewer also observed interactions between the provider and the child.

In Y5 and Y9, the focal child's teachers were also asked to participate in the survey. Teachers who agreed completed a self-administered questionnaire and provided characteristics of their classroom, the school climate, and their assessment of the child's behavior, social skills, and learning, as well as the parents' involvement. The teacher surveys did not include administrative details of the school itself; further information provided on the child's school is provided in the restricted-use file and described in Sect. 2.4.

3.2.3 Medical Records (Restricted Use Only)

Approximately 75% of the mothers interviewed at the FFCWS baseline gave permission for their medical records to be abstracted for analysis. These records contain detailed quantitative and qualitative data on the mother's health and healthcare history, including details of her reproductive history, such as how many previous pregnancies she had had before the focal child was born, and how much weight she gained during the pregnancy. The FFCWS medical records data also contain other anthropomorphic measures (such as the mother's weight and the child's birth weight), indicators of chemical substances in the body at the time of the birth, and diagnoses, including both physical and mental health. The medical records data provides a rich narrative of the mother's health at the time of the birth and serves to identify inconsistencies in maternal self-reports.

3.2.4 School Characteristics File (Restricted Use Only)

At the Y9 follow-up survey, data on the focal child's school was collected by the National Center for Education Statistics (NCES). Although the names and locations of the school are not released in the restricted-use file, a unique identifier is provided for each school in the file, so that children attending the same school can be identified. The NCES data include information on whether the school is a public or private school, the school's grade span (i.e., the grades taught in the school), the racial composition of the student population, Title I funding and eligibility (United States Department of Education 2014), an indicator of socioeconomic disadvantage among the students, and the percent of the student body eligible for free or reduced price lunches.

3.2.5 "Neighborhood" Contextual Data File (Restricted Use Only)

Neighborhood data for both mothers and fathers are measured at each wave. "Neighborhoods" in the FFCWS are defined as each parent's census tract of residence, though to protect respondent privacy, the tract identifiers are coded, and respondents cannot be matched to a specific tract in the restricted-use files. In addition, some random noise has been introduced into the data to ensure that respondents' census tracts cannot be identified from the data. This noise should have no impact on analyses. The contextual data file is based on the US Census and contains information on the tracts' racial composition, local employment and income levels, housing characteristics and rent, and receipt of public assistance.

3.2.6 Macroeconomic Data File (Restricted Use Only)

In addition to tract-level contextual data, the FFCWS has recently released broader contextual data for restricted use. The macroeconomic data file contains information on the national and local economic climate facing both mothers and fathers in the month of their interview. This file is based on MSA-level data from the US Bureau of Labor Statistics, on employment, unemployment, and labor force participation in the MSA containing their sample city, as well as monthly population data in both the MSA and sample state. The file also contains national-level data from the Survey of Consumers on the Consumer Sentiment Index in the month of interview. These data, coupled with the fact that Y9 data collection in the FFCWS took place between August 2007 and March 2010, permit unique analyses of the Great Recession and the effects of economic downturns on families and children (Pilkauskas et al. 2012).

3.2.7 Genetic Data (Restricted Use Only)

In the Y9 wave of data collection, in addition to the survey data collected from parents, children, and teachers, and the administrative data collected to supplement the surveys, the in-home module included the collection of genetic data. More than half of families in the study – and more than 75% of families participating in the Y9 in-home survey – provided noninvasive saliva samples for genotyping. The goal of the genetic data collection was to allow researchers to directly incorporate genetic information into their models of family relationships and child development and to test hypotheses about the relationships between genes, environment, and child health development. Saliva samples were sealed into containers with a liquid preservative and mailed to the survey subcontractor, where they were in turn shipped to the Princeton

University Molecular Biology laboratory, where genetic information was extracted and quantified into genetic markers such as single nucleotide polymorphisms (SNPs) and telomere length (CRCW 2013).

The genetic data file includes results from the genotyping of several candidate polymorphisms hypothesized to influence child health development through their interactions with children's social environments. These candidate polymorphisms include serotonin transporters, dopamine transporter, dopamine D2 receptor, dopamine D4 receptor, catechol-O-methyltransferase, melanocortin 4 receptor, transmembrane protein, and tryptophan hydroxylase. Further information on the specific polymorphisms included in the data file, the genotyping process and quality control mechanisms for each, and valuable references for the study of gene-environment interactions, are available through the Center for Research on Child Wellbeing (2015). At the time of writing, additional data are being developed in conjunction with active research programs, for future release. Data users are encouraged to check the FFCWS home page for up-to-date information.

3.3 Module Participation Rates

Although not all of the data collection modules were completed for each family at each wave, the majority of modules were completed for a substantial majority of families at the waves they were offered. Table 4 provides the participation rates for each of the data collection modules by wave.

4 Using the FFCWS

As noted in Sect. 3.1, FFCWS data can be obtained through two different processes: public access and the contract process for accessing restricted-use data. The access details described in this section apply only to the public-use file. The remainder of this section lays out details of the FFCWS data, which apply to both the public- and restricted-use data.

4.1 Data Access

The FFCWS public-use files can be accessed through a two-step process: users must first register with the data archive at the Princeton University Office of Population Research and then sign up for access to the FFCWS. Registration applications are usually reviewed within one business day. Public-use files, not including Y9, are also available through the Inter-university Consortium for Political and Social Research (ICPSR); however, the Princeton archive has the most current data files and is preferential for scientific research. Access protocols for the

Table 4 Participation rates, FFCWS modules by wave

	Baseline	Year 1	Year 3	Year 5	Year 9
Primary caregiver survey			3258 (67%)	2981 (61%)	3630 (74%)
In-home assessments			2618 (53%)	2376 (49%)	3346 (68%)
Child survey					3375 (69%)
Childcare provider/teacher survey			810 (17%)	1039 (21%)	2254 (46%)
Medical records data file	3684 (75%)				
School data file					3595 (73%)
Neighborhood contextual data file	4725 (96%)	4261 (87%)	4078 (83%)	4251 (87%)	3744 (76%)
Macroeconomic data file	4897 (100%)	4456 (91%)	4365 (89%)	4295 (88%)	3735 (76%)
Genetic data file					2908 (59%)

restricted-use file are available from the Center for Research on Child Wellbeing at Princeton University (CRCW 2009a).

4.2 Data Structure

In both the public- and restricted-use datasets, the FFCWS data are structured with one record per child and identified with a unique family identifier, a string variable called *idnum*. At each wave, mother and father data are stored in separate files and can be merged using the *idnum* variable to match members of the same family. The other modules described in Sect. 3 can also be merged to the core data using the *idnum* variable. Each core dataset has records for all 4898 families, regardless of whether each parent was interviewed. Flag variables indicate whether or not a mother or father was interviewed at a given wave, and cases who didn't participate in a given interview/wave are coded as "not in wave" on all other variables.[4]

4.3 Variable Documentation

The complete merged FFCWS dataset contains more than 10,000 variables, covering a wide variety of domains used in life course health development research. These include parents' demographic information, parental relationships, relationships the parents may form with new partners, relationships between each parent and the focal child, relationships between parents' new partners and the focal child, child wellbeing, health, behavior, and other aspects of health development. The data also contain information on the focal child's physical and social environments, including parental employment, household income and economic wellbeing, parental health and behavior, parental incarceration, social support and other family relationships, housing and neighborhood quality, and access to government programs. Not all domains are covered in each wave of the FFCWS and where each domain appears in the survey varies across waves. Each topic can be located within the five available waves using the FFCWS Core Question Map (CRCW 2009b), which lists in which waves a given topic appears; whether a topic is covered by mothers, fathers, or both; and in which section of the survey. Additionally, there is an In-Home Questionnaire Map for Y3 and Y5. Complete questionnaires are also available on the documentation page of the FFCWS website.

4.3.1 Variable Structure and Construction

Other than the variable *idnum*, which identifies families across data modules, core FFCWS variables are named according to a consistent convention. Core variable names begin with either an *m* or an *f*, depending on whether it was reported by the mother or father, respectively, followed by an indicator of the wave in which it was asked (1 = baseline, 2 = 1 year, 3 = 3 years, 4 = 5 years, and 5 = 9 years), followed by a letter and number to indicate the section and question where it appears in the survey instrument. For example, the variable *m1a12* refers to the mother's baseline survey and the 12th question of section *a*. Variables from the in-home survey are stored in separate modules and are numbered only with a letter and number to indicate section and question.[5] The Y9 dataset includes several additional variable prefixes to accommodate the additional modules described in Sect. 3.2 (CRCW 2011).

Variables in the FFCWS data are also characterized by a consistent schema for responses and

[4] In Y9, there were several types of interviews a PCG may have participated in, so it was possible for them to be coded as "not in wave" for one interview but to participate in a different interview, technically in the same wave. For example, a mother who is the PCG might have participated in the mother core survey but not completed the PCG self-administered questionnaire.

[5] It is important to note that many variable names are used in both the Y3 and Y5 in-home modules, and will need to be renamed for unique identification, usually by adding prefixes (i.e., ih3, ih4), if the variables are used together in a single data file. Future data updates may correct for this by including variable prefixes.

Table 5 Missing data codes in the FFCWS

Numeric code	Meaning	Explanation
-9	Not in wave	Respondent was not interviewed in wave
−8	Out of range	Rare code suggests the response was not appropriate for the question
−7	Did not apply	Also indicated at times by −10 or −14
−6	Skipped question	Question skips are usually dictated by survey design, indicating that a given question did not apply to a given respondent or the answer could be inferred from information already provided
−5	Not asked	This code is most often used when a question was added or taken away following the Oakland and Austin "pilot" interviews. Respondents not receiving the new (or removed) question are coded −5
−3	Missing	Missing for some reason not otherwise listed
−2	Don't know	
−1	Refuse	

Note: In the Y9 survey, a PCG could be coded as "not in wave" for a portion of the survey, but present for other components – if, for example, the PCG participated in the core survey but not the in-home.

missing data. All substantive responses appear in the data as positive numbers. Nonnumeric variables are also coded as positive integers, and their substantive meaning is indicated in the questionnaires and embedded variable labels. (For example, "Yes" answers are usually coded as 1, and "No" answers are usually coded as 2.) Missing responses are indicated with negative numbers, with different negative values indicating different reasons that the data are missing. Details on the missing data codes are provided in Table 5.

The FFCWS dataset also includes numerous variables constructed by CRCW staff to ensure that commonly used concepts are coded consistently by all users. At baseline, examples of constructed variables include the baby's sex, whether or not the birth was of multiple children (i.e., twins), whether the baby had low birth weight (i.e., less than 2500 grams), the ethnicity and race of both parents, and each parent's educational attainment at baseline. At Y1, additional variables were constructed to note the mother's age when she first had a baby and the total number of biological children she had. At Y3, variables were constructed to indicate each parent's cognitive ability (Wechsler 1981). Several other variables were constructed to indicate household composition (along with a second variable to indicate whether the child's grandparents lived in the household), fathers' incarceration histories, whether each parent reported depression and anxiety, and several details of the interview itself – whether it was conducted in Spanish, whether each parent was interviewed, and whether the primary caregiver participated in the in-home study.

4.3.2 Variable Content

The FFCWS data, collected through multiple methods, contains a rich set of child health and behavioral indicators, measures of parental resources and behavior, as well as indicators of parents' physical mental health, health behaviors, incarceration histories, and relationship stability before and since the focal birth. A summary of information collected to date is provided in Table 6, along with the modes of collection used for each class of data.

4.3.3 Tracking Constructs Over Time

One of the strengths of the FFCWS for life course health development research is the consistent measure of multiple substantive constructs across waves of the study. Many of the questions on child health were asked in each wave: parents or primary caregivers are asked to report the focal child's general health status, whether he or she has any physical disabilities, and whether he or she has had any experience with asthma – a diagnosis or an attack, with particular attention to whether the attack required a visit to the emergency room. Parents and caregivers are also asked to report children's medical visits at each wave, including doctor's visits for preventive care, illnesses, and accidents, as well

Table 6 Summary of data collected, FFCWS baseline through year 9 waves

Construct	Data collection method
Child health and development	
Child physical health: health status, developmental milestones, medical conditions, injuries, dental hygiene, exposure to tobacco smoke, physical and developmental disabilities, child height and weight at Y3, Y5, Y9	Interview and assessment
Child mental health: Child Behavioral Checklist (internalizing, externalizing, and various subscales such as aggression, withdrawal, and anxious/depressed) at Y3, Y5, and Y9. Somatic symptoms at Y9, child's report of early delinquency, task completion, sibling relationships, and emotional wellbeing at Y9. Adaptive Social Behavior Inventory at Y9	Interview and assessment
Child's use of medical care: doctor's visits, emergency care, hospitalizations	Interview
Child's health at birth: gestational age, APGAR score, weight and length	Medical records
Child's nutrition: foods consumed, frequency of snacking, use of vitamin supplements	Interview
Daily routines: TV and videogame use, hours of sleep, meals with family	Interview
Cognitive development: Peabody Picture Vocabulary Test (Y3, Y5, Y9), Woodcock-Johnson (Y5, Y9), Forward-Backward Digit Span (Y9)	Assessment
Child relationships: Attachment Q-Sort (Y3), 5-Min Speech Sample (Y5, Y9), mother-child relationship, mothers' perceptions of the father-child relationship	Interview and assessment
Household characteristics	
Household roster: current members, characteristics of new household members	Interview
Child's living arrangements: history between survey waves	Interview
Economic status: employment, earnings, income, public/private transfers, material hardship	Interview
Housing and neighborhoods: Mobility, quality, safety	Interview and observation
Incarceration: current status and history of parents and new partners	Interview
Family relationships	
Bio-parents' relationship and new partners: quality of romantic relationship, cooperation, co-parenting, violence	Interview
Social support: relatives, friends, church attendance, civic participation	Interview
Parental health and cognitive ability	
Physical health: self-rated health, height and weight, smoking, drug and alcohol use, pregnancy risk factors, obstetrical information, and information on delivery of focal child (mothers only)	Medical records
Mental health: anxiety and depression, impulsivity, mental health history, perceived stress	Interview
Cognitive ability: Wechsler Adult Intelligence Scale (Y3); Peabody Picture Vocabulary Test (primary caregiver, English dominant), Testo de Vocabulario en Imagenes Peabody (primary caregiver, Spanish dominant)	Assessment
Parenting	
Nurturance and discipline: HOME, Conflicts Tactics Scales, emotional closeness, supervision	Interview and observation
Cognitive stimulation: reading, materials for cognitive stimulation in home (from HOME assessment)	Interview and observation
Child protective services involvement: whether reported to CPS; disposition of the report	Interview
Childcare/schooling	
Childcare use: time spent in childcare, types and stability of childcare arrangements, cost of care, parents' involvement in childcare centers/kindergarten, connections to other parents	Interview
Childcare/kindergarten: ratings of daycare (Y3), kindergarten (Y5), classroom size, type of instruction, school climate	Observation
Elementary school (Y9): school, classroom, and teacher characteristics, child's behavior, special education services, comparative academic performance, parental involvement, connectedness to school	Interview

as any visits to the hospital or emergency room. Many indicators of the family's social environment were also asked in similar formats across waves, such as parents' reports of relationship quality and co-parenting.

Other family characteristics differ slightly from one wave to the next; for example, parents are asked to report on between 8 and 14 indicators of material hardship in each of the Y1, Y3, and Y5 waves. These measures may be reconciled by analyzing only the eight indicators that appear in all three waves or can be used in their differing format. Still other characteristics, particularly those related to child health development, would be inappropriate to measure in the same way in all waves (e.g., questions on child behavior, cognitive development, and puberty onset). The FFCWS measures are selected and designed to be age-appropriate at the time they are asked. Researchers maintain considerable flexibility in ways to model child cognitive and behavioral health trajectories over time.

5 Looking Ahead

In addition to the rich data that has been collected in the FFCWS to date, the study is currently in the field for a new round of data collection. This data collection is timed around the focal child's 15th birthday (hereafter "Year 15" or "Y15") and designed to improve understanding of how children's experiences in early and middle childhood influence adolescent behaviors. Adolescence is a critical period in human development when children engage in both positive and negative behaviors with lasting consequences for future health and wellbeing. The new wave of the FFCWS will provide new information about how children's adolescent outcomes are influenced by their experiences in infancy and early childhood.

Data in the Y15 wave is being collected through a series of new measures, as well as measures from existing waves that have been expanded to capture children's experiences directly from their self-report. Key areas of expansion include sexual activity (and particularly risky sexual activity), school performance and engagement, delinquency, civic and extracurricular participation, pro-social behaviors, pubertal development, substance use and abuse, sleep, physical activity, eating, multimedia exposure, and a variety of other measures of adolescent health and wellbeing. The Y15 survey is also collecting data on the focal child's relationships with both his or her biological parents, any new partners, and siblings, in order to understand how family complexity and instability influence family interactions and adolescent wellbeing. Finally, the Y15 wave will include new collection of genetic information through additional saliva samples.

The new data will facilitate research on topics related to adolescent risk; the role of the family in shaping adolescent outcomes; racial and ethnic, gender, and income disparities in adolescent health development; and the role of gene-environment interactions in adolescent development. Data collection is scheduled to be completed by 2017, and the data will be cleaned and released for limited and public use in the coming years.

6 Key Resources for Users

In addition to the rich data resources available in the FFCWS, Princeton's Center for Research on Child Wellbeing (CRCW) and the Columbia Population Research Center (CPRC), as the home institutions of the study, devote considerable material and intellectual resources to the community of data users. In addition to the data and extensive documentation available online, CRCW staff maintain an online database of working papers and publications using the FFCWS. Data users are encouraged to publish their working papers and submit their publications for inclusion in the database. CRCW also publishes a series of research briefs based on FFCWS publications, which are both available from the FFCWS website and distributed to a broad audience of researchers, policymakers, and advocates. Finally, CRCW staff are available to answer questions about the study. In addition,

FFCWS researchers host an annual 3-day workshop at CPRC to train new users of the data on the capabilities and use of the dataset. A complete list of FFCWS resources is available in Appendix C.

Fragile Families and Child Wellbeing Study Funders

Government Agencies

R01-HD-36916 from the Eunice Kennedy Shriver National Institute of Child Health and Human Development
5P30-HD-32030 from the Eunice Kennedy Shriver National Institute of Child Health and Human Development through the Office of Population Research, Princeton University
National Science Foundation
US Department of Health and Human Services (ASPE and ACF)

Foundation Support

California HealthCare Foundation
The Center for Research on Religion and Urban Civil Society at the University of Pennsylvania
Commonwealth Fund
Ford Foundation
Foundation for Child Development
Fund for New Jersey
William T. Grant Foundation
Healthcare Foundation of New Jersey
William and Flora Hewlett Foundation
Hogg Foundation
Christian A. Johnson Endeavor Foundation
Kronkosky Charitable Foundation
Leon Lowenstein Foundation
John D. and Catherine T. MacArthur Foundation
A.L. Mailman Family Foundation
Charles Stewart Mott Foundation
David and Lucile Packard Foundation
Public Policy Institute of California
Robert Wood Johnson Foundation
St. David's Hospital Foundation
St. Vincent Hospital and Health Services

Accessing the FFCWS Contract Dataset

The FFCWS restricted-use data includes six add-on files:

- A geographic file with variables for the focal child's birth city, mother's and father's state of residence at each interview, and the family's stratum and primary sampling unit
- Medical records data for mothers and children from the birth hospitalization record (see Sect. 3.2.3 for further information)
- A school characteristic file based on National Center for Education Statistics data (see Sect. 3.2.4 for further information)
- A set of contextual characteristics of each parent's census tract at each wave (see Sect. 3.2.5 for further information)
- A labor market and macroeconomic file with data on local employment and national consumer confidence data (see Sect. 3.2.6 for further information)
- A genetic file for mothers and children drawn from saliva samples (see Sect. 3.2.7 for further information)

To be given access to the contract data, researchers meeting the terms described in Sect. 3.1 must submit two copies of the following items to the Center for Research on Child Wellbeing at Princeton University:

- An extended abstract describing the project and what the Principal Investigator hopes to accomplish, including a one-paragraph justification for why the public-use data will not be sufficient to complete the project.
- Written assurance by the Principal Investigator that his or her institution has an Institutional Review Board (IRB) for Human Subjects which has a Multiple Project Assurance (MPA) or Federalwide Assurance (FWA) from the National Institutes of Health (NIH). The MPA or FWA number must be submitted with the application.
- A data protection plan detailing how the researcher will protect the files while they are

being used, both electronically and any printouts.

- Proof of IRB approval for both the final research plan (the extended abstract in #1) and the final data protection plan (in #3).
- An application fee of $250, payable by check or money order to CRCW.
- A signed Contract Data Agreement by the Principal Investigator.
- A signed Contract Data Agreement by a senior university official who binds the university or institution. This refers to an individual who has the authority to represent the organization in agreements of this sort, such as a Vice President, Dean, Provost, Center Director, or similar official.
- A signed Supplemental Research Agreement with Research Staff for every person who will have access to the data.
- A curriculum vitae for each person who will be accessing the information.
- A copy of the Protecting Human Research Participants web-based training completion certificate from NIH for all research staff who will access the contract data. Proof of equivalent training is also acceptable.

Links to necessary paperwork are available from the Center for Research on Child Wellbeing at Princeton University (CRCW 2009c).

Resources for FFCWS Data Users

Study website

www.fragilefamilies.princeton.edu

Data downloads

www.opr.princeton.edu/archive/ff/

Email questions to

ffdata@princeton.edu

Information on Summer Data Workshops

http://cupop.columbia.edu/research/research-areas/fragile-families-data-workshops

Searchable publications database

http://cupop.columbia.edu/research/research-areas/fragile-families-data-workshops

Includes abstracts, citations, complete working papers, and full articles if the viewing institution has access

Documentation page

www.fragilefamilies.princeton.edu/documentation.asp

Includes questionnaires, guide to the public-use file, core scales documentation, weights documentation and design paper, codebooks including tabulations of all variables, and in-home user's guide

References

Aday, L., & Cornelius, L. J. (2006). *Designing and conducting health surveys* (3rd ed.). San Francisco: Jossey-Bass.

Boutwell, B. B., Beaver, K. M., & Barnes, J. C. (2014). The Association of Parent-Reported Lead Exposure with language skills and externalizing behavioral problems in children. *Journal of Geography & Natural Disasters, 4*(2). doi:10.4172/2167-0587.1000124.

Carlson, B. L. (2008). Fragile families & child wellbeing study: Methodology for constructing mother, father, and couple weights for core telephone public survey data waves 1–4. http://www.fragilefamilies.princeton.edu/documentation/core/weights/const_ffwgts.pdf. Accessed 14 Feb 2015.

Center for Research on Child Wellbeing. (2008a). Fragile families & child wellbeing study: A brief guide to using the mother, father, and couple replicate weights for core telephone surveys waves 1–4. Princeton University Bendheim-Thoman Center for Research on Child Wellbeing. http://www.fragilefamilies.princeton.edu/documentation/core/weights/_vti_cnf/using_ffwgts_rev0709.pdf. Accessed 14 Feb 2015.

Center for Research on Child Wellbeing. (2008b). Fragile families & child wellbeing study: Methodology for constructing mother, father, and couple weights for core telephone public survey data waves 1–4. Princeton University Bendheim-Thoman Center for Research on Child Wellbeing. http://www.fragilefamilies.princeton.edu/documentation/core/weights/const_ffwgts.pdf. Accessed 10 Mar 2015.

Center for Research on Child Wellbeing. (2009a). Fragile families and child wellbeing study restricted use data. http://www.fragilefamilies.princeton.edu/restricted.asp. Princeton University Bendheim-Thoman Center for Research on Child Wellbeing. Accessed 1 Feb 2015.

Center for Research on Child Wellbeing. (2009b). Map of items included in four waves of the fragile families telephone interview. http://www.fragilefamilies.princeton.edu/documentation/core/coreFFqmap.pdf. Princeton University Bendheim-Thoman Center for Research on Child Wellbeing. Accessed 1 Feb 2015.

Center for Research on Child Wellbeing. (2009c). Guide to accessing the fragile families contract data. http://www.fragilefamilies.princeton.edu/documents/restricted_agreement.pdf. Princeton University Bendheim-Thoman Center for Research on Child Wellbeing. Accessed 16 Feb 2015.

Center for Research on Child Wellbeing. (2011). Data user's guide for the nine-year follow-up wave of the fragile families and child wellbeing study. http://www.fragilefamilies.princeton.edu/documentation/year9/year9wave_ff_public.pdf. Princeton University Bendheim-Thoman Center for Research on Child Wellbeing. Accessed 1 Feb 2015.

Center for Research on Child Wellbeing. (2013). *Genetic component of the fragile families and child wellbeing study: Year 9 DNA file*. Princeton: Bendheim-Thoman Center for Research on Child Wellbeing.

Center for Research on Child Wellbeing. (2015). Fragile families genetic component/DNA restricted use data appendage documentation: 9-year follow-up wave. http://www.fragilefamilies.princeton.edu/documentation/collaborative/genetic/ff_gen_9y_pub1.pdf. Princeton University Bendheim-Thoman Center for Research on Child Wellbeing. Accessed 30 June 2015.

Cherlin, A., Frogner, B., Ribar, D., & Moffitt, R. (2009). Welfare reform in the mid-2000s: How African American and Hispanic families in three cities are faring. *Annals of the American Academy of Political and Social Sciences, 621*, 178–201.

Corman, H., Noonan, K., & Reichman, N. E. (2014). Effects of infant health on family food insecurity: Evidence from two US birth cohort studies. *Social Science & Medicine, 123*, 18–25.

Elder, G. H., Jr. (1985). Perspectives on the life course. In G. H. Elder Jr. (Ed.), *Life course dynamics: Trajectories and transitions. 1968–1980* (pp. 23–49). Ithaca: Cornell University Press.

Flanagan, K. D., & West, J. (2004). Children born in 2001: First results from the base year of the Early Childhood Longitudinal Study, Birth Cohort (ECLS-B). http://nces.ed.gov/pubSearch/pubsinfo.asp?pubid=2005036. National Center for Education Statistics. Accessed 14 Feb 2015.

Garfinkel, I., McLanahan, S. S., & Hanson, T. L. (1998). A patchwork portrait of non-resident fathers. In I. Garfinkel, S. S. McLanahan, D. Meyer, & J. Seltzer (Eds.), *Fathers under fire: The revolution in child support enforcement* (pp. 31–60). New York: Russell Sage Foundation.

Geller, A. (2011). Testimony to the New York City Council Committees on General Welfare, Youth Services, Public Safety, Fire and Criminal Justice Services. New York, NY. April 13, 2011.

Graber, J. A., & Brooks-Gunn, J. (1996). Transitions and turning points: Navigating the passage from childhood through adolescence. *Developmental Psychology, 32*(4), 768–776.

Halfon, N., & Forrest, C. B. (2017). The emerging theoretical framework of life course health development. In N. Halfon, C. B. Forrest, R. M. Lerner, & E. Faustman (Eds.), *Handbook of life course health-development science*. Cham: Springer.

Heckman, J. J. (2006). Skill formation and the economics of investing in disadvantaged children. *Science, 312*(5782), 1900–1902.

Holt, E. W., Theall, K. P., & Rabito, F. A. (2013). Individual, housing, and neighborhood correlates of asthma among young urban children. *Journal of Urban Health, 90*(1), 116–129.

Jackson, M., McLanahan, S., & Kiernan, K. (2012). Nativity differences in mothers' health behaviors a cross-national and longitudinal lens. *The Annals of the American Academy of Political and Social Science, 643*(1), 192–218.

Kimbro, R. T., Brooks-Gunn, J., & McLanahan, S. (2007). Racial and ethnic differentials in overweight and obesity among 3-year-old children. *American Journal of Public Health, 97*(2), 298–305. doi:10.2105/AJPH.2005.080812.

Massey, D. S., & Sampson, R. J. (2009). Introduction: Moynihan Redux: Legacies and Lessons. *Annals of the American Academy of Political and Social Sciences, 621*, 6–27.

McLanahan, S. S. (2009). Fragile families and the reproduction of poverty. *Annals of the American Academy of Political and Social Sciences, 621*, 111–131.

McLanahan, S. S., Garfinkel, I., Mincy, R. B., & Donahue, E. (2010). Introducing the issue. *Future of Children, 20*(2), 3–16.

McLanahan, S. S. (2011). Family instability and complexity after a nonmarital birth: Outcomes for children in fragile families. In M. J. Carlson & P. England (Eds.), *Social class and changing families in an unequal America* (pp. 108–133). Stanford, CA: Stanford University Press.

McLanahan, S. S., & Sandefur, G. (1994). *Growing up with a single parent: What hurts, what helps*. Cambridge, MA: Harvard University Press.

Mitchell, C., Hobcraft, J., McLanahan, S. S., Siegel, S. R., Berg, A., Brooks-Gunn, J., Garfinkel, I., & Notterman, D. (2014). Social disadvantage, genetic sensitivity, and children's telomere length. *Proceedings of the National Academy of Sciences, 111*(16), 5944–5949.

Moynihan, D. P. (1965). *The negro family: The case for national action*. Washington, DC: Office of Policy Planning and Research. U.S. Department of Labor.

National Research Council and Institute of Medicine. (2004). *Children's health, the nation's wealth: Assessing and improving child health*. Committee on

Evaluation of Children's Health. Board on Children, Youth, and Families, Division of Behavioral and Social Sciences and Education. Washington, DC: The National Academies Press.

Pilkauskas, N. V. (2014). Breastfeeding initiation and duration in coresident grandparent, mother and infant households. *Maternal and Child Health Journal, 18*(8), 1955–1963.

Pilkauskas, N. P., Currie, J. M., & Garfinkel, I. (2012). The great recession, public transfers, and material hardship. *Social Service Review, 86*(3), 401–427.

Razza, R., Martin, A., & Brooks-Gunn, J. (Forthcoming). Are approaches to learning in Kindergarten associated with academic and social competence similarly? *Child & Youth Care Forum.* doi: 10.1007/s10566-015-9307-0.

Reichman, N. E., & Nepomnyaschy, L. (2008). Maternal pre-pregnancy obesity and diagnosis of asthma in offspring at age 3 years. *Maternal and Child Health Journal, 12*, 725–733.

Reichman, N. E., & Teitler, J. O. (2006). Paternal age as a risk factor for low birthweight. *American Journal of Public Health, 96*(5), 862–866. doi:10.2105/AJPH.2005.066324.

Reichman, N. E., Teitler, J. O., Garfinkel, I., & McLanahan, S. S. (2001). Fragile families: Sample and design. *Children and Youth Services Review, 23*(4/5), 303–326.

Rigby, E., Ryan, R. M., & Brooks-Gunn, J. (2007). Child care quality in different state policy contexts. *Journal of Policy Analysis and Management, 26*(4), 887–908.

Sampson, R. J., & Laub, J. H. (1990). Crime and deviance over the life course: The salience of adult social bonds. *American Sociological Review, 55*(5), 766–779.

Smulian, J., Teitler, J., Nepomnyaschy, L., Anath, C., & Reichman, N. (2005). Intrapartum fever and newborn complications. *American Journal of Obstetrics and Gynecology, 193*(6), S193. doi:10.1016/j.ajog.2005.10.782.

Shonkoff, J. P., & Phillips, D. A. (2000). *From neurons to neighborhoods: The science of early child development.* Washington, DC: National Academy Press.

Sorensen, E., Simms, D. R., Mincy, R. Jones, B., Johnson, J., Garrison, P. J., & Garfinkel, I. (2002). *Recommendations on TANF reauthorization from the strengthening fragile families initiative.* Statement before the U.S. House of Representatives Ways and Means Committee, Subcommittee on Human Resources. http://www.urban.org/publications/900508.html. Accessed 18 Dec 2014.

Suglia, S. F., Solnick, S., & Hemenway, D. (2013). Soft drinks consumption is associated with behavior problems in 5-year-olds. *The Journal of Pediatrics, 163*(5), 1323–1328.

United States Department of Education. (2014). Programs: Improving Basic Programs Offered by Local Educational Agencies (Title I, Part A). http://www2.ed.gov/programs/titleiparta/index.html. Accessed 31 Jan 2014.

Wechsler, D. (1981). *Wechsler adult intelligence scale – Revised (WAIS-R manual).* New York: Harcourt Brace Jovanovich, for the Psychological Corporation.

Wilson, W. J. (1988). *The truly disadvantaged.* Cambridge, MA: Harvard University Press.

9

The Emerging Theoretical Framework of Life Course Health Development

Neal Halfon and Christopher B. Forrest

1 Part 1: Context and Background

Over the last century, we have witnessed the power of the biomedical paradigm to treat the sick and prevent diseases from occurring. Conventional health science, as an applied field, has tried to make sense of what constitutes health by exploring the causes of *disease* in individual patients (medicine) and populations (public health). This approach has created a perspective of health as absence of disease or its risk factors and has been unsuccessful at explaining what it means to be healthy, how health develops over the lifespan, and the impact of health on the lives of individuals.

N. Halfon, MD, MPH (✉)
Department of Pediatrics, David Geffen School of Medicine, UCLA, Los Angeles, CA, USA

Department of Health Policy and Management, Fielding School of Public Health, UCLA, Los Angeles, CA, USA

Department of Public Policy, Luskin School of Public Affairs, UCLA, Los Angeles, CA, USA

Center for Healthier Children, Families, and Communities, UCLA, Los Angeles, CA, USA
e-mail: nhalfon@ucla.edu

C.B. Forrest, MD, PhD
Applied Clinical Research Center, Children's Hospital of Philadelphia, Philadelphia, PA, USA

Concepts of what constitutes health, and theories about how health is produced and optimized, are constantly evolving in response to myriad social and cultural expectations shaped by our contemporary worldview, scientific advances, improvements in health interventions, and the changing capacity of the health system. Stimulated originally by a series of studies demonstrating how growth during early life is related to chronic health conditions that emerge many decades later, an eruption of new research is identifying developmental processes that shape long-term health trajectories (Ben-Shlomo and Kuh 2002; Kuh and Ben-Shlomo 2004; Hanson and Gluckman 2014). This research is demonstrating how complex developmental processes integrate a range of behavioral, social, and environmental influences that modify gene expression, modulate physiologic and behavioral function, and dynamically shape different pathways of health production (Halfon and Hochstein 2002; Kuh and Ben-Shlomo 2004; Halfon et al. 2014). These empirical findings are highlighting the limitations of the more mechanistic biomedical and biopsychosocial models of health, which fail to offer comprehensive explanations about such phenomena as the developmental origins of health, how stress affects current and future health, and the consequences of dynamic interactions between individuals and their environments over time.

Informed by new theoretical perspectives emerging from such fields of study as developmental psychology (Lerner 2012), systems biology (Kitano 2002; Antony et al. 2012; Schadt and Bjorkegren 2012), epigenetics (Egger et al. 2004), the developmental origins of chronic disease (Gluckman and Hanson 2006a), and evolutionary developmental biology (West-Eberhard 2003), a transdisciplinary framework (Gatzweller and Baumuller 2013) is emerging which we call *Life Course Health Development* (*LCHD*) (Halfon and Hochstein 2002, Halfon et al. 2014). As a framework, LCHD organizes several different theories and conceptual models in order to make sense of the enormously challenging question of how health develops over the lifespan.

The LCHD framework addresses the developmental origins of health, the role that biological and behavioral plasticity play in facilitating different levels of adaptation, and how mismatches between biological propensity and environmental context interact to produce breakdowns in health, known as *disease*. As a framework that organizes numerous theories and concepts related to how health develops, LCHD is bridging what have sometimes been assumed to be polar opposites: nature versus nurture, mind versus body, individual versus population, and short-term versus long-term change. By unifying these dichotomies, LCHD offers a new perspective that will guide future scientific inquiry on health development and facilitate a long overdue and needed synthesis of medicine and public health—a synthesis that links treatment, prevention, and health promotion and catalyzes more integrated and networked strategies for designing, organizing, and implementing multilevel health interventions that transcend individual and population dichotomies. The LCHD framework will be increasingly useful as the human ecological footprint expands and influences the health development of Earth itself, creating new threats to human health via rapid and disruptive changes in physical environments, geographic dispersion of populations, and changes in social development.

This emergence of LCHD is reflective of larger scientific trends that are transforming research in the physical, natural, and social sciences. The comfort and certainty of simple, linear, and deterministic causal pathways are giving way to the uncomfortable uncertainty of nonlinear causal clusters that are networked together into complex, multilevel, interactive, and relational systems. LCHD embraces this complexity as the salient target of inquiry and requires research to be conducted with teams that are multidisciplinary, often large, networked, and highly collaborative. These shifts in scientific approach are helping us understand how our modern interdependent world is organized, how it functions, and how it contributes to the production of human health.

Given the explosion of life course-focused research in many scientific fields—including chronic disease epidemiology, developmental neuroscience, developmental psychology, evolutionary biology, genetics, epigenetics, environmental health sciences, economics, sociology, and many more—there is a growing need to provide a systematic framework for understanding and organizing this emerging knowledge base (i.e., sense making) so that it can be more effectively applied to solving health problems and guiding new and productive streams of exploration and discovery.

Our intent is not to provide a grand theory of Life Course Health Development. Rather, we seek to establish a set of principles that describe the contours of the rapidly emerging health development knowledge base by organizing many theories and conceptual models into a coherent synthesis. We recognize that LCHD is a work in progress. Our aim is to create conceptual coherence by contextualizing the meaning of disparate research findings, identifying gaps and uncertainties—including how concepts are defined, operationalized, and interpreted—and moving inquiry, application, and implementation forward. We hope that the principles of LCHD presented here, coupled with our explanatory narrative, will encourage theory building and testing, inspire innovative transdisciplinary research, and mature the framework into a scientific model with descriptive, explanatory, and predictive utility. Furthermore, we hope that LCHD will shine a light on the conundrum of how little attributable risk is explained in many studies of chronic disease, how early experience conditions future biological response patterns, and how these early experiences play through complex, environmentally influenced, and developmentally plastic health development pathways (Table 1).

In Part 2 of this chapter, we describe the ontological pathways—including theories, empirical findings, and concepts—that led to the LCHD framework, thereby orienting our view of health development from simple, mechanistic, and reductionist models to contemporary models that are holistic, complex, dynamically relational, and adaptive. In Part 3, we summarize the principles of the LCHD framework, grounding them in a set of transdisciplinary theories, models, and perspectives and addressing their implications for future inquiry (Fig. 1).

Beginning with the simple, mechanical, and mostly linear biomedical model, we chart how it was transformed into a more hierarchical, dynamic, and multiply determined biopsychosocial model, as the result of scientific breakthroughs in the understanding of the contribution of behavioral, social factors and their influence on individuals during specific life stages. This biopsychosocial model has now evolved into a more complex, relational, adaptive, dynamic, and developmental model of Life Course Health Development (LCHD) as result of the influence of scientific breakthroughs in epigenetics, neurodevelopment, and life course chronic disease epidemiology.

Table 1 Principles of the Life Course Health Development Framework

Principle	Brief description
1. Health Development	Health development integrates the concepts of health and developmental processes into a unified whole
2. Unfolding	Health development unfolds continuously over the lifespan, from conception to death, and is shaped by prior experiences and environmental interactions
3. Complexity	Health development results from adaptive, multilevel, and reciprocal interactions between individuals and their physical, natural, and social environments
4. Timing	Health development is sensitive to the timing and social structuring of environmental exposures and experiences
5. Plasticity	Health development phenotypes are systematically malleable and enabled and constrained by evolution to enhance adaptability to diverse environments
6. Thriving	Optimal health development promotes survival, enhances well-being, and protects against disease
7. Harmony	Health development results from the balanced interactions of molecular, physiological, behavioral, cultural, and evolutionary processes

2 Part 2: Emergence of the Life Course Health Development Framework

The LCHD framework has emerged from a network of theories, conceptual models, and empirical findings and provides a more comprehensive description of how health develops over the life course than any single component part. In this section, we describe the streams of scientific inquiry, the key theories and models, and the seminal scientific insights that are brought together by the LCHD framework. Figure 1 provides an epistemological schematic, charting the changing paradigms of health and how different streams of research and their findings influenced the flow of conceptual models.

A few decades ago, research linked fetal development with degenerative diseases of old age (Ben-Shlomo and Kuh 2002), stimulating new ways of thinking about the mechanisms underlying what was originally termed "fetal programming" and other environmentally induced modifications in gene expression that presumably take place early in life. These insights pointed out the need to better characterize interactions between genes and the environment, to better understand gene regulation that occurs in response to environmental signal transduction, and to better integrate into explanatory models the importance of the timing and phasing of these developmental processes. The prevailing epidemiological framework, with its simple additive, exposure-response models of risk accumulation

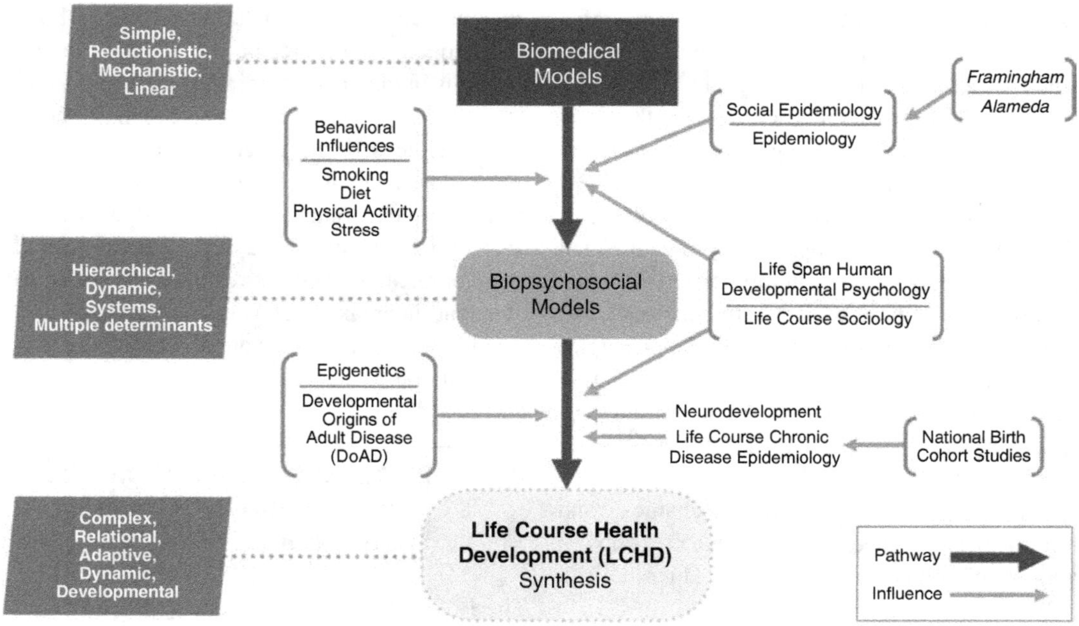

Fig. 1 The evolution of conceptual models of health development

as the etiology for chronic disease in adult life, could not satisfactorily explain these more complex time-dependent phenomena. Instead, a theoretical framework was needed to explain the processes of translating an individual's experiences and exposures into the development of health over the life course.

Two converging streams of biological research and conceptual constructs have contributed to the LCHD framework. The first stream represents the basic biology of human development, informed by the neo-Darwinian synthesis that resulted from the convergence of Darwin's theory of evolution and Mendel's notion of genes as the building blocks of heredity. Although the central dogma of "*genes/DNA → mRNA → proteins*" has served as a foundational construct for modern molecular biology, it led to overly deterministic genotype-to-phenotype models (Huang 2012). Recent advances in panomics (e.g., genomics, epigenomics, proteomics, metabolomics) and systems biology are redefining our understanding of how gene networks are regulated and dynamically interact with each other and the environment, resulting in a new synthesis of biological systems development and functioning (Huang 2012; Forrest 2014; Davila-Velderrain et al. 2015). Breakthroughs in understanding the relationships between evolutionary processes and biological development, and advances in the use of life history theory to explain how mismatches between biological propensities and modern environments influence the onset of disease, have also provided a new way of considering the relationship of an individual's or a population's genetic endowment and the phenotypes that emerge (Del Giudice et al. 2015; Green et al. 2015; Hanson and Gluckman 2014; Lieberman 2014; Gluckman and Hanson 2006a).

The second stream of inquiry, which interacted with genetic concepts and models, represents the evolution of models of disease causation, informed by contributions from basic, clinical, epidemiologic, social, and psychological research disciplines. In the first era of health science, scientific methods applied to medicine resulted in the development of a biomedical framework in which anatomical-pathological disease models, along with other mechanistic constructs, were used to explain why disease develops. One prototypical theoretical construct was germ theory (i.e., germs as the unique causes of infectious diseases) (Stewart 1968). Others included theories of inheritance that were informed by simple and mechanistic notions of genes as the unique causes of inherited disorders and risk status. Several decades of research on the "upstream" social and behavioral determinants of health were stimulated by epidemiologic studies like the Framingham Study and Alameda County Study that highlighted how cardiovascular and other chronic diseases were not caused by bad germs, bad genes, or bad luck, but were related to behaviors like smoking, diet, exercise, and other social factors as well as the metabolic changes that these social and behavioral risk factors induced (Dawber et al. 1974; Haynes 1980; Berkman and Syme 1979). This led to a more dynamic ecological analysis of the multiple risk factors that lead to disease causation, informing the creation of a multi-causal, biopsychosocial framework of disease (Engel 1977). Over the last 20 years, this biopsychosocial model of health has continued to evolve as a result of the integration of concepts from life course research in sociology (Elder 1995; Elder and Shanahan 2007), lifespan developmental research in psychology (Lerner 2012), systems biology (Schadt and Bjorkegren 2012), and longitudinal studies on the origins of chronic disease (Gluckman and Hanson 2004b). The biopsychosocial model undergirds much of the current focus on the social determinants of health and the important role that contextual factors play in shaping health outcomes (McMichael 1999; Krieger 2001).

Midway through the twentieth century, social scientists started examining how the rapidly changing social circumstances of the second industrial revolution were transforming the developmental pathways of different generations. Separate yet related streams of research emerged, converging around notions of the life course, the lifespan, and the human life cycle development. Two lines of investigation in particular have informed recent notions of health development: life course sociology and lifespan human developmental psychology (Diewald and Mayer 2009).

Life course theories emerged in sociology research in the 1960s, championed by Elder, Clausen, and others. These theories distinguished how social institutions and history shape the roles, personal events, transitions, and trajectories of individuals who follow different developmental pathways (Clausen 1986; Elder et al. 2003). Macro-level social processes and social relationships influence interweaving trajectories at different ages, stages, and transitions of development (Elder 1995). Untangling age, period, and cohort effects and understanding the cumulative impact of experience on socially and institutionally constructed life pathways form the basis of life course sociology. For example, the experience of low socioeconomic status, discrimination, and racial segregation may have different effects on health for different cohorts (i.e., groups born at different times), based on prevailing (period effects), compensatory, and mediating factors such as the availability of healthcare or the impact of different social policies (Chen et al. 2010; Masters et al. 2012).

Building on the work of Glen Elder, Duane Alwin (2012) suggested five ways that the term "life course" was used to describe etiologic processes in social and behavioral sciences: (1) lifespan development, humans develop over the life course; (2) agency, individuals construct their lives through choices and actions they take within social structures that provide opportunities and impose constraints; (3) cohort and geographic variation, lives of individuals are embedded and shaped by historical time and place where they live; (4) timing, impact of events, experiences, and transitions are conditional on their timing in a person's life; and, (5) linked lives, people's lives are lived interdependently (e.g., husband and wife, siblings).

Lifespan human developmental psychologists attempt to explain how individual differences emerge at different ages and stages (Lerner 1984; Lerner 2012). These differences are, in part, determined by endogenous characteristics (i.e., each individual's personal adaptability, plasticity, resilience, and reactivity) interacting with exogenous factors (i.e., external physical, social, and psychological environments that promote adaptation). These interactions cause human behavior to continuously change from conception to death (Lerner 1984, 2012). By focusing on the individual's capacity to adapt to events and experiences (Dannefer 1984; Alwin 2012), developmental psychologists have suggested that lifespan human development research concentrates on the plasticity associated with individual development (ontogenesis), whereas life course social sciences researchers emphasize "sociogenesis" or how life pathways are informed and structured by socially constructed developmental scaffolding and constraints. In short, psychologists have tended to focus on how *endogenous or constitutional* ontogenetic processes influence lifelong developmental trajectories, while sociologists have been more concerned with *contextual or exogenous* factors.

Over the past 30 years, there has growing convergence between life course sociology and lifespan human developmental psychology. Research on "linked lives," where the common and differential impact of shared exposures is experienced by individuals whose lives are linked geographically or socially (e.g., spouses, workers in a town, friendship networks) and work on transitions and turning points that are biologically (menarche, menopause) or socially determined (e.g., transitions from preschool to kindergarten, school to work, work to retirement), have each benefited from consideration of endogenous and exogenous factors. As the sociological approaches to life course and psychological approaches to lifespan research converge into a more integrated discipline of developmental science (Cairns et al. 1996; Bornstein and Lamb 2005; Diewald and Mayer 2009), ongoing conceptual and empirical integration is increasingly influenced by the study of nonlinear dynamic systems, including complex adaptive systems theory (Greenberg and Partridge 2010).

Many researchers and thought leaders have contributed to the conceptual evolution and empirical evidence supporting a more integrated developmental systems theory (Sameroff 1975; Bronfenbrenner 1976; Baltes et al. 1980; Lerner 1984; Cicchetti and Cohen 1995; Magnusson 1995; Cairns et al. 1996; Bronfenbrenner and Morris 2006; Sameroff 2010) which built upon earlier behavioral and biological theories (Greenberg and Partridge 2010; Marshall 2014). Overton and Lerner have proposed a theoretical construct that they call "relational developmental systems theory (RDST)" (Lerner 2006; Lerner and Overton 2008). Rejecting what they consider a false dichotomy between individual and context, they suggest that a person's development is embedded in, organized by, and co-regulated by his or her surrounding environments. Developmental regulatory functions are best understood as mutually influential, bidirectional, person-context interactions. RDST sees individuals as active co-developers of their own developmental pathways, adaptively responding to different biological, social, cultural, and physical environmental contexts that they influence and are also influenced by. RDST has been used as a theoretical foundation for research on self-regulation and positive youth development and has added a stronger relational dimension to life course thinking.

Like the converging influences of life course sociology and lifespan human developmental psychology, many fields of the life sciences have also informed this transition toward a life course developmental view of health. Embryologists and teratologists in the first part of the twentieth century understood that environmental insults could disrupt the normal processes of development leading to malformation and other "genetic" abnormalities, and some scientists began to consider how childhood conditions might directly influence adult mortality (Kuh and Davey Smith 2004). But it was not until the 1970s—when Forsdahl suggested a relationship between childhood socioeconomic status and later cardiovascular disease, Barker studied the relationship between birth weight and cardiovascular disease, and Wadsworth observed that other early childhood factors influenced a range of adult health outcomes—that a focus on what is called the developmental origins of adult health and disease (DOHaD) began to emerge (Forsdahl 1977; Arnesen and Forsdahl 1985; Barker et al. 1989a,b; Kuh and Wadsworth 1993).

The receptivity to this new perspective was heightened by a growing number of challenges to the biomedical model of causation. Echoing George Engel and others, social epidemiologists like John Cassel, Leonard Syme, Lisa Berkman, and Michael Marmot and health service researchers like Barbara Starfield began to adopt a more complex, multidimensional "web of causation" construct to explain the origins of disease (Cassel 1964; Starfield 1973; Starfield et al. 1984; Marmot and Syme 1976; Syme and Berkman 1976; Marmot et al. 1978a, b). At the same time, a growing body of new research in psychoneuroimmunology described the "embodiment of disease risk" by demonstrating how different social, cultural, and psychological exposures quite literally "get under the skin" and are encoded or embedded into developing biobehavioral systems (Sapolsky et al. 1985; Maier et al. 1994; Cohen and Herbert 1996; McEwan 1998; Repetti et al. 2002).

Over the past two decades, the Barker hypothesis, as it was commonly referred to, was further elaborated by a series of studies examining the impact of birth weight, fetal growth, placental size, and weight gain in the first year of life on metabolic regulation and cardiovascular disease (Barker et al. 1989a,b, 1993; McMillen and Robinson 2005; Barker et al. 2010). An entire field of life course epidemiology was spawned that has not only confirmed Barker's findings in several other cohorts and settings but vastly expanded the empirical base linking fetal and early childhood growth and nutrition to a growing array of adult health conditions. This work has also gone beyond examining fetal and early childhood origins to explore the developmental origins of health and disease more broadly and has generated various conceptual models to analyze and synthesize results (Schlotz and Phillips 2009; Gluckman et al. 2010; Entringer et al. 2012). A new generation of recent epigenetic studies have begun to provide a stronger biological and theoretical basis for understanding how developmental plasticity is manifested, how gene expression may be modified in response to environmental cues, and how biological and behavioral traits can be perpetuated across multiple generations (Hochberg et al. 2010; Gluckman 2014; Thayer and Kuzawa 2011; Davey Smith 2012; Lillycrop and Burdge 2012; Relton and Davey Smith 2012; Gilbert et al. 2015; Cunliffe 2015).

Complementary studies of the developing brain demonstrated how stress and social adversity influence the biology of human development during sensitive periods (Hertzman 1999; Boyce et al. 2012; Hertzman 2012). Building on earlier studies of experience-dependent and experience-expectant[1] neuronal development, neurodevelopmental research demonstrated how development is guided by the combined and interactive influences of genes and experience (Boyce et al. 2012). Animal models of experience-modified neural development demonstrated how early behavioral experiences of adversity or comfort can lead to different DNA methylation patterns, which are believed to affect gene regulation and result in different functional levels of neurotransmission capacity (Meaney 2001; Szyf et al. 2005; Meaney et al. 2007). Similar methylation alterations have been demonstrated in children who have experienced adversity associated with maternal stress in the early years (Essex et al. 2011). Research on the neurobiology of stress and on the role that cumulative physiologic stress can have on the function of neuroendocrine and neuroimmunologic pathways has provided direct evidence for how exposure to risk and/or highly adverse environments is embedded in lifelong biobehavioral function (Seeman 1997; McEwan 1998; Seeman et al. 2001; Repetti et al. 2011; McEwen 2012). This research on neural development, stress, and biological priming provides an important empirical and conceptual bridge between observed social gradients in health and the experience-dependent conditioning of biobe-

[1] Experience-dependent neuronal development refers to the role that experience plays in fortifying neuronal connections (e.g., a violin player who shows increased synaptic density in the area of the brain corresponding to the motor cortex controlling the fingers, or the hypertrophy of hippocampus in London cab drivers that is associated with improved spatial navigation and spatial memory). Experience-expectant neuronal development refers to brain development that is contingent on experiences that are expected to occur as part of normal development. For example, typical development of the visual cortex occurs in response to visual stimuli that are available in everyday life. If vision is obstructed and the brain does not receive these expected stimuli, the relevant synapses will either not form or will atrophy.

havioral systems that occurs during the process of human development (Hertzman 1999; Keating and Hertzman 1999; Halfon and Hochstein 2002).

In several ways, the converging relationship between life course chronic disease epidemiology, neurodevelopmental, and DOHaD research is analogous to the converging relationship between life course sociology and lifespan human developmental psychology. DOHaD and neurodevelopmental research have focused more on the individual differences in developmental plasticity from early development through old age (ontogenesis), leading to a growing understanding that epigenetic factors influence non-germline heredity. For example, the exposures grandparents experience can influence adaptive responses two generations later. In contrast, life course chronic disease epidemiology has focused more on social class, social gradients, and the social scaffolding of exposures (sociogenesis). New longitudinal cohort studies integrate both perspectives, including not only measures of phenotype but also genetic, epigenetic, and other biobehavioral adaptations (Alfred et al. 2012; Borghol et al. 2012; Elks et al. 2012).

3 Part 3: Principles of the Life Course Health Development Framework

In this section, we present the seven principles of the Life Course Health Development framework that emerged from our analysis of the network of theories, concepts, models, and research findings related to how health develops over the life course.

Each principle is described, connected to relevant theories, models, and perspectives, and discussed in terms of its implications for future research. Together, the principles constitute the LCHD framework, which is proposed as a way of systematically organizing the breadth of theories and conceptual models that help to explain and predict empirical findings on the production of health and disease causation over the life course.

4 Principle 1: Health Development

4.1 What We Mean by "Health Development"

Health development integrates the concepts of health and developmental processes into a unified whole.

We use the term "health development" to signify the framework's central focus, which is the linkage of health and development into a single construct. Health is often understood as a set of instrumental attributes that are employed when individuals pursue goal-directed behavior (Richman 2004; Forrest 2014). These attributes can be thought of as "assets" that are desirable, acquired, optimized, and maintained during the life course, enabling growth of an individual, survival, and adaptation to manifold environments. Examples of health assets that emerge at the level of an individual include motor function (capacity for movement), emotional regulation (capacity to manage emotions during challenges or stressful events), and cognitive function (capacity to perceive, process, and act on information leading to the acquisition of knowledge).

Development, in this context, refers to the processes by which health attributes change (i.e., mature, weather, degrade) during the lifespan. If health is a set of attributes that emerge at the level of the whole individual, development refers to the evolutionarily informed processes by which these attributes enable adaptation to changing social-environmental conditions. Health is the "what" (i.e., what changes) and development is the "how" (i.e., how health attributes change over time) of health development.

As an expression of an organism's livingness and essential adaptive nature, health development is an emergent property of a living system (Forrest 2014). Importantly, because this principle combines both health and development, it blends a temporal dimension into our conceptualization of human health. Health development has time-dependent and transactional connotations and is therefore dynamic.

The health development of an individual at the level of "self" cannot be understood by isolating the biological function (or dysfunction) of an organ system or a particular behavior of an individual—although of course these subsystems have their own unique health development trajectories. The health development of an individual is comprised of an integrated set of capacities that dynamically mature and are involved in managing energy flows; processing and acting on information; recovering from, adapting to, and growing with environmental challenges; learning and forming capabilities; and producing offspring (Forrest 2014). Health development is a life course-informed phenomenon that results from transactions between the organism and its internal (i.e., gene, panomic, organ system, and physiologic networks) and external environments (i.e., family, social, cultural, and physical networks and environments).

4.2 Theories and Frameworks Relevant to Health Development

This principle combines a rich set of theories and conceptual frameworks related to health and development. Conceptualizing health development as an emergent property of an organism differs from earlier linear and reductionistic biomedical models of health and even from multilevel biopsychosocial models. It also sets the stage for considering health development as complex adaptive processes that emerge from living systems interacting with their environments. Its relational ontology implies that other principles contribute to the understanding of this complex emergent process.

The optimization of health development is codependent on several contributing developmental processes and resulting propensities that are highlighted in the other LCHD principles and drawn from relational developmental systems theory (Lerner 2006; Overton 2007), developmental systems theory (Oyama 1985), dynamic systems theory (Spencer et al. 2009), and the unified theory of development (Sameroff 2010)

4.3 Implications of the Health Development Principle

The *health development* principle signals the importance of context and our inability to reduce health to its component parts divorced from the contexts within which they develop. This type of developmental systems thinking requires new typologies to describe health development phenotypes. In effect, a new set of concepts is needed to convey a language of health development as observed and experienced at the level of whole persons in dynamic interaction with their environments. As our understanding of the interrelationships between health development and a range of influential environmental variables matures, health development typologies can become full-fledged ontologies that help explain and predict which relational influences are important and have measurable consequences on health development.

The creation of "whole person" health development metrics that operationalize health development concepts is necessary to capture developmentally influenced continuity, consistency, and variability. To distinguish "health development" from other fields in the developmental sciences, we will need to specify the unique concepts that constitute it and the measures that assess health development's multidimensional functionality (adaptation, energy management, reproduction, information processing, capacity to execute tasks in response, and restoration and their integration) as well as its multilevel (from the molecular to the individual to the environmental) nature. Measures of health development will also need to be informed and reflective of the other LCHD principles outlined below. Such measures will be particularly important in enabling and measuring the contribution of health-producing social systems to the optimization of health development.

5 Principle 2: Unfolding

5.1 What We Mean by "Unfolding"

Health development occurs continuously over the lifespan, from conception to death, and is shaped by prior experiences and environmental interactions.

The *unfolding* principle describes the developmental processes by which expression of a few thousand genes—none of which has a blueprint or roadmap for constituting a viable, living human body—can unfold in an ordered, coherent pattern that has been shaped by the adaptive success of what has worked before. The nonlinear, self-organizing process of development that is made possible by molecule-to-molecule, cell-to-cell, tissue-to-tissue, and human-to-human sensing and communication processes means that health development is neither linear, passive, nor static; rather, it is adaptive, self-organizing, and autocatalytic (Davies 2014).

By "adaptive," we mean those biological, behavioral, and cultural differences that are privileged, prioritized, or selected for because of the advantage they imbue on reproductive fitness and success. Adaptive change occurs at multiple levels, from the biochemical and cellular to behavioral change at the level of individuals to environmental change. For some biological systems, such as neural networks, adaptation occurs quite rapidly, enabling real-time responses to acute environmental challenges and acquisition of novel information. However, some biological and behavioral subsystems change slowly responding to gradual shifts in the intensity and quality of ecological exposures. Thus, the adaptation that characterizes health development transpires over multiple time scales enabling response to both fast- and slow-changing variables. The principles of *complexity* and *timing* will further elaborate on these features of adaptation.

By "self-organizing," we mean the dynamic nonlinear process of self-assembly and self-perpetuation that emerges through multiple relational coactions between the components of a system and its environments. In the case of human health development, it describes how internally determined structures emerge from a genetic code that is regulated by layers of sensing, signaling, and feedback loops that organize the expression of the code based on chemical self-assembly into variable levels and forms of differentiation. Simple differences in external environments (at the cellular, tissue, organ system, organism, or cultural levels) transform the pathways of development from dull uniformity to autocatalytic diversity of forms and function (Davies 2014).

By "autocatalytic," we mean that health development produces the "fuel" that propels it forward (Henrich 2015). Health development dynamically shapes and is shaped by environmental contexts. Today's health development serves as substrate for the emergence of future health development states. The person-environmental transactions that unfold during the life course can influence gene regulation of biobehavioral processes through epigenetic changes. Better characterization of this set of mechanisms is helping to explain how physical and social exposures during childhood affect health and disease during adulthood.

The adaptive, self-organizing, autocatalytic processes of unfolding can help to explain how genes and culture have coevolved. According to Henrich (2015), as humans evolved, cultural information and practices began to accumulate and produce cultural adaptations. These new cultural adaptations feed forward and produce significant selection pressure on genes to improve psychological capacities to further acquire, store, process, and organize an array of fitness-enhancing skills and practices. These new adaptive capacities in turn become increasingly available to others in the same cultural group. So as genetic evolution improves the ability of our brains to learn from others, cultural evolution can generate adaptations (i.e., religions, markets, science) that both enhance function and increase the selective pressure on our brains to effectively navigate these increasingly complex cultural forms.

Life history theory suggests that variation in the process of unfolding result in part from the optimization of fitness that occurs during functionally organized phases of the lifespan. Borrowing from Paul Baltes' lifespan theory (Baltes, Lindenberger, Staudinger 2006), the *unfolding* principle offers a conceptualization of human health development as having four major functional phases:

(1) *Generativity*—the preconception, prenatal, and perinatal periods are dedicated to the formation of the organism.

(2) *Acquisition of capacity*—the early years are dedicated to the acquisition, maturation, and optimization of specific health development capacities.

(3) *Maintenance of capacity*—the middle years are dedicated to maintaining health development capacities in the face of accumulating risks and ongoing weathering.

(4) *Managing decline*—the later years are devoted to managing, adjusting, and adapting to functional decline of various body and regulatory systems, even as other aspects of health development such as stress management and positive psychological functioning may improve with age.

Each of these phases is conceptually distinct but can contain overlapping elements, as is the case when an older individual who is mostly in the process of managing decline can also be acquiring new capacities (e.g., learning to play piano at 70). This becomes an adaptive process of maintaining optimal function in the face of declining capacities.

By reflecting evolutionarily defined developmental processes, levels of plasticity, and variation in expression within and across individuals (and within and across biobehavioral systems in the same individual), these four phases help us to see and understand the patterns and coherence of health development. For example, evolution has ensured that the anatomic and metabolic process of bone development in women produces strong bones that enable additional weight carrying associated with pregnancy, until the age of the fourth and fifth decade when menopause emerges. This is an anticipatory developmental process whereby early anticipatory changes prepare the individual to meet future developmental needs. Optimizing bone metabolism and preventing osteoporosis can take several forms, such as physical activity (particularly on hard surfaces), and include different strategies that can be employed during the phases of acquisition and maintenance of bone metabolism and strength and during the management of decline after menopause.

5.2 Theories and Frameworks Relevant to Unfolding

The concept of health development as a continuously unfolding adaptive and self-organizing process comprised of distinct yet overlapping functional phases provides a framework for considering how evolutionarily defined stages from life history theory (Stearns 1992; Worthman and Kuzara 2005; Del Giudice et al. 2015), psychological constructs from lifespan human development theory (Baltes 1983; Featherman 1983; Lerner et al. 2010), and sociological constructs from life course sociology (Elder 2000; Mayer 2009; Alwin 2012) can be aligned, compared, and potentially integrated. It also provides a better way of articulating and assessing the alignment between biologically, psychologically, socially, and culturally determined transitions and turning points and understanding how they impact health development over the lifespan (Davies 2014; Henrich 2015) (see Principle 4--Timing). For example, the alignment among the biological processes of menarche, the behavioral maturation of reproduction behaviors, and the culturally created process of mating and marriage has dramatically changed as the age of menarche has declined, the age of marriage has increased, and the introduction of sexualized behavioral stimuli has increased through a variety of different media and information platforms.

5.3 Implications of the Unfolding Principle

The adaptive, self-organizing, and autocatalytic way that health development unfolds via complex sensing, communication, and regulatory processes implies that our basic, clinical, and translational research needs to elucidate how these processes influence the adaptive capacity of individuals and populations. A clearer understanding of how similar self-organizing processes unfold from the cellular level to the cultural level could point to new ways of integrating preventive, health promoting and therapeutic interventions designed to optimize health development by embracing a "cells to society" perspective.

We have proposed that there are four major functional phases of LCHD: generativity, acquisition of capacity, maintenance of capacity, and managing decline. Do these four phases provide a logical staging for all aspects of health development? Are there subphases that need to be articulated to help us better understand the dynamics of health development? To address these questions, we need better measurement of the flow of health development, both continuities and discontinuities, and its variation across and within individuals.

Childhood obesity provides a useful example to illustrate the research implications of the *unfolding* principle. To evaluate obesity risk, body mass index (BMI) is assessed at a fixed point in time and contrasted with values obtained with population age-sex-specific norms. Newer statistical methods have been developed that enable analysis of intraindividual trajectories to more accurately characterize the pattern of childhood growth and uncover new associations between the functional form of growth trajectories and future obesity and obesity-related comorbidities (Wen et al. 2012). To apply this sort of methodology to health development more broadly requires precise definitions and frequent assessments of health development measures, as well as an understanding of the expected trajectory of health development for the population. These types of assessments are being made available by electronic health records and other digitized health data collected by healthcare organizations, which are a new and ready data source for health development research.

The interaction between various forms of adversity and health development provides another example. Understanding the effects of social adversity and other environmental exposures on the unfolding of health development entails not only connecting the specific types of adversity to different outcomes but also developing a better understanding of the adaptive and self-organizing neuronal and behavioral processes, pathways, and mechanisms by which these outcomes are affected. These include assessing the relationships between neurodevelopmental correlates of socioeconomic adversity and differential structural and functional changes in different regions of the brain (as measured using functional MRIs) and understanding how these changes feed forward and potentially compound or dissipate over time (Caspi et al. 2003; Evans and Schamberg 2009; Hackman and Farah 2009; Noble et al. 2012; Power et al. 2005a, b; Evans et al. 2012).

The short- and long-term effects of adverse in utero exposures on health development are an area of inquiry that is producing a wealth of information and ripe for expansion (Gluckman et al. 2008). This research includes studies regarding epigenetic programming associated with fetal exposure to chemical compounds, environmental toxicants, and smoking (Skinner et al. 2008; Launay et al. 2009; Perera et al. 2009; Martino and Prescott 2011), as well as studies examining the impact of nutritional stresses on metabolic function and future disease (Li et al. 2010).

Research on the epigenetic effects of adversity on neurodevelopment has exploded in recent years. Beginning with Meaney's pathbreaking work on the impact of maternal behavior on epigenetic mechanisms that influence gene expression and regulation of the endocrine response to stress (including the glucocorticoid receptor and the corticotropin-releasing factor (CRF) systems that regulate the hypothalamic-pituitary-adrenal axis), there have been a large number of studies examining how different experiences, exposures, and influences can lead to epigenetic alterations affecting a wide range of biobehavioral functions (Meaney 2001, 2010; Turecki and Meaney 2016; Lester et al. 2016). One of the most interesting and challenging areas of epigenetic research concerns the trans-generational transmission of exposures and risk through non-germline alterations of genetic information and the persistence of these influences across subsequent generations (Bale 2015).

6 Principle 3: Complexity

6.1 What We Mean by "Complexity"

Health development results from adaptive, multilevel, and reciprocal relations between individuals and their physical, natural, and social environments.

This principle indicates that health development occurs within living systems that are not only adaptive, self-organizing, and autocatalytic but also complex and hierarchically arranged. The topologies of health development phenotypes cannot be fully understood using a traditional biomedical reductionist approach that relies on an analysis and assembly of the parts of subunits. Health development emanates from the hierarchical and relational coactions of the biological and behavioral subsystems and their individual and collective relations with each other and various interconnected external suprasystems (i.e., familial, social, cultural, ecological). Health development phenotypes result from the interplay between the individual and multiple physical, biochemical, psychological, social, and cultural networks that dynamically coact. As in many complex adaptive systems, the directionality of these influences is often context dependent, reciprocal, and influenced by feedback and feed-forward influences. On the other hand, small changes in particularly vulnerable parts of a biobehavioral system—or at a specific time-sensitive junction in a cascading process of developmental change—can have profound nonlinear effects on the emergence of a capability or health asset or on the overall robustness or fragility of the health development process.

Transactions between different environments can influence gene expression, and gene expression and resultant phenotype can also influence various environments, which will in turn influence additional gene expression. Processes at the molecular level can dynamically coact with each other, as well as with processes at the social and ecological levels, and everywhere in between. These are not simply hierarchical relationships of dependent parts, but are *holarchical* in the sense that each level is both a part and a whole, nested and hierarchically aligned in the common purpose. In some cases, common purposes are optimizing health development, and in other circumstances, they are aligned to ensure reproductive fitness at the expense of optimal health development (Günther and Folke 1993).

6.2 Theories and Frameworks Relevant to Complexity

The *complexity* principle adds the systems-oriented concepts of complexity, adaptation, emergence, nonlinear change (i.e., small changes can produce large effects and vice versa), and multilevel person-environmental coactions. Key theories, frameworks, and perspectives that support the conceptualization of this principle include general systems theory (von Bertalanffy 1968), chaos theory (Gleick 1987; Lorenz 1993), living systems theory (Miller 1978), human-system framework (Brody 1973; Seeman 1989), and complex adaptive systems theory (Holland 1998). The systems orientation to health development suggests a holistic, integrated view that there is a need to understand the interdependence of the parts that constitute the whole, which is embedded in its natural and social environments.

6.3 Implications of the Complexity Principle

Progress in genomics and network analysis is enabling researchers to interrogate all known gene-disease associations simultaneously and to create a network view of patterns and principles of human disease that would not be apparent by examining genetic associations' one disease at a time (Goh et al. 2007). Extending this approach to health development suggests the need to add environmental exposures, or what has been called the "exposome," to analytic models to engender a better understanding of how networks of genes and networks of environments produce health development phenotypes.

The time-honored scientific approach uses the hypothetico-deductive method that derives its cogency from the certainty of deductive inference and the plausibility of abductive inference. Children exposed to the same interacting family, school, and neighborhood environments experience patterns of risk, protective, and health-promoting influences that emerge out of the complex topography of those person-environmental interactions. By statistically categorizing and analyzing children by their ethnicity, family income, and family structure, the rich interactions of different environmental factors are often lost (Molenaar et al. 2003). Health development is non-ergodic, meaning that each individual's experiences, environmental interactions, and health development phenotypes are unique and that within a population there is marked heterogeneity. Averaging effects across groups tells us something about population effects, but little about individual effects (Molenaar and Campbell 2009). Furthermore, even though individuals may have different life course experiences, they can experience the same health development phenotype, a phenomenon called *equifinality* (Cicchetti and Rogosch 1996).

Systems biology and other systems-oriented sciences offer a set of methods that can address the non-ergodic attribute of health development (Huang 2009). Rather than being hypothesis driven, these methods are systems driven and require a research strategy of interrogating the system at the level of the whole (EA Roberts 2015, 2012). This more complex way of experimenting and generating scientifically valid information bears further discussion and explication. New approaches to study design generation and statistical analysis will be needed to understand how patterns of health development are produced by complex coactions of networks over time. Identifying characteristic health development phenotypes will require nonlinear models that recognize and embrace the complexity of health development. The focus should be on measuring patterns of intraindividual health development, which will require study designs that collect detailed and large volumes of health and environmental information on individuals, forming *big health development data* resources.

Environments coact with individual constitutional factors to produce health development phenotypes within a person. We have only a vague understanding of the specific environmental variables responsible for these interactions. There is an urgent need to create scientifically useful typologies of environmental variables. This will enable research to better understand how health development signals are transduced from the environment to the individual, altering biobehavioral system configuration and function. Better characterization—and, ultimately, standardization—of environmental variables (the exposome) will accelerate research on how an individual's contexts affect the epigenetic topography and organize what complex systems science might refer to as health development attractor[2] states. Standardization of concepts and measures enables synthesis and meta-analyses across studies.

[2]An attractor is the end state of a dynamic system as it moves over time. Once the object or data point goes into the basin of attraction, it does not leave unless a strong force is applied. The set of one or more attractors of a dynamic system can be represented visually or graphically as trajectories in state space, where state space represents the multidimensional, abstract space of all possible system behavior. There are four types of possible attractors: fixed points, limit cycles, toroidal attractors, and chaotic (or strange) attractors. Point attractors are regular, terminating in a single point in state space. Cycle attractors are also regular, sometimes oscillating between two or more fixed points or exhibiting a sinusoidal pattern over time. Toroidal attractors are semi-regular, representing coupled rhythms whose ratio of periodicities terminates in an irrational rather than a rational number and appearing in state space as a donut. Chaotic attractors are fully irregular, represented by an aperiodic trajectory in state space that never repeats or settles to a stable pattern, whose basin of attraction is often fractal in shape; see chaos. Regular point and cycle attractors are characteristics of relatively simple systems. Irregular toroidal and chaotic attractors are more characteristics of complex systems.

We have almost no idea at present how to map or represent multilevel emergence, because the transactional nature of health development is not well specified, measured, analyzed, or interpreted. For example, a child exposed to a stressful stimulus that is repeated in unpredictable and unanticipated ways may experience epigenetic changes in neurotransmitter metabolism that cannot be explained just by measuring the stressful stimulus. The developmental timing of these stressful events, their unpredictable repetition, and the temporal rhythms of restorative processes (e.g., sleep) are also at play, which brings us to the next principle.

7 Principle 4: Timing

7.1 What We Mean by "Timing"

Health development is sensitive to the timing and social structuring of environmental exposures and experiences.

Health development is not a linear process in which exposures to environmental stimuli or internalized experiences have equal effects, regardless of when in the life course they occur. Instead, health development results from nonlinear interactions that are both time-specific and time-dependent. There are sensitive periods of a child's life when the impact of certain exposures can be greater than during other periods (Halfon et al. 2014). Time-specific health development pathways refer to biological conditioning that occurs during these sensitive periods, when developing systems are most adaptable and plastic and exogenous and endogenous influences can result in different adaptive responses. In other words, the same exposures can have very different effects depending on when during the life course they occur. Because childhood is a phase of life when biological and behavioral systems are shaped by environmental exposures and social experiences, the *timing* principle emphasizes the importance of nurturing children when they are most sensitive to these influences (Conti and Heckman 2013). For example, exposure to a rich set of words during the early years of life can greatly improve a child's subsequent language development, with cascading effects on subsequent school performance, health behaviors, and future health status (Hart and Risley 2003).

Time-specific transitions and turning points in health development also result from socially structured pathways that link experiences and exposures in time-influenced ways that create recursive and mutually reinforcing patterns of risk, protection, and promotion. Socially structured pathways have both period-specific and time-dependent (cumulative) characteristics. By arraying risk, protective, and promoting factors into socially constructed and institutionally reinforced pathways that interact with sensitive periods of health development, societies can either support the emergence of positive health development phenotypes or reinforce negative ones. The role, relative dose, duration, and coaction of risk, protective, and promoting factors during formative, maintenance, and declining phases of the life course all influence the slope, shape, and contours of health development trajectories.

Thus, the *timing* principle summarizes a set of models and constructs that elaborate the importance of the time dimension on health development. There are time-specific pathways that refer to sensitive periods when environmental exposures and experiences can influence health development, and there are time-dependent pathways that refer to the accumulation of repeated exposures to the same environmental stimuli that can result in a weathering process that accelerates aging (Geronimus 2013).

7.2 Theories and Frameworks Relevant to Timing

The *unfolding* principle introduced the concept of functional phases or epochs that organize the historical foundations of health development. The *timing* principle adds the concepts of time-dependent and time-sensitive health development pathways that create periods of vulnerability and robustness, as well as social structuring of environmental exposures and experiences. These concepts are drawn from several theories, frameworks, and perspectives including developmental origins of health and disease (Gluckman and Hanson 2006a), life course perspective (Elder 2000; Mayer 2009; Alwin 2012), biological embedding (Hertzman and Boyce 2010), chronobiology (Kreitzman and Foster 2004), developmental time (Kuzawa and Thayer 2011), and adaptive developmental plasticity (Gluckman et al. 2009).

7.3 Implications of the Timing Principle

Scientists have accumulated tantalizing but as yet limited evidence for time-sensitive health development (Hanson and Gluckman 2014; Hertzman 2012; Boyce and Kobor 2015). Progress in this area has been slow in part because of a lack of data systems that integrate large volumes of biological (especially patterns of gene response and epigenetic changes), clinical (such as electronic health records and biosensors), behavioral (self-report questionnaires), and environmental data. Each of these data sources exists in isolation. What is needed is a new field of health development informatics that is devoted to assembling large, integrated, longitudinal data resources and mining them for novel associations between time, environment, and health development outcomes.

Another challenge is the lack of research that establishes the specific time-dependent pathways by which human health development phenotypes are altered or protected by various internal and external factors. A variety of studies suggest that physical and social environments can alter a person's biology via epigenetic pathways that influence regulation of genetic pathways (Hertzman and Boyce 2010). This "embedding" of experience seems to have its largest impact during specific sensitive periods of development. Why the same experience engenders different outcomes among individuals is one of the great mysteries of health development. More work is needed to elucidate these iterative and dynamic pathways that connect environment to gene regulation to physiological states to environmental impact.

8 Principle 5: Plasticity

8.1 What We Mean by "Plasticity"

Health development phenotypes are systematically malleable and are enabled and constrained by evolution to enhance adaptability to diverse environments.

The relative plasticity of these phenotypes is responsive to transactions between evolutionarily selected biological and behavioral conditioning and supportive, challenging, and constraining environments. These phenotypes have evolved to provide adaptive capacity, plasticity (i.e., ability of the organism to systematically alter its phenotype in response to environmental challenges, opportunities, barriers, and constraints), and growth potential, which in aggregate refer to the robustness of an individual's health development. Heredity transmits these evolutionary signals through genetic, epigenetic, behavioral, and cultural dimensions (Jablonka and Lamb 2006), which establish the set of health development phenotypes that, depending on environmental circumstances, may or may not be selected and optimized to produce desirable outcomes. At the microlevel, there are a range of strategies to introduce variable types and levels of plasticity to optimize adaptability from the molecular to the behavioral level. At a macro-level, there are social and cultural strategies that organize the phases and life stages of health development into functionally productive entities.

Because developmental plasticity enables the genome to produce a repertoire of possible phenotypes based on environmental cues, an individual begins their life with the capacity to develop in different ways. Different exposures and experiences select and instruct a developmental pathway to respond based on these evolutionary determined strategies. Underlying many forms of plasticity are epigenetic process and resulting cascades of secondary and tertiary responses. Because plasticity can manifest at different levels, behavioral plasticity may be influenced by neural plasticity, and neural plasticity in turn may be influenced by molecular plasticity influenced by epigenetic mechanisms (Bateson and Gluckman 2011).

8.2 Theories and Frameworks Relevant to Plasticity

Evolution both enables and constrains the portfolio of adaptive plastic responses that an individual may experience in response to environmental interactions. Therefore, plasticity is relative, not absolute. Although Darwin's theory of evolution (Darwin 1859; Huxley 1942) laid the foundation for understanding the principle of *plasticity*, more recent syntheses have expanded our understanding of heredity as including not just genetic change but also epigenetic, behavioral, and cultural phenomena that are transmitted across generations (Waddington 1942; West-Eberhard 2003; Richardson and Boyd 2005; Jablonka and Lamb 2006; Konner 2011; Henrich 2015). These evolutionary forces act at the individual and group level, a perspective known as multilevel selection theory (Okasha 2006).

In some cases, health development outcomes result from the developing individual "predicting" likely future environmental stimuli based on the cues received during sensitive periods of health development. This has been called "predictive adaptive responses" (Gluckman and Hanson 2004). If the developing organism predicts incorrectly—that is, if the environment experienced in the future is not compatible with the cues received during periods of developmental plasticity—health development "mismatches" will occur. This phenomenon can be observed among individuals exposed in utero to maternal malnutrition who later become obese and glucose intolerant, a result of being born into an energy-rich environment (Hales and Barker 1992).

8.3 Implications of the Plasticity Principle

Evolution has acted on body systems in different ways to encode various types and levels of health development plasticity. The formation of some biological subsystems is tightly controlled by time and gene regulation (e.g., cardiovascular), whereas others seem to have a range of phenotypes that can emerge as a result of interactions with the environment (e.g., stress response, executive function). New models are needed to explain the deep archeology of evolution as it relates to the emergence of health development. Fields like comparative biology can test some of these hypotheses by examining the degree to which specific processes and pathways of health development vary or are preserved across species. For example, patterns of sleep have been selected for and preserved across species in ways that affect how sleep is regulated (Tamaki et al. 2016). Moreover, the success of human civilization has removed much of the selection pressure exerted by mortality, so optimization of specific pathways may be more strongly influenced by culture, behavioral, and epigenetic heredity rather than genetic forces (Enriquez and Gullans 2015). This hypothesis should be tested.

The predictive adaptive response hypothesis has accumulated a substantial amount of animal and human evidence for energy regulation (Gluckman and Hanson 2004a,b). This work should be extended to other domains—for example, behavioral health. Just as childhood obesity may result from mismatches between children's energy regulation and exposure to energy-dense environments, it is possible that the proliferation of childhood disorders like attention deficit hyperactivity disorder, anxiety, and learning disabilities may be a consequence of mismatches between predictive adaptive behavioral responses and the demands children face in terms of executive functioning, emotional functioning, and learning in their home, school, and other environments.

9 Principle 6: Thriving

9.1 What We Mean by "Thriving"

Optimal health development promotes survival, enhances well-being, and protects against disease.

Health development bestows upon the individual resources that have instrumental value, enabling an individual to pursue goals and thrive (Seedhouse 2001; Blaxter 2004; Richman 2004; Forrest 2014).

It provides assets that individuals employ to pursue the beings and doings (Sen 1999) that characterize each person's lived experiences. Thus, health development phenotypes are instrumental resources that enable individuals to pursue desired goals and live long, flourishing lives.

Health development phenotypes can be considered optimal according to the degree to which they improve the chances of survival of individuals and groups of individuals, the degree to which they support transmission of heritable information to successor generations, and the degree to which they support physical robustness and psychological flourishing (what we term thriving) across time and within the contexts of its environments.

On the other hand, the pathways by which health development phenotypes are formed can be perturbed to create suboptimal states that are precursors to fully formed disease phenotypes. These so-called endophenotypes represent intermediate, subclinical-phased transitions toward a fully manifest phenotypic expression of a disease or disorder (John and Lewis 1966; Gottesman and Gould 2003). For example, the exposure to unpredictable and uncontrollable stressors during sensitive periods of neural development can influence midbrain development and the functional development of attachment relationships, the prefrontal cortex and the functional development of executive function, and the hypothalamic pituitary axis and the regulation of stress responses (Castellanos and Tannock 2002; Boyce 2016). Endophenotypes characterized by anxious attachment, poor impulse control, and hyperactive stress response can impact health behaviors and mental health and contribute to the development of many different chronic diseases including obesity, diabetes, and cardiovascular disease (Duric et al. 2016).

9.2 Theories and Frameworks Relevant to Thriving

The principle of *health development* articulated the singularity of the concepts of health and development. The principle of *thriving* further clarifies the nature of health development by explicitly characterizing its instrumental nature. That is, health development provides a set of resources that organisms draw on in order to pursue goals, such as surviving, achieving a state of physical robustness and resilience, and psychological flourishing (Seedhouse 2001; Blaxter 2004; Committee on Evaluation of Children's Health 2004; Richman 2004; Forrest 2014). Health development therefore enables the attainment of various beings (states of happiness, life satisfaction, and meaning and purpose) and doings (desired activities that an individual pursues) as individuals pursue their goals over the life course (Sen 1999).

9.3 Implications of the Thriving Principle

LCHD recognizes that phenotype is produced by the continuous coactions of at least five factors: genome, epigenome, environment, developmental time, and life course stage. These coactions do not merely produce single outcomes; instead they produce landscapes of possibilities with peaks and valleys shaped by an individual's life history, evolutionary determined possibilities and constraints, and the five-way interaction. Which "attractor" state (i.e., health development phenotype) an individual settles in is the result of this complex, nonlinear process. We know very little about which attractor states are most likely to produce desirable outcomes (i.e., thriving) for which individuals under which circumstances. As we learn more about the interrelationships among these variables, we will begin to forge an *ontology* that specifies how health development variables interrelate with one another, their subsystems and suprasystem environmental influences, and their consequences. Research is needed that links health development phenotypes, singularly and collectively, that enable individuals with varying personal characteristics and environmental exposures to lead long lives, avoid debilitating disease, and achieve desirable goals and an optimal lived experience.

10 Principle 7: Harmony

10.1 What We Mean by "Harmony"

Health development results from the balanced and coherent relations among molecular, physiological, behavioral, cultural, and evolutionary processes.

Genetic modulations that occur in molecular time frames measured in nanoseconds are linked to biochemical modulation measured in milliseconds, homeostatic mechanisms measured in seconds to days, social norms that evolve or years and decades, cultural processes that change from years to centuries, and ecological processes that until recently took millennia. Harmonious synchronization of these processes produces the rhythms and variability that characterize health development. Loss of coordination of these processes results in less robustness of the human system, with resultant negative consequences. For example, the age of menarche has decreased in response to a variety of environmental changes that have resulted in better health and nutrition. In traditional societies, and until about 100 years ago, menarche coincided with maturation of a repertoire of psychological capabilities. Now, menarche precedes this process of psychological maturation, which has also been altered and extended by other cultural and environmental changes (Gluckman and Hanson 2006b). So the adaptive response of menarche to better nutrition and health has led to a temporal and functional uncoupling of biological and psychological capabilities that had previously been harmonized. This has been associated with a range of maladaptive outcomes (Mendle et al. 2007; Ellis and Essex 2007).

10.2 Theories and Frameworks Relevant to Harmony

The *timing* principle introduced the concepts of time dependence, time sensitivity, and social structuring of exposures. The *harmony* principle extends these concepts by adding the notions of harmonious and balanced relations of the various biological, behavioral, environmental, and cultural systems that an individual is embedded within. Extension of the classic evolutionary modern synthesis—which assumes that phenotypic transitions occur through a series of small steps that result in gradual evolutionary change—has questioned and advanced core assumption about pace of such change. Gradualism has given way in the extended evolutionary synthesis to the notion that evolution can manifest variable rates of change, especially when mutations occur in major regulatory control genes or when developmental process responds to environmental challenges with change in coordinated suites of traits or via nonlinear threshold effects (Laland et al. 2015). Although key theories, frameworks, and models in support of this principle come from chronobiology (Kreitzman and Foster 2004), developmental time (Kuzawa and Thayer 2011), and adaptive developmental plasticity (Gluckman et al. 2009), there is much more theoretical work needed for this principle.

10.3 Implication of the Harmony Principle

According to the principles of *timing* and *plasticity*, we know that there are periods of the life course when environmental influences can have particularly large effects on health development plasticity. The tremendous plasticity of humans contributes to the robustness and the ordinary magic of child health development (Masten 2001). We need better descriptions and conceptualizations of developmental time as it affects all levels and dimensions of health development and how different time frames nest together to produce coherent developmental pathways and robustness and variability in phenotypic expression. This includes a better understanding of how molecular, physiologic, developmental, historical, cultural, and evolutionary time frames independently and in harmony influence phenotypic variation, through genetic, epigenetic, and yet to be determined mechanisms and pathways. Because developmental time is uneven in its potency, intensity of change, and accessibility to environmental influences, there is a great need to better characterize and measure these temporal parameters (Boyce et al. 2012).

11 Summary

Health and development are unified into a single construct (*health development* principle) that adaptively unfolds over the life course (*unfolding* principle) according to the principles of complex adaptive systems (*complexity* principle). Change in health development results from time-specific processes (*timing* principle) that influence biobehavioral systems during sensitive periods when they are most susceptible (*plasticity* principle), and the balanced alignment of molecular, biological, behavioral, cultural, and evolutionary process (*harmony* principle) can result in developmental coherence. Health development provides instrumental assets that enable individuals and populations to pursue desired lived experiences (*thriving* principle).

The Life Course Health Development framework organizes its seven principles into a coherent whole to enable the emergence of a new field of science. The principles should not be viewed as static, independent statements or claims. Instead, they should be considered a set of nodes within a highly interconnected knowledge producing and testing network. We anticipate that these principles will change and evolve as the many fields subsumed by the health development framework themselves mature. Ultimately, we anticipate that the framework will transform into a fully formed theoretical model that enables explanation and prediction of health development phenomena.

References

Alfred, T., Ben-Shlomo, Y., et al. (2012). A multi-cohort study of polymorphisms in the GH/IGF Axis and physical capability: The HALCyon Programme. *PloS One, 7*(1), e29883.

Alwin, D. F. (2012). Integrating varieties of life course concepts. *The Journals of Gerontology. Series B, Psychological Sciences and Social Sciences, 67*(2), 206–220.

Antony, P. M., Balling, R., et al. (2012). From systems biology to systems biomedicine. *Current Opinion in Biotechnology, 23*(4), 604–608.

Arnesen, E., & Forsdahl, A. (1985). The Tromsø heart study: Coronary risk factors and their association with living conditions during childhood. *Journal of Epidemiology and Community Health, 39*(3), 210–214.

Bale, T. L. (2015). Epigenetic and transgenerational reprogramming of brain development. *Nature Reviews Neuroscience, 16*(6), 332–344.

Baltes, P. B. (1983). Life-span developmental psychology: Observations on history and theory revisited. In R. M. Lerner (Ed.), *Developmental Psychology: Historical and philosophical perspectives* (pp. 79–111). Hillsdale: Erlbaum.

Baltes, P. B., Lindenberger, U., & Staudinger, U. M. (2006). *Life span theory in developmental psychology*. New York: John Wiley & Sons, Inc..

Baltes, P. B., Reese, H. W., et al. (1980). Life-span Developmental Psychology. *Annual Review of Psychology, 31*(1), 65–110.

Barker, D. J., Gluckman, P. D., et al. (1993). Fetal nutrition and cardiovascular disease in adult life. *Lancet, 341*(8850), 938–941.

Barker, D. J., Osmond, C., et al. (1989a). Growth in utero, blood pressure in childhood and adult life, and mortality from cardiovascular disease. *BMJ, 298*(6673), 564–567.

Barker, D. J., Osmond, C., et al. (1989b). The intrauterine and early postnatal origins of cardiovascular disease and chronic bronchitis. *Journal of Epidemiology and Community Health, 43*(3), 237–240.

Barker, D. J. P., Thornburg, K. L., et al. (2010). Beyond birthweight: The maternal and placental origins of chronic disease. *Journal of Developmental Origins of Health and Disease, 1*(6), 360–364.

Bateson, P., & Gluckman, P. (2011). *Plasticity, robustness, development and evolution*. Cambridge: Cambridge University Press.

Ben-Shlomo, Y., & Kuh, D. (2002). A life course approach to chronic disease epidemiology: Conceptual models, empirical challenges and interdisciplinary perspectives. *International Journal of Epidemiology, 31*(2), 285–293.

Berkman, L. F., & Syme, S. L. (1979). Social networks, host resistance, and mortality: A nine-year follow-up study of Alameda County residents. *American Journal of Epidemiology, 109*(2), 186–204.

Blaxter, M. (2004). *Health*. Cambridge: Polity Press.

Borghol, N., Suderman, M., et al. (2012). Associations with early-life socio-economic position in adult DNA methylation. *International Journal of Epidemiology, 41*(1), 62–74.

Bornstein, M. H., & Lamb, M. E. (Eds.). (2005). *Developmental science: An advanced textbook* (5th ed.). New York: Psychology Press.

Boyce, W. T., & Kobor, M. S. (2015). Development and the epigenome: the 'synapse'of gene–environment interplay. *Developmental science, 18*(1), 1–23.

Boyce, W. T. (2016). Differential susceptibility of the developing brain to contextual adversity and stress.

Neuropsychopharmacology: Official Publication of the American College of Neuropsychopharmacology, 41(1), 142–162.

Boyce, W. T., Sokolowski, M. B., et al. (2012). Toward a new biology of social adversity. *Proceedings of the National Academy of Sciences of the United States of America, 109*(Suppl 2), 17143–17148.

Brody, H. (1973). The systems view of man: Implications for medicine, science, and ethics. *Perspectives in Biology and Medicine, 17*, 71–92.

Bronfenbrenner, U. (1976). The ecology of human development: History and perspectives [The ecology of human development: History and perspectives]. *Psychologia Wychowawcza 19*(5), 537–549.

Bronfenbrenner, U., & Morris, P. A. (2006). The Bioecological model of human development. In R. M. Lerner & W. Damon (Eds.), *Handbook of child psychology: Theoretical models of human development* (Vol. 1, 6th ed., pp. 793–828). Hoboken: John Wiley & Sons, Inc..

Cairns, R. B., Elder, G. H., et al. (1996). *Developmental science: Cambridge studies in social and emotional development*. New York: Cambridge University Press.

Caspi, A., Sugden, K., et al. (2003). Influence of life stress on depression: Moderation by a polymorphism in the 5-HTT gene. *Science, 301*(5631), 386–389.

Cassel, J. (1964). Social science theory as a source of hypotheses in epidemiological research. *American Journal of Public Health and the Nation's Health, 54*(9), 1482–1488.

Castellanos, F. X., & Tannock, R. (2002). Neuroscience of attention-deficit/hyperactivity disorder: The search for endophenotypes. *Nature Reviews Neuroscience, 3*(8), 617–628.

Chen, F., Yang, Y., et al. (2010). Social change and socioeconomic disparities in health over the life course in China a cohort analysis. *American Sociological Review, 75*(1), 126–150.

Cicchetti, D., & Cohen, D. J. (1995). *Developmental psychopathology: Theory and methods* (Vol. 1). Oxford, UK: John Wiley & Sons.

Cicchetti, D., & Rogosch, F. A. (1996). Equifinality and multifinality in developmental psychopathology. *Development and Psychopathology, 8*(04), 597–600.

Clausen, J. A. (1986). *The life course: A sociological perspective*. Englewood Cliffs: Prentice-Hall.

Cohen, S., & Herbert, T. B. (1996). Health psychology: Psychological factors and physical disease from the perspective of human psychoneuroimmunology. *Annual Review of Psychology, 47*, 113–142.

Committee on Evaluation of Children's Health, N. R. C. (2004). *Children's health, the Nation's wealth: Assessing and improving child health*. Washington, DC: National Academies Press.

Conti, G., & Heckman, J. J. (2013). The developmental approach to child and adult health. *Pediatrics, 131*(Suppl 2), S133–S141.

Cunliffe, V. T. (2015). Experience-sensitive epigenetic mechanisms, developmental plasticity, and the biological embedding of chronic disease risk. *Wiley Interdisciplinary Reviews: Systems Biology and Medicine, 7*(2), 53–71.

Dannefer, D. (1984). The role of the social in life-span developmental psychology, past and future: Rejoinder to Baltes and Nesselroade. *American Sociological Review, 49*(6), 847–850.

Darwin, C. (1859). *On the origin of species by means of natural selection, or the preservation of Favoured races in the struggle for life*. London, UK: John Murray.

Davey Smith, G. (2012). Epigenesis for epidemiologists: Does evo-devo have implications for population health research and practice? *International Journal of Epidemiology, 41*(1), 236–247.

Davies, J. (2014). *Life unfolding: How the human body creates itself*. Oxford, UK: Oxford University Press.

Davila-Velderrain, J., Martinez-Garcia, J. C., & Alvarez-Buylla, E. R. (2015). Modeling the epigenetic attractors landscape: Toward a post-genomic mechanistic understanding of development. *Frontiers in Genetics, 6*, 160.

Dawber, T. R., Kannel, W. B., & Gordon, T. (1974). Coffee and cardiovascular disease: Observations from the Framingham study. *New England Journal of Medicine, 291*(17), 871–874.

Del Giudice, M., Gangestad, S. W., & Kaplan, H. S. (2015). Life history theory and evolutionary psychology. The handbook of evolutionary psychology. John Wiley & Sons, Inc.

Diewald, M., & Mayer, K. U. (2009). The sociology of the life course and life span psychology: Integrated paradigm or complementing pathways? *Advances in Life Course Research, 14*(1), 5–14.

Duric, V., Clayton, S., Leong, M. L., & Yuan, L. L. (2016). Comorbidity factors and brain mechanisms linking chronic stress and systemic illness. *Neural Plasticity, 8*, 2016.

Egger, G., Liang, G., et al. (2004). Epigenetics in human disease and prospects for epigenetic therapy. *Nature, 429*(6990), 457–463.

Elder, G. H., Jr. (1995). The life course paradigm: Social change and individual development. In P. Moen, G. H. Elder Jr., & K. Luscher (Eds.), *Examining lives in context: Perspectives on the ecology of human development* (pp. 101–139). Washington, DC: American Psychological Association.

Elder, G. H., Jr. (2000). The life course. In E. F. Borgatta & R. J. V. Montgomery (Eds.), *Encyclopedia of sociology* (Vol. 3, pp. 1614–1622). New York: Macmillan Reference.

Elder, G. H., & Shanahan, M. J. (2007). The life course and human development. In *Handbook of child psychology*. New York: John Wiley & Sons, Inc.

Elder, G. H., Johnson, M. K., & Crosnoe, R. (2003). The emergence and development of life course theory. *In Handbook of the life course* (pp. 3–19). New York: Springer US.

Elks, C. E., Loos, R. J. F., et al. (2012). Adult obesity susceptibility variants are associated with greater childhood weight gain and a faster tempo of growth: The

1946 British birth cohort study. *American Journal of Clinical Nutrition, 95*(5), 1150–1156.

Ellis, B. J., & Essex, M. J. (2007). Family environments, adrenarche, and sexual maturation: A longitudinal test of a life history model. *Child Development, 78*(6), 1799–1817.

Engel, G. L. (1977). The need for a new medical model: A challenge for biomedicine. *Science, 196*(4286), 129–136.

Enriquez, J., & Gullans, S. (2015). *Evolving ourselves: How unnatural selection and nonrandom mutation are changing life on earth*. New York: Penguin.

Entringer, S., Buss, C., et al. (2012). Fetal programming of body composition, obesity, and metabolic function: The role of intrauterine stress and stress biology. *Journal of Nutrition and Metabolism, 2012*, 632548.

Essex, M. J., Thomas Boyce, W., et al. (2011). Epigenetic vestiges of early developmental adversity: Childhood stress exposure and DNA methylation in adolescence. *Child Development, 84*, 58–75.

Evans, G. W., & Schamberg, M. A. (2009). Childhood poverty, chronic stress, and adult working memory. *Proceedings of the National Academy of Sciences of the United States of America, 106*(16), 6545–6549.

Evans, G. W., Chen, E., et al. (2012). How poverty gets under the skin: A life course perspective. In V. Maholmes & R. B. King (Eds.), *The Oxford handbook of poverty and child development* (pp. 13–100). New York: Oxford University Press.

Featherman, D. L. (1983). Life span perspectives in social science research. In P. B. Baltes & G. Brim (Eds.), *Life-span development and behavior* (Vol. 5, pp. 1–57). New York: Academic Press.

Forrest, C. B. (2014). A living systems perspective on health. *Medical Hypotheses, 82*, 209–214.

Forsdahl, A. (1977). Are poor living conditions in childhood and adolescence an important risk factor for arteriosclerotic heart disease? *British Journal of Preventive & Social Medicine, 31*(2), 91–95.

Gatzweiler, F. W., & Baumüller, H. (2013). Marginality—A framework for analyzing causal complexities of poverty. In J. Braun von & F. W. Gatzweiler (Eds.), *Marginality: Addressing the nexus of poverty, exclusion and ecology* (pp. 27–40). Dordrecht: Springer.

Geronimus, A. T. (2013). Deep integration: Letting the epigenome out of the bottle without losing sight of the structural origins of population health. *American Journal of Public Health, 103*(S1), S56–S63.

Gilbert, S. F., Bosch, T. C., & Ledón-Rettig, C. (2015 Oct 1). Eco-Evo-Devo: Developmental symbiosis and developmental plasticity as evolutionary agents. *Nature Reviews Genetics, 16*(10), 611–622.

Gleick, J. (1987). *Chaos: Making a new science*. New York: Penguin Books.

Gluckman, P. D., & Hanson, M. A. (2004a). Developmental origins of disease paradigm: A mechanistic and evolutionary perspective. *Pediatric Research, 56*(3), 311–317.

Gluckman, P. D., & Hanson, M. A. (2004b). Living with the past: Evolution, development, and patterns of disease. *Science, 305*(5691), 1733–1736.

Gluckman, P. D., & Hanson, M. A. (2004c). The developmental origins of the metabolic syndrome. *Trends in Endocrinology and Metabolism, 15*(4), 183–187.

Gluckman, P. D., & Hanson, M. A. (2006a). *Developmental origins of health and disease*. Cambridge, UK: Cambridge University Press.

Gluckman, P. D., & Hanson, M. A. (2006b). Evolution, development and timing of puberty. *Trends in Endocrinology and Metabolism, 17*(1), 7–12.

Gluckman, P. D., Hanson, M. A., et al. (2008). Effect of in utero and early-life conditions on adult health and disease. *New England Journal of Medicine, 359*(1), 61–73.

Gluckman, P. D., Hanson, M. A., et al. (2009). Towards a new developmental synthesis: Adaptive developmental plasticity and human disease. *The Lancet, 373*(9675), 1654–1657.

Gluckman, P. D., Hanson, M. A., et al. (2010). A conceptual framework for the developmental origins of health and disease. *Journal of Developmental Origins of Health and Disease, 1*(1), 6–18.

Goh, K. I., Cusick, M. E., et al. (2007). The human disease network. *Proceedings of the National Academy of Sciences, 104*(21), 8685–8690.

Gottesman, I. I., & Gould, T. D. (2003). The endophenotype concept in psychiatry: Etymology and strategic intentions. *The American Journal of Psychiatry, 160*(4), 636–645.

Green, S., Fagan, M., & Jaeger, J. (2015). Explanatory integration challenges in evolutionary systems biology. *Biological Theory, 10*(1), 18–35.

Greenberg, G., & Partridge, T. (2010). *Biology, evolution, and psychological development, In The Handbook of life-span development* (pp. 115–148). Hoboken: John Wiley & Sons.

Günther, F., & Folke, C. (1993 Sep). Characteristics of nested living systems. *Journal of Biological Systems, 1*(03), 257–274.

Hackman, D. A., & Farah, M. J. (2009). Socioeconomic status and the developing brain. *Trends in Cognitive Sciences, 13*(2), 65–73.

Hales, C. N., & Barker, D. J. P. (1992). Type 2 (non-insulin dependent) diabetes mellitus: The thrifty phenotype hypothesis. *Diabetologia, 35*, 595–601.

Halfon, N., & Hochstein, M. (2002). Life course health-development: An integrated framework for developing health, policy, and research. *The Milbank Quarterly, 80*(3), 433–479. iii.

Halfon, N., Larson, K., Lu, M., Tullis, E., & Russ, S. (2014). Lifecourse health development: Past, present and future. *Maternal and Child Health Journal, 18*(2), 344–365.

Hanson, M. A., & Gluckman, P. D. (2014). Early developmental conditioning of later health and disease: physiology or pathophysiology? *Physiological Reviews, 94*(4), 1027–1076.

Hart, B., & Risley, T. R. (2003). The early catastrophe: The 30 million word gap by age 3. *American Educator, 27*(1), 4–9.

Haynes, S., Feinleib, M., & Kannel, W. B. (1980). The relationship of psychosocial factors to coronary heart disease in the Framingham Study. III. Eight-year incidence of coronary heart disease. *American Journal of Epidemiology, 111*(1), 37–58.

Henrich, J. (2015). *The secret of our success: how culture is driving human evolution, domesticating our species, and making us smarter*. Princeton: Princeton University Press.

Hertzman, C. (1999). The biological embedding of early experience and its effects on health in adulthood. *Annals of the New York Academy of Sciences, 896*, 85–95.

Hertzman, C. (2012). Putting the concept of biological embedding in historical perspective. *Proceedings of the National Academy of Sciences of the United States of America, 109*(Suppl 2), 17160–17167.

Hertzman, C., & Boyce, T. (2010). How experience gets under the skin to create gradients in developmental health. *Annual Review of Public Health, 31*, 329–347.

Hochberg, Z. E., Feil, R., Constancia, M., Fraga, M., Junien, C., Carel, J. C., Boileau, P., Le Bouc, Y., Deal, C. L., Lillycrop, K., & Scharfmann, R. (2010). Child health, developmental plasticity, and epigenetic programming. *Endocrine Reviews, 32*(2), 159–224.

Holland, J. H. (1998). *Emergence: From chaos to order*. Cambridge, MA: Perseus Books.

Huang, S. (2009). Non-genetic heterogeneity of cells in development: More than just noise. *Development, 136*(23), 3853–3862.

Huang, S. (2012). The molecular and mathematical basis of Waddington's epigenetic landscape: A framework for post-Darwinian biology? *BioEssays: News and Reviews in Molecular, Cellular and Developmental Biology, 34*(2), 149–157.

Huxley, J. (1942). *Evolution: The modern synthesis*. London, UK: Allen & Unwin.

Jablonka, E., & Lamb, K. J. (2006). *Evolution in four dimensions: Genetic, epigenetic, behavioral, and symbolic variation in the history of life*. Cambridge, MA: MIT Press.

John, B., & Lewis, K. R. (1966). Chromosome variability and geographic distribution in insects. *Science, 152*(3723), 711–721.

Keating, D. P., & Hertzman, C. (Eds.). (1999). *Developmental health and the wealth of nations: Social, biological, and educational dynamics*. New York: Guilford Publications.

Kitano, H. (2002). Systems biology: A brief overview. *Science, 295*(5560), 1662–1664.

Konner, M. (2011). *The evolution of childhood: Relationships, emotion, mind*. Cambridge, MA: Belknap Press of Harvard University Press.

Kreitzman, L., & Foster, R. G. (2004). *Rhythms of life: The biological clocks that control the daily lives of every living thing*. New Haven: Yale University Press.

Krieger, N. (2001). Theories for social epidemiology in the 21st century: An ecosocial perspective. *International Journal of Epidemiology, 30*(4), 668–677.

Kuh, D., & Ben-Shlomo, Y. (2004). Introduction. In D. Kuh & Y. Ben-Shlomo (Eds.), *A life course approach to chronic disease epidemiology* (pp. 3–14). New York: Oxford University Press.

Kuh, D., & Davey Smith, G. (2004). The life course and adult chronic disease: An historical perspective with particular reference to coronary heart disease. In *Life course approach to chronic disease epidemiology* (pp. 15–37). Oxford University Press.

Kuh, D. J. L., & Wadsworth, M. E. J. (1993). Physical health status at 36 years in a British national birth cohort. *Social Science & Medicine, 37*(7), 905–916.

Kuzawa, C. W., & Thayer, Z. M. (2011). Timescales of human adaptation: The role of epigenetic processes. *Epigenomics, 3*(2), 221–234.

Laland, K. N., Uller, T., Feldman, M. W., Sterelny, K., Müller, G. B., Moczek, A., Jablonka, E., & Odling-Smee, J. (2015). The extended evolutionary synthesis: Its structure, assumptions and predictions. *Proceedings. Royal Society B, 282*(1813), 20151019.

Launay, J. M., Del Pino, M., et al. (2009). Smoking induces long-lasting effects through a monoamine-oxidase epigenetic regulation. *PloS One, 4*(11), e7959.

Lerner, D. R. M. (1984). *On the nature of human plasticity*. Cambridge: Cambridge University Press.

Lerner, R. M. (2006). Developmental science, developmental systems, and contemporary theories of human development. In W. Damon & R. M. Lerner (Eds.), *Handbook of child psychology, Vol. 1: Theoretical models of human development* (pp. 1–17). Hoboken: Wiley.

Lerner, R. M. (2012). Developmental science: Past, present, and future. *International Journal of Developmental Science, 6*(1), 29–36.

Lerner, R. M., & Overton, W. F. (2008). Exemplifying the integrations of the relational developmental system synthesizing theory, research, and application to promote positive development and social justice. *Journal of Adolescent Research, 23*(3), 245–255.

Lerner, R. M., Overton, W., et al. (2010). Life-span development: Concepts and issues. In *The Handbook of life-span development* (pp. 1–29). Hoboken: Wiley.

Lester, B. M., Conradt, E., & Marsit, C. (2016). Introduction to the special section on epigenetics. *Child Development, 87*(1), 29–37.

Li, C. C., Maloney, C. A., et al. (2010). Epigenetic programming by maternal nutrition: Shaping future generations. *Epigenomics, 2*(4), 539–549.

Lillycrop, K. A., & Burdge, G. C. (2012). Epigenetic mechanisms linking early nutrition to long term health. *Best Practice & Research Clinical Endocrinology & Metabolism, 26*(5), 667–676.

Lieberman, D. (2014). *The story of the human body: evolution, health, and disease*. New York: Vintage Books.

Lorenz, E. (1993). *The essence of chaos*. Seattle: University of Washington Press.

Magnusson, D. (1995). Individual development: A holistic, integrated model. In A. Holistic, P. Moen, G. H. Elder Jr., & K. Luscher (Eds.), *Examining lives in context: Perspectives on the ecology of human development* (pp. 19–60). Washington, DC: American Psychological Association.

Maier, S. F., Watkins, L. R., et al. (1994). Psychoneuroimmunology - the Interface between behavior, brain, and immunity. *American Psychologist, 49*(12), 1004–1017.

Marshall, P. J. (2014). Beyond different levels: embodiment and the developmental system. *Frontiers in Psychology, 5*, 929.

Marmot, M. G., & Syme, S. L. (1976). Acculturation and coronary heart disease in Japanese- Americans. *American Journal of Epidemiology, 104*(3), 225–247.

Marmot, M. G., Adelstein, A. M., et al. (1978a). Changing social-class distribution of heart disease. *British Medical Journal, 2*(6145), 1109–1112.

Marmot, M. G., Rose, G., et al. (1978b). Employment grade and coronary heart disease in British civil servants. *Journal of Epidemiology and Community Health, 32*(4), 244–249.

Martino, D., & Prescott, S. (2011). Epigenetics and prenatal influences on asthma and allergic airways disease. *Chest, 139*(3), 640–647.

Masten, A. S. (2001). Ordinary magic. Resilience processes in development. *The American Psychologist, 56*(3), 227–238.

Masters, R. K., Hummer, R. A., et al. (2012). Educational differences in U.S. adult mortality a cohort perspective. *American Sociological Review, 77*(4), 548–572.

Mayer, K. U. (2009). New Directions in life course research. *Annual Review of Sociology, 35*, 413–433.

McEwan, B. S. (1998). Protective and damaging effects of stress mediators. *New England Journal of Medicine, 338*(3), 171–179.

McEwen, B. S. (2012). Brain on stress: How the social environment gets under the skin. *Proceedings of the National Academy of Sciences of the United States of America, 109*(Suppl 2), 17180–17185.

McMichael, A. J. (1999). Prisoners of the proximate: Loosening the constraints on epidemiology in an age of change. *American Journal of Epidemiology, 149*(10), 887–897.

McMillen, I. C., & Robinson, J. S. (2005). Developmental origins of the metabolic syndrome: Prediction, plasticity, and programming. *Physiological Reviews, 85*(2), 571–633.

Meaney, M. J. (2001). Maternal care, gene expression, and the transmission of individual differences in stress reactivity across generations. *Annual Review of Neuroscience, 24*, 1161–1192.

Meaney, M. J. (2010). Epigenetics and the biological definition of gene x environment interactions. *Child Development, 81*(1), 41–79.

Meaney, M. J., Szyf, M., et al. (2007). Epigenetic mechanisms of perinatal programming of hypothalamic-pituitary-adrenal function and health. *Trends in Molecular Medicine, 13*(7), 269–277.

Mendle, J., Turkheimer, E., & Emery, R. E. (2007). Detrimental psychological outcomes associated with early pubertal timing in adolescent girls. *Developmental Review, 27*(2), 151–171.

Miller, J. G. (1978). *Living systems*. New York: McGraw-Hill.

Molenaar, P. C. M., & Campbell, C. G. (2009). The new person-specific paradigm in psychology. *Current Directions in Psychological Science, 18*(2), 112–117.

Molenaar, P. C. M., Huizenga, H. M., & Nesselroade, J. R. (2003). The relationship between the structure of interindividual and intraindividual variability: A theoretical and empirical vindication of developmental systems theory. In *Understanding Human Development* (pp. 339–360). New York: Springer.

Mortimer, J. T., & Shanahan, M. J. (2007). *Handbook of the life course* New York: Springer Science & Business Media.

Noble, K. G., Houston, S. M., et al. (2012). Neural correlates of socioeconomic status in the developing human brain. *Developmental Science, 15*(4), 516–527.

Okasha, S. (2006). *Evolution and the levels of selection*. New York: NY, Oxford University Press.

Overton, W. F. (2007). A coherent Metatheory for dynamic systems: Relational Organicism- Contextualism. *Human Development, 50*(2–3), 154–159.

Oyama, S. (1985). *The ontogeny of information: Developmental systems and evolution*. Cambridge, UK: Cambridge University Press.

Perera, F., Tang, W. Y., et al. (2009). Relation of DNA methylation of 5′-CpG island of ACSL3 to transplacental exposure to airborne polycyclic aromatic hydrocarbons and childhood asthma. *PloS One, 4*(2), e4488.

Power, C., Graham, H., et al. (2005a). The contribution of childhood and adult socioeconomic position to adult obesity and smoking behaviour: An international comparison. *International Journal of Epidemiology, 34*(2), 335–344.

Power, C., Hypponen, E., et al. (2005b). Socioeconomic position in childhood and early adult life and risk of mortality: A prospective study of the mothers of the 1958 British birth cohort. *American Journal of Public Health, 95*(8), 1396–1402.

Relton, C. L., & Davey Smith, G. (2012). Is epidemiology ready for epigenetics? *International Journal of Epidemiology, 41*(1), 5–9.

Roberts, E. A. (2012). Using metalloproteomics to investigate the cellular physiology of copper in hepatocytes. *Metallomics, 4*(7), 633–640.

Roberts, E. (2015). System-driven research: Legitimate experimental design for biological/biomedical research. Accessed 2017 https://dalspace.library.dal.ca/bitstream/handle/10222/56275/Roberts-Eve-PhD-PHIL-May-2015.pdf?sequence=1&isAllowed=y

Relton, C. L., & Davey Smith, G. (2012). Is epidemiology ready for epigenetics? *International Journal of Epidemiology, 41*(1), 5–9.

Repetti, R. L., Robles, T. F., et al. (2011). Allostatic processes in the family. *Development and Psychopathology, 23*(3), 921–938.

Repetti, R. L., Taylor, S. E., et al. (2002). Risky families: Family social environments and the mental and physical health of offspring. *Psychological Bulletin, 128*(2), 330–366.

Richman, K. A. (2004). *Ethics and the metaphysics of medicine*. Cambridge, MA: The MIT Press.

Richardson, P. J., & Boyd, R. (2005). *Not by genes alone: How culture transformed human evolution*. University of Chicago Press.

Sameroff, A. (1975). Transactional models in early social relations. *Human Development, 18*(1–2), 65–79.

Sameroff, A. (2010). A unified theory of development: A dialectic integration of nature and nurture. *Child Development, 81*(1), 6–22.

Sapolsky, R. M., Krey, L. C., & McEWEN, B. R. U. C. E. S. (1985). Prolonged glucocorticoid exposure reduces hippocampal neuron number: Implications for aging. *The Journal of Neuroscience, 5*(5), 1222–1227.

Schadt, E. E., & Bjorkegren, J. L. (2012). NEW: Network-enabled wisdom in biology, medicine, and health care. *Science Translational Medicine, 4*(115), 115rv111.

Schlotz, W., & Phillips, D. I. (2009). Fetal origins of mental health: Evidence and mechanisms. *Brain, Behavior, and Immunity, 23*(7), 905–916.

Seedhouse, D. D. (2001). *Health: The foundations for achievement*. Hoboken: Wiley.

Seeman, J. (1989). Toward a model of positive health. *The American Psychologist, 44*(8), 1099–1109.

Seeman, T. E. (1997). Price of adaptation--allostatic load and its health consequences. MacArthur studies of successful aging. *Archives of Internal Medicine, 157*(19), 2259–2268.

Seeman, T. E., McEwen, B. S., et al. (2001). Allostatic load as a marker of cumulative biological risk: MacArthur studies of successful aging. *Proceedings of the National Academy of Sciences, 98*(8), 4770–4775.

Sen, A. (1999). *Commodities and capabilities*. Oxford: Oxford University Press.

Skinner, M. K., Anway, M. D., et al. (2008). Transgenerational epigenetic programming of the brain transcriptome and anxiety behavior. *PloS One, 3*(11), e3745.

Spencer, J. P., Thomas, M. S. C., et al. (Eds.). (2009). *Toward a unified theory of development: Connectionism and dynamic systems theory re-considered*. New York: Oxford University Press.

Starfield, B. (1973). Health services research: A working model. *The New England Journal of Medicine, 289*(3), 132–136.

Starfield, B., Katz, H., Gabriel, A., et al. (1984). Morbidity in childhood - a longitudinal view. *The New England Journal of Medicine, 310*(13), 824–829.

Stearns, S. (1992). *The evolution of life histories*. New York: Oxford.

Stewart, G. T. (1968). Limitations of the germ theory. *The Lancet, 291*(7551), 1077–1081.

Syme, S. L., & Berkman, L. F. (1976). Social class, susceptibility and sickness. *American Journal of Epidemiology, 104*(1), 1–8.

Szyf, M., Weaver, I. C. G., et al. (2005). Maternal programming of steroid receptor expression and phenotype through DNA methylation in the rat. *Frontiers in Neuroendocrinology, 26*(3–4), 139–162.

Tamaki, M., Bang, J. W., Watanabe, T., & Sasaki, Y. (2016). Night watch in one brain hemisphere during sleep associated with the first-night effect in humans. *Current Biology, 26*(9), 1190–1194.

Thayer, Z. M., & Kuzawa, C. W. (2011). Biological memories of past environments: Epigenetic pathways to health disparities. *Epigenetics: Official Journal of the DNA Methylation Society, 6*(7), 798–803.

Turecki, G., & Meaney, M. J. (2016). Effects of the social environment and stress on glucocorticoid receptor gene methylation: A systematic review. *Biological Psychiatry, 79*(2), 87–96.

von Bertalanffy, L. (1968). *General system theory: Foundations, development, application*. New York, NY: George Braziller.

Waddington, C. H. (1942). The Epigenotype. *Endeavour, 1*, 18–20.

Wen, X., Kleinman, K., et al. (2012). Childhood body mass index trajectories: Modeling, characterizing, pairwise correlations and socio-demographic predictors of trajectory characteristics. *BMC Medical Research Methodology, 12*, 38.

West-Eberhard, M. J. (2003). *Developmental plasticity and evolution*. New York: Oxford University Press.

Worthman, C. M., & Kuzara, J. (2005). Life history and the early origins of health differentials. *American Journal of Human Biology: The Official Journal of the Human Biology Council, 17*(1), 95–112.

10

Preconception and Prenatal Factors and Metabolic Risk

Guoying Wang, Tami R. Bartell, and Xiaobin Wang

1 Introduction

There is growing evidence that early life may have a profound impact on health and disease in later life (Gluckman et al. 2008; Hales et al. 1991). Because this growing evidence about the prenatal and preconception origins of health and disease is vast, this chapter will primarily focused on early life origins of metabolic risk for obesity and type 2 diabetes (T2DM). Obesity and type 2 diabetes affect all age groups including mothers and young children (International Diabetes Federation 2013), especially in poor minority populations (Al-Rubeaan 2015). Increasing evidence points to a profound impact of early life factors (e.g., maternal obesity, diabetes, and unhealthy diet) on offspring metabolic risk (Barbour 2014a), leading to a transgenerational amplification of obesity and diabetes. The period from conception to birth is a time of very rapid growth, cellular differentiation, and functional maturation of organ systems. This early life period is particularly sensitive to alterations of the intrauterine environment including the metabolic milieu. Epigenomic variations (regulation of gene expression) are largely established in utero (Bogdarina et al. 2004) and are particularly sensitive to prenatal environmental factors that may have a lifelong impact on health and disease. Moreover, babies that are large at birth are more likely to be overweight or obese in childhood, with these conditions persisting into adulthood (Knittle et al. 1979; Rolland-Cachera et al. 2006). Recent data suggest that elevated insulin levels may also originate in utero and persist into early childhood (Wang et al. 2014a). Taken together, the prenatal period is a critical developmental stage for obesity and metabolic outcomes (Wang et al. 2014b; Dietz 2004). In light of the global obesity and T2DM epidemic and growing evidence of early life origins of obesity and diabetes, early identification of individuals at high risk and early prevention of obesity and metabolic syndrome are a key to achieve primary prevention and reverse the trends of the obesity and T2DM epidemics.

As illustrated in Fig. 1, human health is interconnected from conception to fetal life to childhood and on into adulthood and influenced by multilevel factors from gene to society. This

G. Wang, MD, PhD
Department of Population, Family and Reproductive Health, Center on the Early Life Origins of Disease, Johns Hopkins University Bloomberg School of Public Health, Baltimore, MD, USA

T.R. Bartell, BA
Stanley Manne Children's Research Institute, Ann & Robert H Lurie Children's Hospital of Chicago, Chicago, IL, USA

X. Wang, MD, MPH, ScD (✉)
Center on the Early Life Origins of Disease, Department of Population, Family and Reproductive Health, Johns Hopkins University Bloomberg School of Public Health, Baltimore, MD, USA
e-mail: xwang82@jhu.edu

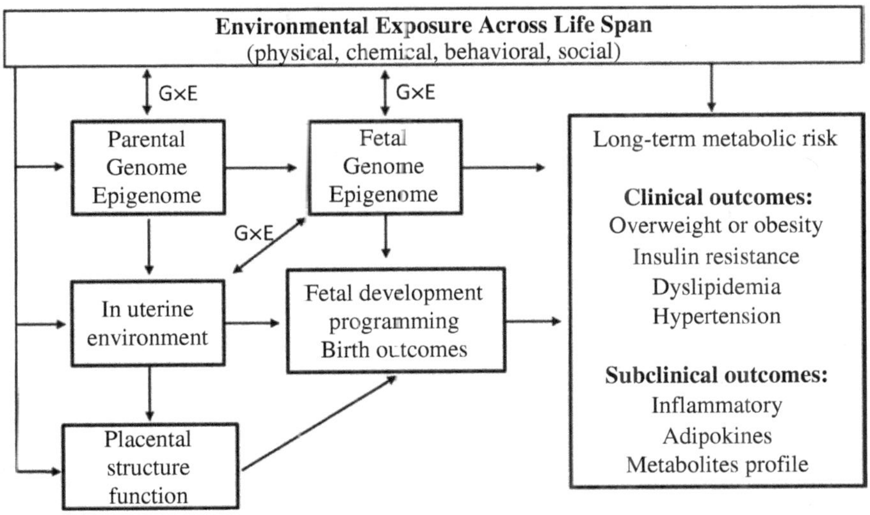

Fig. 1 Conceptual framework for preconceptional and prenatal factors and metabolic risk

chapter will discuss the impact of important preconceptional and prenatal factors, including maternal obesity and/or diabetes, gestational weight gain, and maternal micronutrient status, on in utero and lifelong metabolic outcomes and the possible gene–environment interactions and epigenetic mechanisms underlying early life origins of metabolic risk. Finally, it will provide perspectives on current knowledge gaps and recommendations to advance the field.

2 The Effects of Maternal Preconceptional Obesity and/or Diabetes and Micronutrient Status on Offspring Metabolic Outcomes

Evidence is growing about the associations between early life exposures and later health. Major exposures encompass multilevel and multifactorial influences from the societal level through to individual lifestyle and biological factors. While a discussion of all of the possible risks or protective factors is beyond the scope of this chapter, below we highlight some important preconceptional and prenatal factors, including prepregnancy obesity, excessive weight gain during pregnancy, preexistent or gestational diabetes, and maternal micronutrient status.

2.1 Maternal Prepregnancy Obesity and Gestational Weight Gain

In parallel with the global obesity epidemic, the prevalence of obesity among women of childbearing age has also increased. In 2009–2010, the National Health and Nutrition Examination Survey (NHANES) found that 56% of US women aged 20–39 were overweight or obese (body mass index (BMI) ≥ 25 kg/m^2), and in particular, 32% were obese (BMI ≥ 30.0 kg/m^2) (Flegal et al. 2012). Thus, more than half of women starting their pregnancy are already overweight or obese, and most of them remain overweight or obese during their entire pregnancy. To further complicate things, women who are overweight or obese going into pregnancy are at an increased risk for developing metabolic disorders, such as gestational diabetes mellitus (GDM) (Torloni et al. 2009), hypertensive disorders of pregnancy (Bautista-Castano et al. 2013), and excessive gestational weight gain (GWG) (Chu et al.

2009). More important, maternal obesity and its relevant metabolic disorders may impact offspring metabolic risk in later life.

Excessive maternal prepregnancy weight and GWG are consistent risk factors for offspring obesity and cardiometabolic risk (Lawlor 2013; Hochner et al. 2012). In the Jerusalem Perinatal Family Follow-Up Study, greater maternal prepregnancy BMI, independent of GWG and confounders, was significantly associated with higher offspring blood pressures, serum insulin and triglyceride concentrations, BMI, waist circumference, and lower high-density lipoprotein cholesterol (Hochner et al. 2012). Of note, the associations between maternal BMI and offspring BP, insulin, and lipids appeared to be largely mediated by offspring concurrent body size (both BMI and waist circumference) (Hochner et al. 2012). This finding emphasizes the impact that maternal adiposity may have through offspring adiposity on various predictors of subclinical and clinical disease, including diabetes mellitus and cardiovascular diseases. A large US cohort study reported that excessive maternal GWG was independently associated with a 46% increased risk of overweight or obesity in offspring at 2–5 years of age (Sridhar et al. 2014). In a retrospective cohort study, excessive maternal GWG had an adverse impact on the risk of childhood overweight and abdominal adiposity (Ensenauer et al. 2013). Kaar et al. further reported that maternal prepregnancy BMI was not only associated with increased general adiposity (BMI) and abdominal adiposity (waist circumference) in offspring but visceral adipose tissue at age 10 years (Kaar et al. 2014). A recent study points to an association between maternal excess weight in pregnancy and offspring BMI increase from adolescence to adulthood (Lawrence et al. 2014). Early pregnancy obesity has also been associated with an increased risk of premature death in adult offspring (Reynolds et al. 2013a). To further the negative impact, maternal prepregnancy BMI was also associated with increased offspring insulin resistance at age 10 years (Kaar et al. 2014) and an increased risk of developing T2DM (Dabelea et al. 2008).

2.2 Preexistent and Gestational Diabetes

In parallel with the obesity epidemic is a diabetes pandemic, which includes an increasing number of women with type 1 diabetes (T1D), T2DM, and GDM (Torloni et al. 2009). A body of studies has established a link between exposure to maternal diabetes in utero and metabolic risk in later life. In a multiethnic population aged 6–13 years, exposure to maternal GDM was associated with higher BMI, waist circumference, and more abdominal fat (Crume et al. 2011). Adjustment for socioeconomic factors, birthweight, gestational age, maternal smoking during pregnancy, diet, and physical activity did not alter the associations; however, adjustment for maternal prepregnancy BMI attenuated all associations (Crume et al. 2011), suggesting that maternal obesity is an important mediator. The studies in Pima Indians of the long-term effects of diabetic pregnancy on offspring revealed that the offspring of women with preexistent diabetes and GDM were more obese and had higher glucose concentrations and more diabetes than the offspring of nondiabetic women or women who developed diabetes after pregnancy (Pettitt et al. 1993). In the Chicago Diabetes in Pregnancy study, offspring of mothers with preexistent diabetes and GDM had significantly higher 2-h blood glucose and insulin levels and rate of impaired glucose tolerance than the control group of nondiabetic mothers (Silverman et al. 1995). In the SEARCH Case–Control Study (Dabelea et al. 2008), maternal diabetes and obesity were associated with 5.7 times and 2.8 times the risk of T2DM in young offspring aged 10–22 years, respectively. Notably, combined prenatal exposure to maternal diabetes and obesity could explain about 47% of the offspring risk of T2DM (Dabelea et al. 2008). Among Pima Indian adults, individuals whose mothers had diabetes during pregnancy had a 40% lower acute insulin response to a 25 g intravenous glucose challenge than those whose mothers developed diabetes at an early age but after the birth of the child (Gautier et al. 2001).

One important mediator is maternal blood glucose level during pregnancy. The Hyperglycemia and Adverse Pregnancy Outcome (HAPO) study demonstrated that maternal glucose levels below those diagnostic of diabetes were positively associated with increased birthweight and cord blood C-peptide levels (Metzger et al. 2008). Poor glycemic control in women with pregestational diabetes increased the risk of congenital malformations and spontaneous abortions (Kendrick 2004; Miller et al. 1981). Although T1D and T2DM have different pathogeneses, the rates of pregnancy loss were similar (Cundy et al. 2007). Another factor related to diabetes is the comorbidities. Diabetic gastropathy, a form of diabetic neuropathy, not only worsens nausea and vomiting but also can cause difficulty with glucose control during pregnancy (Kitzmiller et al. 2008). Reece et al. reviewed the literature and reported that maternal diabetic nephropathy is complicated by hypertension (60%), preeclampsia (41%), premature delivery (22–30%), and fetal growth restriction (16%) (Reece et al. 1998). Taken together, better control of blood glucose levels and diabetic complications may improve prenatal outcomes.

2.3 Maternal Micronutrient Status

Growing evidence suggests that maternal nutrition, through its impact on the fetal intrauterine environment, has a profound and lifelong influence on later health (Barker et al. 1993). Among a number of specific nutrients that have been implicated, folate is particularly important. Folate is an essential vitamin B involved in nucleic acid synthesis, DNA methylation, cellular growth, differentiation, and repair (Crider et al. 2012; Kim 2000). The demand for folate increases during pregnancy due to the need for fetal and placental growth and uterus enlargement (Greenberg et al. 2011). The causal role of folate deficiency in fetal neural tube defects (NTDs) is well established (De Wals et al. 2007). A recent study showed that low maternal folate concentration was associated with higher BMI in offspring at 5–6 years (Krikke et al. 2016). Our study also showed that maternal low folate was not only independently associated with offspring overweight or obesity but also worsened the adverse effects of maternal prepregnancy obesity on offspring metabolic risk (Wang et al. 2016). On the other hand, excess maternal folate status may also link to offspring adverse metabolic outcomes. A study in an Indian population reported a positive association between maternal folate level and offspring homeostatic model assessment-insulin resistance (HOMA-IR) (Krishnaveni et al. 2014). What we gather from the combined results of these studies is that optimizing folate nutrition in women, and especially OWO women, may offer a safe, simple, and effective way to decrease the risk of transgenerational obesity and diabetes.

2.4 Adverse Birth Outcomes

Birthweight reflects cumulative growth in utero. A body of studies has suggested that maternal obesity is associated with a risk for large for gestational age (LGA) or macrosomia in the offspring (Bautista-Castano et al. 2013). In addition, Brumbaugh et al. demonstrated that newborns of obese mothers with GDM showed increased intrahepatic fat at birth (Brumbaugh et al. 2013). Prepregnancy obesity also has been shown to increase the risk of Cesarean section (Martin et al. 2015; Dzakpasu et al. 2014) and preterm birth (Cnattingius et al. 2013). In a case–control study of 914 women with pregestational diabetes and 4000 controls, diabetes was associated with an increased risk of preterm birth (Cnattingius et al. 1994). Maternal diabetes has also been linked to macrosomia and Cesarean section (Barbour 2014b; Koyanagi et al. 2013)

These adverse birth outcomes are also associated with obesity and metabolic syndrome (including hypertension, dyslipidemia, obesity, and insulin resistance/diabetes) in later life. *Hypertension:* Previous studies demonstrated that preterm birth was associated with hypertension in childhood (Sipola-Leppanen et al. 2014) and adulthood (Irving et al. 2000; Johansson et al. 2005). In a prospective study, Irving et al. found that preterm birth was associated with the risk of hypertension and hyperglycemia in adulthood (Irving et al. 2000). A meta-analysis of 27 studies further confirmed that preterm birth was associated with cardiovascular risk factors, such as higher systolic and diastolic blood pressure and low-density lipoprotein cholesterol in adulthood (Parkinson et al. 2013). Even more interesting is that the difference in blood pressure between those born preterm and those born at term may be greater in women than in men (Parkinson et al. 2013). *Dyslipidemia:* A large cohort study reported that boys born early preterm had 6.7% higher total cholesterol, 11.7% higher low-density lipoprotein cholesterol (LDL-C), and 12.3% higher apolipoprotein B concentrations than their term peers (Sipola-Leppanen et al. 2014). *Obesity*: As fat deposition occurs largely during the third trimester of pregnancy, preterm babies are born with low levels of body fat (Rigo et al. 1998; Uthaya et al. 2005). Postnatally, preterm babies are more likely to gain excessive weight, a known risk factor of childhood obesity (Ong et al. 2000), and tend to have a higher proportion of central adiposity (Uthaya et al. 2005). *Insulin resistance/diabetes:* Like children who were born at term and small for gestational age (SGA), children born preterm have lower insulin sensitivity (Wang et al. 2014a; Hofman et al. 2004). Hovi et al. reported that preterm birth itself, independent of birth size, may contribute to insulin resistance, elevated blood glucose, and higher blood pressure (BP) in young adulthood (Hovi et al. 2007). In addition, a Swedish study found that preterm birth was associated with later T2DM: the hazard ratio for T2DM comparing very preterm (≤32 weeks of gestation) with term birth was 1.67 (Kaijser et al. 2009). There is a particular lack of large-scale longitudinal birth cohort studies to examine the effects of preterm birth on metabolic outcomes over critical developmental windows. One prospective birth cohort study found that preterm birth is associated with elevated plasma insulin levels (indirect evidence of insulin resistance) at birth that persist to age 6.5 years (Wang et al. 2014a), suggesting that insulin resistance originates in utero and persists into later life. There is also evidence from a mechanistic study, which revealed that preterm birth increased the risk of T2DM via diminished insulin sensitivity (Pilgaard et al. 2010), and yet another study showed that preterm birth was associated with changes in the cord blood adipokine profile that may contribute to the impairment of glucose metabolism (Bhargava et al. 2004).

3 Mechanisms/Pathways Underlying Early Life Origins of Metabolic Risk

Compelling evidence suggests that prenatal experiences influence metabolic alterations in late life via multiple pathways, including genetic, in utero environment, gene–environment interaction, and epigenetic and shared familial socioeconomic and lifestyle factors (Fig. 1).

3.1 Genetics

Several lines of evidence support that genetics play a key role in the long-term effects of maternal obesity and diabetes on offspring metabolic risk. First, obesity and diabetes tend to aggregate among families. We also know that GDM is associated with a history of T2DM. One study showed that, compared to women with nondiabetic parents, women with any parental history of T2DM experienced a 2.3-fold increased risk of GDM, suggesting that the risk of GDM was positively associated with parental history of T2DM (Williams et al. 2003). Second, the extensive study of genetic variation in obesity and diabetes has led to the identification of numerous candidate genes. Although currently identified genetic markers only explain a small proportion of metabolic risks, twin studies reveal that BMI, body fat, and insulin sensitivity are all highly heritable (Zhang et al. 2009; Ouyang et al. 2010). Finally, some gene variants related to adult diseases have been linked to offspring outcomes. A epidemiological study showed that a genetic risk score (GRS) comprised of SNPs associated with adult obesity-related traits may provide an approach for predicting LGA birth and newborn adiposity beyond established risk factors (Chawla et al. 2014). A genome-wide association study of women of European descent established that common variants near the melanocortin-4 receptor (*MC4R*) influence fat mass, weight and obesity risk and over transmission of the risk allele to obese offspring (Loos et al. 2008). GDM is not only associated with later risk of diabetes in mothers but also with metabolic changes that may lead to the development of diabetes in their offspring (Silverman et al. 1998). Some genes and their interactions in functional networks between the mother and fetus may also play a role in organ development (Charalambous et al. 2007).

Additionally related is the fetal insulin hypothesis proposed by Drs. Hattersley and Tooke, which highlights that fetal genetic factors affect not only insulin-mediated fetal growth by regulating either fetal insulin secretion or insulin sensitivity but also insulin resistance in childhood and adulthood (Hattersley and Tooke 1999). One example is the case in which a mother transmits mutations and pleiotropic effects in the glucokinase gene to her child. The glucokinase gene codes for the glycolytic enzyme glucokinase, which acts as the pancreatic beta-cell glucose sensor (Matschinsky et al. 1993). Such mutations result in mild beta-cell dysfunction with slightly elevated fasting blood glucose concentrations, which is present in early childhood and shows little change with age (Hattersley 1998).

3.2 Intrauterine Environment

Based on observational research, Barker et al. proposed the fetal programming hypothesis, which conceptualized that intrauterine experiences modify fetal systems and influence health in later life (Hales and Barker 1992). Fetal development responds to changes in the in utero environment in response to changing metabolism, hormone production, and tissue sensitivity to hormones (Gluckman et al. 2008). These adaptive changes may influence the relative development of various organs, leading to persistent alterations in physiologic and metabolic homeostasis. *Maternal prepregnancy BMI*: In a large cohort of 4,091 mother–father–offspring trios in Britain, researchers found that the association between parental prepregnancy BMI and offspring adiposity at ages 9–11 years was stronger among mother–offspring pairs than among father–offspring pairs (Lawlor et al. 2008). Given that maternal and paternal prepregnancy BMI are markers of genetic, behavioral, and environmental factors but that only the maternal prepregnancy BMI was reflected in the intrauterine environment, this finding provides some support for the role of the in utero environment in lifelong metabolic risk beyond genetic and shared environmental contributions. *Pregestational and Gestational Diabetes:* A sibling study of Pima Indians showed that the BMI of siblings born after the mother developed T2DM was significantly higher than that of siblings born before their mother developed T2DM (Dabelea et al. 2000). Offspring born to mothers with T2DM or GDM had up to a sixfold higher risk of developing T2DM as young adults compared to offspring born to mothers before they developed T2DM (Dabelea and Crume 2011). Other strong evidence comes from a study in which comparisons were made between sibling groups where one sibling was born before the mother experienced dramatic weight loss after bariatric surgery and the other was born after the surgery (Kral et al. 2006). Siblings born before maternal bariatric surgery were at a much greater risk for obesity than siblings born after the weight loss surgery (Kral et al. 2006). Moreover, infants of mothers who had bariatric surgery before pregnancy were at a reduced risk of being LGA at birth (Johansson et al. 2015) and developing obesity and insulin resistance in childhood and adolescence (Smith et al. 2009). Collectively, these findings support the role of the intrauterine environment in transmitting a risk for obesity beyond that of genetics.

3.3 Gene and Environment Interaction and Epigenetics

Epigenetic mechanisms are critical to normal human development and play an important role in complex human diseases (O'Neill et al. 2014;

Reynolds et al. 2013b; Dolinoy et al. 2007). Both animal models and human studies implicate the intrauterine period as a sensitive time for the establishment of epigenetic variability (Heijmans et al. 2008; Cook et al. 2007; Tang et al. 2012; Radford et al. 2014; Janssen et al. 2013), which in turn influences risk for a range of disorders that develop later in life. In the Boston Birth Cohort, we observed a wide range of interindividual variations in genome-wide methylation at birth (Wang et al. 2012). One possible mechanism by which maternal obesity affects offspring OWO is via alterations in fetal DNA methylation induced by maternal obesity.

Animal studies have shown that certain transient environmental influences in utero can produce persistent changes in epigenetic marks that have lifelong consequences (Sinclair et al. 2007; Anway et al. 2005). In humans, our previous study showed an association between maternal prepregnancy BMI and alterations in fetal DNA methylation (Liu et al. 2014). Other studies also showed the link between maternal obesity and fetal epigenome alterations (Lesseur et al. 2013; Yang et al. 2013). In addition, the use of methyl donor supplementation has been shown to prevent transgenerational obesity (Waterland et al. 2008). A recent study indicated lower DNA methylation plasticity in skeletal muscle among low birthweight vs. normal birthweight men, which potentially contributes to our understanding of the link between low birthweight and an increased risk of T2DM (Jacobsen et al. 2014).

Genes related to metabolic risk are regulated by epigenetic alteration: Evidence suggests that epigenetic mechanisms are involved in the risk of obesity. Current evidence supports the important role of epigenetic regulation in key genes involved in the control of adipogenesis, glucose homeostasis, inflammation, and/or insulin signaling, including *leptin* (Milagro et al. 2009), *peroxisome proliferator-activated receptor gamma* (Noer et al. 2007), *insulin* (Yang et al. 2011), *glucose transporter* (Yokomori et al. 1999), *proliferator-activated receptor-γ* (Fujiki et al. 2009), *lipoprotein lipase* (Noer et al. 2007), and *fatty acid-binding protein 4* (Noer et al. 2007). In addition, greater methylation in the promoter region of the *retinoid X receptor-a* gene was also related to greater adiposity in childhood (Godfrey et al. 2011).

Genes subject to genomic imprinting are predominantly expressed from one of the two parental chromosomes and are often clustered in the genome and epigenetically regulated. The role of imprinted genes in growth control has been apparent since the discovery of imprinting in the early 1980s. A related study found altered methylation at multiple imprint regulatory regions in children born to obese parents compared with children born to nonobese parents (Soubry et al. 2015).

4 Preconception and Prenatal Care

Maternal health is not only important for the mother but also for the fetus and neonate, which makes it critical for women to be and stay healthy during their reproductive years. It is well recognized that optimizing a woman's health and knowledge before planning and conceiving a pregnancy may eliminate or reduce health risks to her and her baby. As emerging clinical and scientific advances come to be realized through a life course health development approach to health optimization, the AAP/ACOG Guidelines for Perinatal Care have shifted from framing preconceptional care as appropriately targeted toward prospective parents who are contemplating pregnancy to an emphasis on the integration of preconception health promotion throughout the lifespan. Taking this approach, all women and men can benefit from preconception health, whether or not they plan to have a baby one day. The implementation of effective interventions that prioritize risk factors and the provision of quality health services during prepregnancy and pregnancy are recommended (Bilano et al. 2014). In a multicenter randomized trial, 1108 overweight (BMI ≥ 25 kg/m^2) women were randomized to a comprehensive dietary and lifestyle intervention. Infants born to women who had received lifestyle advice were significantly less likely to have a birthweight above 4000 g; treatment effect (95%CI):0.82, 0.68–0.99; $P = 0.04$) (Dodd et al. 2014). All women with T2DM should be advised regarding safe, effective contraception and the benefits of optimal glycemic control, folic acid supplementation, and avoidance of potentially harmful medications before attempting pregnancy. Adequate glucose control in a woman with diabetes before conception and throughout pregnancy can decrease maternal morbidity, spontaneous abortion, fetal malformation, fetal macrosomia, intrauterine fetal death, and neonatal morbidity (American College of Obstetricians and Gynecologists 2005).

5 Recommendations for Future Study and Perspectives

5.1 Major Themes and Findings

Growing evidence indicates that preconception and prenatal risk factors may play an important role both in fetal metabolic reprogramming and long-term metabolic disorders in later life. Although the onset of obesity and diabetes may begin later in childhood or adulthood, programming at the earliest ages may contribute a latent susceptibility. In addition to genetic susceptibility, epigenetic alterations may be important molecular mechanisms underlying gene–environment interactions in early life origins of disease. Early identification and intervention may improve long-term health outcomes and help to reverse the obesity and diabetes epidemics during the most sensitive developmental stages, when interventions are likely to be most cost-efficient. Particular attention is required for US urban low-income minority populations that have been disproportionally affected by the obesity and diabetes epidemics, and most likely fall into vicious cycle of transgenerational obesity and diabetes.

5.2 Research Priorities

5.2.1 Epidemiologic research

Despite the notion of early life origins of obesity and T2DM, there is a particular lack of well-powered prospective birth cohort studies to examine to what degree and how early life factors affect pregnancy and infant and child health outcomes across multiple developmental windows in a life course framework, particularly in high-risk US urban low-income minority populations. Findings from this line of research will have important research, clinical, and public health implications.

5.2.2 Mechanism research

In light of growing recognition that epigenetic mechanisms may play an important role in mediating early life origins of diseases and that epigenome is potentially modifiable and reversible, well-designed large-scale prospective birth cohort studies are needed to trace the pathways from early life factors to adverse pregnancy outcomes to postnatal long-term metabolic outcomes and to better understand how epigenome changes from fetal to childhood to adolescence in response to environmental exposures. The role of social and environmental adversity in obesity and diabetes among urban low-income minorities has taken on new urgency given that these populations are disproportionally affected by the obesity and diabetes epidemics. In addition to genetics and epigenetics, the field may also leverage and benefit from the latest advances in other "omics" such as metabolomics and microbiome as well as system sciences and bioinformatics.

5.2.3 Translational research

A particular challenge in preventing childhood obesity is to identify important and modifiable early life risk and protective factors to design safe, effective, and sustainable interventions. Evidence is needed to inform clinical guidelines regarding the optimal age to screen for obesity in children. Conflicting recommendations have been proposed for the starting age: age 5 by the US Preventive Services Task Force (Barton 2010) vs. age 2 by the Expert Committee (Barlow 2007). While low birthweight has been included in current clinical assessment of future metabolic risk, there is a need to consider preterm birth as an important risk factor of future metabolic risk. The American Diabetes Association included histories of SGA and maternal history of diabetes or GDM during the child's gestation as part of their diabetes risk assessment for children

(American Diabetes Association 2014). To date, preterm birth has not been included in the diabetes risk assessment guidelines in children and adults, an area that requires more research given growing evidence linking preterm with subsequent metabolic risk.

5.3 Data and Methods Development Priorities

Advanced analytical methods are needed to comprehensively examine temporal and causal links of multilevel early life factors with metabolic outcomes. Future studies need to fully capture the complex interplay of broad environmental factors, genome, epigenome, metabolome, and microbiome that affect metabolic outcomes across lifespan and generations. While some systems models exist to help characterize particular sub-systems of the complex set of factors that influences children's bodyweight, none have tried to comprehensively represent the relationship between early life factors and the subsequent development of childhood metabolic risk across critical developmental stages.

6 Conclusions

There is growing evidence that preconceptional and prenatal factors play an important role in fetal metabolic programming and metabolic risk in later life. More research is needed to identify important and modifiable early life risk and protective factors and underlying mechanisms, which will pave the road for developing cost-effective early screening, prevention, and treatment strategies to halt and reverse the obesity and T2DM epidemics in the US, in particular among the most vulnerable populations (urban low-income minorities).

7 Source of Funding

Drs. Xiaobin Wang and Guoying Wang are supported in part by the National Institutes of Health (NIH) grant R01HD086013 (PI: X Wang).

References

Al-Rubeaan, K. (2015). National surveillance for type 1, type 2 diabetes and prediabetes among children and adolescents: A population-based study (SAUDI-DM). *Journal of Epidemiology and Community Health.* doi:10.1136/jech-2015-205710.

American College of Obstetricians and Gynecologists. (2005). ACOG Practice Bulletin. Clinical Management Guidelines for Obstetrician-Gynecologists. Number 60, March 2005. Pregestational diabetes mellitus. *Obstetrics and Gynecology, 105*(3), 675–685.

American Diabetes Association. (2014). Diagnosis and classification of diabetes mellitus. *Diabetes Care, 37*(Suppl 1), S81–S90.

Anway, M. D., Cupp, A. S., Uzumcu, M., & Skinner, M. K. (2005). Epigenetic transgenerational actions of endocrine disruptors and male fertility. *Science, 308*(5727), 1466–1469.

Barbour, L. A. (2014a). Changing perspectives in pre-existing diabetes and obesity in pregnancy: Maternal and infant short- and long-term outcomes. *Current Opinion in Endocrinology, Diabetes, and Obesity, 21*(4), 257–263.

Barbour, L. A. (2014b). Changing perspectives in pre-existing diabetes and obesity in pregnancy: Maternal and infant short- and long-term outcomes. *Current Opinion in Endocrinology, Diabetes, and Obesity, 21*(4), 257–263.

Barker, D. J., Gluckman, P. D., Godfrey, K. M., Harding, J. E., Owens, J. A., & Robinson, J. S. (1993). Fetal nutrition and cardiovascular disease in adult life. *Lancet, 341*(8850), 938–941.

Barlow, S. E. (2007). Expert committee recommendations regarding the prevention, assessment, and treatment of child and adolescent overweight and obesity: Summary report. *Pediatrics, 120*(Suppl 4), S164–S192.

Barton, M. (2010). Screening for obesity in children and adolescents: US Preventive Services Task Force recommendation statement. *Pediatrics, 125*(2), 361–367.

Bautista-Castano, I., Henriquez-Sanchez, P., Aleman-Perez, N., et al. (2013). Maternal obesity in early pregnancy and risk of adverse outcomes. *PLoS One, 8*(11), e80410.

Bhargava, S. K., Sachdev, H. S., Fall, C. H., et al. (2004). Relation of serial changes in childhood body-mass index to impaired glucose tolerance in young adulthood. *The New England Journal of Medicine, 350*(9), 865–875.

Bilano, V. L., Ota, E., Ganchimeg, T., Mori, R., & Souza, J. P. (2014). Risk factors of pre-eclampsia/eclampsia and its adverse outcomes in low- and middle-income countries: A WHO secondary analysis. *PLoS One, 9*(3), e91198.

Bogdarina, I., Murphy, H. C., Burns, S. P., & Clark, A. J. (2004). Investigation of the role of epigenetic modification of the rat glucokinase gene in fetal programming. *Life Sciences, 74*(11), 1407–1415.

Brumbaugh, D. E., Tearse, P., Cree-Green, M., et al. (2013). Intrahepatic fat is increased in the neonatal offspring of obese women with gestational diabetes. *The Journal of Pediatrics, 162*(5), 930–936; e931.

Charalambous, M., da Rocha, S. T., & Ferguson-Smith, A. C. (2007). Genomic imprinting, growth control and the allocation of nutritional resources: Consequences for postnatal life. *Current Opinion in Endocrinology, Diabetes, and Obesity, 14*(1), 3–12.

Chawla, R., Badon, S. E., Rangarajan, J., et al. (2014). Genetic risk score for prediction of newborn adiposity and large-for-gestational-age birth. *The Journal of Clinical Endocrinology and Metabolism, 99*(11), E2377–E2386.

Chu, S. Y., Callaghan, W. M., Bish, C. L., D'Angelo, D. (2009). Gestational weight gain by body mass index among US women delivering live births, 2004-2005: Fueling future obesity. *American Journal of Obstetrics and Gynecology,. 200*(3), 271; e271–277.

Cnattingius, S., Berne, C., & Nordstrom, M. L. (1994). Pregnancy outcome and infant mortality in diabetic patients in Sweden. *Diabetic Medicine, 11*(7), 696–700.

Cnattingius, S., Villamor, E., Johansson, S., et al. (2013). Maternal obesity and risk of preterm delivery. *JAMA, 309*(22), 2362–2370.

Cook, J. D., Davis, B. J., Goewey, J. A., Berry, T. D., & Walker, C. L. (2007). Identification of a sensitive period for developmental programming that increases risk for uterine leiomyoma in Eker rats. *Reproductive Sciences, 14*(2), 121–136.

Crider, K. S., Yang, T. P., Berry, R. J., & Bailey, L. B. (2012). Folate and DNA methylation A review of molecular mechanisms and the evidence for folate's role. *Advances in Nutrition, 3*(1), 21–38.

Crume, T. L., Ogden, L., West, N. A., et al. (2011). Association of exposure to diabetes in utero with adiposity and fat distribution in a multiethnic population of youth: The Exploring Perinatal Outcomes among Children (EPOCH) Study. *Diabetologia, 54*(1), 87–92.

Cundy, T., Gamble, G., Neale, L., et al. (2007). Differing causes of pregnancy loss in type 1 and type 2 diabetes. *Diabetes Care, 30*(10), 2603–2607.

Dabelea, D., & Crume, T. (2011). Maternal environment and the transgenerational cycle of obesity and diabetes. *Diabetes, 60*(7), 1849–1855.

Dabelea, D., Hanson, R. L., Lindsay, R. S., et al. (2000). Intrauterine exposure to diabetes conveys risks for type 2 diabetes and obesity: A study of discordant sibships. *Diabetes, 49*(12), 2208–2211.

Dabelea, D., Mayer-Davis, E. J., Lamichhane, A. P., et al. (2008). Association of intrauterine exposure to maternal diabetes and obesity with type 2 diabetes in youth: The SEARCH Case-Control Study. *Diabetes Care, 31*(7), 1422–1426.

De Wals, P., Tairou, F., Van Allen, M. I., et al. (2007). Reduction in neural-tube defects after folic acid fortification in Canada. *The New England Journal of Medicine, 357*(2), 135–142.

Dietz, W. H. (2004). Overweight in childhood and adolescence. *The New England Journal of Medicine, 350*(9), 855–857.

Dodd, J. M., Turnbull, D., McPhee, A. J., et al. (2014). Antenatal lifestyle advice for women who are overweight or obese: LIMIT randomised trial. *BMJ, 348*, g1285.

Dolinoy, D. C., Weidman, J. R., & Jirtle, R. L. (2007). Epigenetic gene regulation: Linking early developmental environment to adult disease. *Reproductive Toxicology, 23*(3), 297–307.

Dzakpasu, S., Fahey, J., Kirby, R. S., et al. (2014). Contribution of prepregnancy body mass index and gestational weight gain to caesarean birth in Canada. *BMC Pregnancy and Childbirth, 14*, 106.

Ensenauer, R., Chmitorz, A., Riedel, C., et al. (2013). Effects of suboptimal or excessive gestational weight gain on childhood overweight and abdominal adiposity: Results from a retrospective cohort study. *International Journal of Obesity, 37*(4), 505–512.

Flegal, K. M., Carroll, M. D., Kit, B. K., & Ogden, C. L. (2012). Prevalence of obesity and trends in the distribution of body mass index among US adults, 1999-2010. *JAMA, 307*(5), 491–497.

Fujiki, K., Kano, F., Shiota, K., & Murata, M. (2009). Expression of the peroxisome proliferator activated receptor gamma gene is repressed by DNA methylation in visceral adipose tissue of mouse models of diabetes. *BMC Biology, 7*, 38.

Gautier, J. F., Wilson, C., Weyer, C., et al. (2001). Low acute insulin secretory responses in adult offspring of people with early onset type 2 diabetes. *Diabetes, 50*(8), 1828–1833.

Gluckman, P. D., Hanson, M. A., Cooper, C., & Thornburg, K. L. (2008). Effect of in utero and early-life conditions on adult health and disease. *The New England Journal of Medicine, 359*(1), 61–73.

Godfrey, K. M., Sheppard, A., Gluckman, P. D., et al. (2011). Epigenetic gene promoter methylation at birth is associated with child's later adiposity. *Diabetes, 60*(5), 1528–1534.

Greenberg, J. A., Bell, S. J., Guan, Y., & Yu, Y. H. (2011). Folic Acid supplementation and pregnancy: More than just neural tube defect prevention. *Reviews in Obstetrics & Gynecology, 4*(2), 52–59.

Hales, C. N., & Barker, D. J. (1992). Type 2 (non-insulin-dependent) diabetes mellitus: The thrifty phenotype hypothesis. *Diabetologia, 35*(7), 595–601.

Hales, C. N., Barker, D. J., Clark, P. M., et al. (1991). Fetal and infant growth and impaired glucose tolerance at age 64. *BMJ, 303*(6809), 1019–1022.

Hattersley, A. T. (1998). Maturity-onset diabetes of the young: Clinical heterogeneity explained by genetic heterogeneity. *Diabetic Medicine, 15*(1), 15–24.

Hattersley, A. T., & Tooke, J. E. (1999). The fetal insulin hypothesis: An alternative explanation of the association of low birthweight with diabetes and vascular disease. *Lancet, 353*(9166), 1789–1792.

Heijmans, B. T., Tobi, E. W., Stein, A. D., et al. (2008). Persistent epigenetic differences associated with prenatal exposure to famine in humans. *Proceedings of the National Academy of Sciences of the United States of America, 105*(44), 17046–17049.

Hochner, H., Friedlander, Y., Calderon-Margalit, R., et al. (2012). Associations of maternal prepregnancy body mass index and gestational weight gain with adult offspring cardiometabolic risk factors: The Jerusalem Perinatal Family Follow-up Study. *Circulation, 125*(11), 1381–1389.

Hofman, P. L., Regan, F., Jackson, W. E., et al. (2004). Premature birth and later insulin resistance. *The New England Journal of Medicine, 351*(21), 2179–2186.

Hovi, P., Andersson, S., Eriksson, J. G., et al. (2007). Glucose regulation in young adults with very low birth weight. *The New England Journal of Medicine, 356*(20), 2053–2063.

International Diabetes Federation. IDF Diabetes Atlas, 5th ed. 2013.; http://www.idf.org/diabetesatlas. Accessed July 19, 2013.

Irving, R. J., Belton, N. R., Elton, R. A., & Walker, B. R. (2000). Adult cardiovascular risk factors in premature babies. *Lancet, 355*(9221), 2135–2136.

Jacobsen, S. C., Gillberg, L., Bork-Jensen, J., et al. (2014). Young men with low birthweight exhibit decreased plasticity of genome-wide muscle DNA methylation by high-fat overfeeding. *Diabetologia, 57*(6), 1154–1158.

Janssen, B. G., Godderis, L., Pieters, N., et al. (2013). Placental DNA hypomethylation in association with particulate air pollution in early life. *Particle and Fibre Toxicology, 10*, 22.

Johansson, S., Iliadou, A., Bergvall, N., Tuvemo, T., Norman, M., & Cnattingius, S. (2005). Risk of high blood pressure among young men increases with the degree of immaturity at birth. *Circulation, 112*(22), 3430–3436.

Johansson, K., Cnattingius, S., Naslund, I., et al. (2015). Outcomes of pregnancy after bariatric surgery. *The New England Journal of Medicine, 372*(9), 814–824.

Kaar, J. L., Crume, T., Brinton, J. T., Bischoff, K. J., McDuffie, R., & Dabelea, D. (2014). Maternal obesity, gestational weight gain, and offspring adiposity: The exploring perinatal outcomes among children study. *The Journal of Pediatrics, 165*(3), 509–515.

Kaijser, M., Bonamy, A. K., Akre, O., et al. (2009). Perinatal risk factors for diabetes in later life. *Diabetes, 58*(3), 523–526.

Kendrick, J. M. (2004). Preconception care of women with diabetes. *The Journal of Perinatal & Neonatal Nursing, 18*(1):14–25; quiz 26–17.

Kim, Y. I. (2000). Methylenetetrahydrofolate reductase polymorphisms, folate, and cancer risk: A paradigm of gene-nutrient interactions in carcinogenesis. *Nutrition Reviews, 58*(7), 205–209.

Kitzmiller, J. L., Block, J. M., Brown, F. M., et al. (2008). Managing preexisting diabetes for pregnancy: Summary of evidence and consensus recommendations for care. *Diabetes Care, 31*(5), 1060–1079.

Knittle, J. L., Timmers, K., Ginsberg-Fellner, F., Brown, R. E., & Katz, D. P. (1979). The growth of adipose tissue in children and adolescents. Cross-sectional and longitudinal studies of adipose cell number and size. *The Journal of Clinical Investigation, 63*(2), 239–246.

Koyanagi, A., Zhang, J., Dagvadorj, A., et al. (2013). Macrosomia in 23 developing countries: An analysis of a multicountry, facility-based, cross-sectional survey. *Lancet, 381*(9865), 476–483.

Kral, J. G., Biron, S., Simard, S., et al. (2006). Large maternal weight loss from obesity surgery prevents transmission of obesity to children who were followed for 2 to 18 years. *Pediatrics, 118*(6), e1644–e1649.

Krikke, G. G., Grooten, I. J., Vrijkotte, T., van Eijsden, M., Roseboom, T. J., & Painter, R. C. (2016). Vitamin B12 and folate status in early pregnancy and cardiometabolic risk factors in the offspring at age 5-6 years: Findings from the ABCD multi-ethnic birth cohort. *BJOG, 123*(3), 384–392.

Krishnaveni, G. V., Veena, S. R., Karat, S. C., Yajnik, C. S., & Fall, C. H. (2014). Association between maternal folate concentrations during pregnancy and insulin resistance in Indian children. *Diabetologia, 57*(1), 110–121.

Lawlor, D. A. (2013). The Society for Social Medicine John Pemberton Lecture 2011. Developmental overnutrition--an old hypothesis with new importance? *International Journal of Epidemiology, 42*(1), 7–29.

Lawlor, D. A., Timpson, N. J., Harbord, R. M., et al. (2008). Exploring the developmental overnutrition hypothesis using parental-offspring associations and FTO as an instrumental variable. *PLoS Medicine, 5*(3), e33.

Lawrence, G. M., Shulman, S., Friedlander, Y., et al. (2014). Associations of maternal pre-pregnancy and gestational body size with offspring longitudinal change in BMI. *Obesity (Silver Spring), 22*(4), 1165–1171.

Lesseur, C., Armstrong, D. A., Paquette, A. G., Koestler, D. C., Padbury, J. F., & Marsit, C. J. (2013). Tissue-specific Leptin promoter DNA methylation is associated with maternal and infant perinatal factors. *Molecular and Cellular Endocrinology, 381*(1–2), 160–167.

Liu, X., Chen, Q., Tsai, H. J., et al. (2014). Maternal preconception body mass index and offspring cord blood DNA methylation: Exploration of early life origins of disease. *Environmental and Molecular Mutagenesis, 55*(3), 223–230.

Loos, R. J., Lindgren, C. M., Li, S., et al. (2008). Common variants near MC4R are associated with fat mass, weight and risk of obesity. *Nature Genetics, 40*(6), 768–775.

Martin, K. E., Grivell, R. M., Yelland, L. N., & Dodd, J. M. (2015). The influence of maternal BMI and gestational diabetes on pregnancy outcome. *Diabetes Research and Clinical Practice, 108*(3), 508–513.

Matschinsky, F., Liang, Y., Kesavan, P., et al. (1993). Glucokinase as pancreatic beta cell glucose sensor and diabetes gene. *The Journal of Clinical Investigation, 92*(5), 2092–2098.

Metzger, B. E., Lowe, L. P., Dyer, A. R., et al. (2008). Hyperglycemia and adverse pregnancy outcomes. *The New England Journal of Medicine, 358*(19), 1991–2002.

Milagro, F. I., Campion, J., Garcia-Diaz, D. F., Goyenechea, E., Paternain, L., & Martinez, J. A. (2009). High fat diet-induced obesity modifies the methylation pattern of leptin promoter in rats. *Journal of Physiology and Biochemistry, 65*(1), 1–9.

Miller, E., Hare, J. W., Cloherty, J. P., et al. (1981). Elevated maternal hemoglobin A1c in early pregnancy and major congenital anomalies in infants of diabetic mothers. *The New England Journal of Medicine, 304*(22), 1331–1334.

Noer, A., Boquest, A. C., & Collas, P. (2007). Dynamics of adipogenic promoter DNA methylation during clonal culture of human adipose stem cells to senescence. *BMC Cell Biology, 8*, 18.

O'Neill, R. J., Vrana, P. B., & Rosenfeld, C. S. (2014). Maternal methyl supplemented diets and effects on offspring health. *Frontiers in Genetics, 5*, 289.

Ong, K. K. L., Ahmed, M. L., Emmett, P. M., Preece, M. A., Dunger, D. B., & Pregnancy, A. L. S. (2000). Association between postnatal catch-up growth and obesity in childhood: Prospective cohort study. *British Medical Journal, 320*(7240), 967–971.

Ouyang, F., Christoffel, K. K., Brickman, W. J., et al. (2010). Adiposity is inversely related to insulin sensitivity in relatively lean Chinese adolescents: A population-based twin study. *The American Journal of Clinical Nutrition, 91*(3), 662–671.

Parkinson, J. R., Hyde, M. J., Gale, C., Santhakumaran, S., & Modi, N. (2013). Preterm birth and the metabolic syndrome in adult life: A systematic review and meta-analysis. *Pediatrics, 131*(4), e1240–e1263.

Pettitt, D. J., Nelson, R. G., Saad, M. F., Bennett, P. H., & Knowler, W. C. (1993). Diabetes and obesity in the offspring of Pima Indian women with diabetes during pregnancy. *Diabetes Care, 16*(1), 310–314.

Pilgaard, K., Faerch, K., Carstensen, B., et al. (2010). Low birthweight and premature birth are both associated with type 2 diabetes in a random sample of middle-aged Danes. *Diabetologia, 53*(12), 2526–2530.

Radford, E. J., Ito, M., Shi, H., et al. (2014). In utero effects. In utero undernourishment perturbs the adult sperm methylome and intergenerational metabolism. *Science, 345*(6198), 1255903.

Reece, E. A., Leguizamon, G., & Homko, C. (1998). Pregnancy performance and outcomes associated with diabetic nephropathy. *American Journal of Perinatology, 15*(7), 413–421.

Reynolds, R. M., Allan, K. M., Raja, E. A., et al. (2013a). Maternal obesity during pregnancy and premature mortality from cardiovascular event in adult offspring: Follow-up of 1 323 275 person years. *BMJ, 347*, f4539.

Reynolds, R. M., Jacobsen, G. H., & Drake, A. J. (2013b). What is the evidence in humans that DNA methylation changes link events in utero and later life disease? *Clinical Endocrinology, 78*(6), 814–822.

Rigo, J., Nyamugabo, K., Picaud, J. C., Gerard, P., Pieltain, C., & De Curtis, M. (1998). Reference values of body composition obtained by dual energy X-ray absorptiometry in preterm and term neonates. *Journal of Pediatric Gastroenterology and Nutrition, 27*(2), 184–190.

Rolland-Cachera, M. F., Deheeger, M., Maillot, M., & Bellisle, F. (2006). Early adiposity rebound: Causes and consequences for obesity in children and adults. *International Journal of Obesity, 30*(Suppl 4), S11–S17.

Silverman, B. L., Metzger, B. E., Cho, N. H., & Loeb, C. A. (1995). Impaired glucose tolerance in adolescent offspring of diabetic mothers. Relationship to fetal hyperinsulinism. *Diabetes Care, 18*(5), 611–617.

Silverman, B. L., Rizzo, T. A., Cho, N. H., & Metzger, B. E. (1998). Long-term effects of the intrauterine environment. The Northwestern University Diabetes in Pregnancy Center. *Diabetes Care, 21*(Suppl 2), B142–B149.

Sinclair, K. D., Allegrucci, C., Singh, R., et al. (2007). DNA methylation, insulin resistance, and blood pressure in offspring determined by maternal periconceptional B vitamin and methionine status. *Proceedings of the National Academy of Sciences of the United States of America, 104*(49), 19351–19356.

Sipola-Leppanen, M., Vaarasmaki, M., Tikanmaki, M., et al. (2014). Cardiovascular risk factors in adolescents born preterm. *Pediatrics, 134*(4), e1072–e1081.

Smith, J., Cianflone, K., Biron, S., et al. (2009). Effects of maternal surgical weight loss in mothers on intergenerational transmission of obesity. *The Journal of Clinical Endocrinology and Metabolism, 94*(11), 4275–4283.

Soubry, A., Murphy, S. K., Wang, F., et al. (2015). Newborns of obese parents have altered DNA methylation patterns at imprinted genes. *International Journal of Obesity, 39*(4), 650–657.

Sridhar, S. B., Darbinian, J., Ehrlich, S. F., et al. (2014). Maternal gestational weight gain and offspring risk for childhood overweight or obesity. *American Journal of Obstetrics and Gynecology, 211*(3):259; e251–258.

Tang, W. Y., Morey, L. M., Cheung, Y. Y., Birch, L., Prins, G. S., & Ho, S. M. (2012). Neonatal exposure to estradiol/bisphenol A alters promoter methylation and expression of Nsbp1 and Hpcal1 genes and transcriptional programs of Dnmt3a/b and Mbd2/4 in the rat prostate gland throughout life. *Endocrinology, 153*(1), 42–55.

Torloni, M. R., Betran, A. P., Horta, B. L., et al. (2009). Prepregnancy BMI and the risk of gestational diabetes: A systematic review of the literature with meta-analysis. *Obesity Reviews, 10*(2), 194–203.

Uthaya, S., Thomas, E. L., Hamilton, G., Dore, C. J., Bell, J., & Modi, N. (2005). Altered adiposity after extremely preterm birth. *Pediatric Research, 57*(2), 211–215.

Wang, D., Liu, X., Zhou, Y., et al. (2012). Individual variation and longitudinal pattern of genome-wide DNA methylation from birth to the first two years of life. *Epigenetics: Official Journal of the DNA Methylation Society, 7*(6), 594–605.

Wang, G., Divall, S., Radovick, S., et al. (2014a). Preterm birth and random plasma insulin levels at birth and in early childhood. *JAMA, 311*(6), 587–596.

Wang, G., Chen, Z., Bartell, T., & Wang, X. (2014b). Early Life Origins of Metabolic Syndrome: The Role of Environmental Toxicants. *Current Environmental Health Reports*. doi:10.1007/s40572-013-0004-6.

Wang, G., Hu, F., Mistry, K., et al. (2016). Maternal Prepregnancy BMI, Plasma Folate Level and Child Metabolic Risk. *JAMA Pediatrics. 170*(8), e160845.

Waterland, R. A., Travisano, M., Tahiliani, K. G., Rached, M. T., & Mirza, S. (2008). Methyl donor supplementation prevents transgenerational amplification of obesity. *International Journal of Obesity, 32*(9), 1373–1379.

Williams, M. A., Qiu, C., Dempsey, J. C., & Luthy, D. A. (2003). Familial aggregation of type 2 diabetes and chronic hypertension in women with gestational diabetes mellitus. *The Journal of Reproductive Medicine, 48*(12), 955–962.

Yang, B. T., Dayeh, T. A., Kirkpatrick, C. L., et al. (2011). Insulin promoter DNA methylation correlates negatively with insulin gene expression and positively with HbA(1c) levels in human pancreatic islets. *Diabetologia, 54*(2), 360–367.

Yang, Q. Y., Liang, J. F., Rogers, C. J., Zhao, J. X., Zhu, M. J., & Du, M. (2013). Maternal obesity induces epigenetic modifications to facilitate Zfp423 expression and enhance adipogenic differentiation in fetal mice. *Diabetes, 62*(11), 3727–3735.

Yokomori, N., Tawata, M., & Onaya, T. (1999). DNA demethylation during the differentiation of 3T3-L1 cells affects the expression of the mouse GLUT4 gene. *Diabetes, 48*(4), 685–690.

Zhang, S., Liu, X., Brickman, W. J., et al. (2009). Association of plasma leptin concentrations with adiposity measurements in rural Chinese adolescents. *The Journal of Clinical Endocrinology and Metabolism, 94*(9), 3497–3504.

Permissions

All chapters in this book were first published in HLCHD, by Springer; hereby published with permission under the Creative Commons Attribution License or equivalent. Every chapter published in this book has been scrutinized by our experts. Their significance has been extensively debated. The topics covered herein carry significant findings which will fuel the growth of the discipline. They may even be implemented as practical applications or may be referred to as a beginning point for another development.

The contributors of this book come from diverse backgrounds, making this book a truly international effort. This book will bring forth new frontiers with its revolutionizing research information and detailed analysis of the nascent developments around the world.

We would like to thank all the contributing authors for lending their expertise to make the book truly unique. They have played a crucial role in the development of this book. Without their invaluable contributions this book wouldn't have been possible. They have made vital efforts to compile up to date information on the varied aspects of this subject to make this book a valuable addition to the collection of many professionals and students.

This book was conceptualized with the vision of imparting up-to-date information and advanced data in this field. To ensure the same, a matchless editorial board was set up. Every individual on the board went through rigorous rounds of assessment to prove their worth. After which they invested a large part of their time researching and compiling the most relevant data for our readers.

The editorial board has been involved in producing this book since its inception. They have spent rigorous hours researching and exploring the diverse topics which have resulted in the successful publishing of this book. They have passed on their knowledge of decades through this book. To expedite this challenging task, the publisher supported the team at every step. A small team of assistant editors was also appointed to further simplify the editing procedure and attain best results for the readers.

Apart from the editorial board, the designing team has also invested a significant amount of their time in understanding the subject and creating the most relevant covers. They scrutinized every image to scout for the most suitable representation of the subject and create an appropriate cover for the book.

The publishing team has been an ardent support to the editorial, designing and production team. Their endless efforts to recruit the best for this project, has resulted in the accomplishment of this book. They are a veteran in the field of academics and their pool of knowledge is as vast as their experience in printing. Their expertise and guidance has proved useful at every step. Their uncompromising quality standards have made this book an exceptional effort. Their encouragement from time to time has been an inspiration for everyone.

The publisher and the editorial board hope that this book will prove to be a valuable piece of knowledge for researchers, students, practitioners and scholars across the globe.

List of Contributors

W. Thomas Boyce
Departments of Pediatrics and Psychiatry, University of California San Francisco, San Francisco, CA, USA

Clyde Hertzman
Human Early Learning Partnership, School of Population and Public Health, University of British Columbia, Vancouver, BC, Canada

Marco DelGiudice
Department of Psychology, University of New Mexico, Logan Hall, 2001 Redondo Dr. NE, Albuquerque, NM 87131, USA

Richard M. Lerner
Tufts University, Medford, MA, USA

Claire D. Brindis
University of California-San Francisco (UCSF), Philip R. Lee Institute for Health Policy Studies and the Adolescent and Young Adult Health National Resource Center, San Francisco, CA, USA

Milena Batanova
Institute for Applied Research in Youth Development, Tufts University, Medford, MA, USA

Robert Wm. Blum
Johns Hopkins Bloomberg School of Public Health, Baltimore, MD, USA

David Wood
Department of Pediatrics, ETSU College of Medicine, Johnson City, TN 37614, USA

Tara Crapnell, Lynette Lau, Debra Lotstein, Maria Ferris and Alice Kuo
UCLA, Department of Pediatrics, Los Angeles, CA, USA

Ashley Bennett
Department of Pediatrics, USC, Los Angeles, CA, USA

James J. Crall
Division of Public Health and Community Dentistry, University of California Los Angeles (UCLA) School of Dentistry, Los Angeles, CA, USA

Christopher B. Forrest
Applied Clinical Research Center, Children's Hospital of Pennsylvania, Philadelphia, PA, USA

Michael E. Msall
Developmental and Behavioral Pediatrics University of Chicago, Comer and LaRabida Children's Hospitals, Chicago, IL, USA
JP Kennedy Research Center on Intellectual and Developmental Disabilities, University of Chicago Comer Children's Hospital, Section of Developmental and Behavioral Pediatrics, 950 East 61St Street, SSC Room 207, Chicago, IL 60637, USA

Sarah A. Sobotka and Amelia Dmowska
Section of Developmental and Behavioral Pediatrics, University of Chicago Comer Children's Hospitals, Chicago, IL, USA

Dennis Hogan
Sociology and Demography, Population Research and Training Center, Brown University, Providence, RI, USA

Mary Sullivan
University of Rhode Island, College of Nursing, Women and Infants Hospital, Providence, RI, USA

Summer Sherburne Hawkins
Boston College, Chestnut Hill, MA, USA

Emily Oken and Matthew W. Gillman
Harvard Medical School and Harvard Pilgrim Health Care Institute, Boston, MA, USA

Amanda Geller
New York University, New York, NY, USA

Kate Jaeger
Princeton University, Princeton, NJ, USA

Garrett Pace
Doctoral Student, School of Social Work, Department of Sociology, University of Michigan, Ann Arbor, MI, USA

Neal Halfon
Department of Pediatrics, David Geffen School of Medicine, UCLA, Los Angeles, CA, USA
Department of Health Policy and Management, Fielding School of Public Health, UCLA, Los Angeles, CA, USA
Department of Public Policy, Luskin School of Public Affairs, UCLA, Los Angeles, CA, USA
Center for Healthier Children, Families and Communities, UCLA, Los Angeles, CA, USA

Christopher B. Forrest
Applied Clinical Research Center, Children's Hospital of Philadelphia, Philadelphia, PA, USA

Guoying Wang
Department of Population, Family and Reproductive Health, Center on the Early Life Origins of Disease, Johns Hopkins University Bloomberg School of Public Health, Baltimore, MD, USA

Tami R. Bartell
Stanley Manne Children's Research Institute, Ann & Robert H Lurie Children's Hospital of Chicago, Chicago, IL, USA

Xiaobin Wang
Center on the Early Life Origins of Disease, Department of Population, Family and Reproductive Health, Johns Hopkins University Bloomberg School of Public Health, Baltimore, MD, USA

Index

A

Adiposity, 13, 26, 30, 58, 64, 67, 83, 87, 126, 130-131, 136, 139, 186, 203

Adolescence, 33, 45, 48, 56, 60-66, 70, 73, 75-76, 78, 80-82, 85, 88, 99, 105-107, 109, 112-113, 136, 146, 151, 154, 170, 174-175, 181, 185, 190, 193, 196-197, 201, 203, 208-212, 216, 226-227, 229

Adult Oral Health, 46-47, 50

Anticonvulsants, 110

Anxiety, 21, 26, 50, 57, 62, 72, 85-86, 94, 102-103, 112, 115, 196-197

Autism, 14, 21, 29-30, 100-101, 111, 115, 160

Autism Spectrum Disorder (asd), 100

B

Bariatric Surgery, 26

Birth Cohorts, 48, 64

Birth Outcomes, 12, 29, 85, 102-103, 114, 116, 134, 140, 178, 184

Body Mass Index (bmi), 64

Breastfeeding, 7, 21, 125, 132, 134, 138, 142, 174

C

Child Health, 1, 22-24, 27-29, 33, 53, 61, 64, 77, 80, 87, 110, 114, 116, 139, 169, 173, 175-176, 182-187, 190

Childhood Overweight, 139

Cognitive Processes, 98, 193

Commensurate, 157

Cross-sectional Studies, 159, 177, 180

D

Depression, 21, 56-57, 70, 77, 80, 84-87, 94, 96, 103, 112, 140, 145, 166, 170, 172-174, 184, 187, 196-198

E

Early Childhood, 12-14, 26, 33, 35, 38, 46, 51, 53, 62, 73, 78, 87, 89, 91, 96, 105, 110, 114, 119, 121, 134, 139, 146, 151, 169, 173, 176, 178-181, 183-184, 188, 195-196, 198, 206-208, 210-213

Educational Attainment, 66-67, 85-86, 99, 105-107, 127, 171, 198, 200-201

Epidemiologic, 23, 49, 80, 118, 121, 123-124, 133, 139, 161, 170, 173, 181, 186

Epigenetic, 2, 4-6, 8-9, 15, 21-23, 26-29, 36, 73, 89, 94, 102-103, 110, 112-113, 116, 123, 130, 134, 148, 159, 163, 165, 172-173, 178, 183, 188, 223, 231-233

F

Family Relationships, 174

Fertility, 138, 142

Fetal Nutrition, 183

Food Insecurity, 22, 24

G

Genetic Factors, 45, 150, 232

Genetics, 2, 4, 12, 20, 23, 28, 31-32, 121, 135, 138-139, 142, 147, 159, 161, 164, 166, 184, 208, 225, 230-231, 234, 238-239

Gestation Length, 104

H

Health Development, 1, 7, 13, 16, 21, 27, 33, 41, 49, 51, 55, 59, 70, 74, 82, 90, 110, 113, 118, 126, 129, 133, 137, 145, 153, 158, 160, 165, 168, 173, 177, 185, 190, 203, 209, 214, 219, 225, 227, 235

Health Disparities, 33, 51, 76, 111, 113, 128, 168-169, 171-178, 180-184, 186-188

Health-care Utilization, 109

Human Health, 30, 35, 118-119, 121, 128, 182

Hypotheses, 122, 159

I

Impaired Glucose Tolerance, 9, 172

Incarceration, 198

Infancy, 9, 24, 56, 59, 62, 80, 88, 100, 116, 118, 121, 124-126, 129-130, 134-135, 139-141, 148-149, 154, 173, 193, 208, 212, 216, 218-219, 225

Insulin Resistance, 74, 84, 104, 114, 139, 220, 227

L

Leptin, 27, 129-130, 134, 136, 140

Life Course Epidemiology, 34, 45-46

Life Course Perspective, 27, 33, 53, 169, 184
Low Birth Weight, 6-8, 12, 27, 29, 51-52, 64, 90-92, 102-104, 107-109, 111, 113-114, 116, 124, 172-174, 184, 217-220, 222, 229, 234, 236, 238-240

M
Maternal Overnutrition, 125
Maternal Stress, 80, 103, 128, 134
Mental Health, 21, 43, 46, 78, 80, 91, 94, 100, 103, 108-109, 111-114, 122-123, 140, 155-156, 162, 167, 173, 187, 200, 209
Microbiome, 2, 12, 20-23, 25-27, 30-32, 35, 43, 129, 134, 138, 141, 216
Middle Childhood, 60-63, 65, 105, 107, 112, 146

N
Neighborhood Effects, 186

O
Offspring, 5, 9, 11, 13-14, 24, 26, 30-32, 73, 84, 87, 89, 112, 120-121, 123-125, 127-128, 134-135, 139, 171, 178, 184, 186, 216, 222, 228, 235
Oral Cancers, 36, 38, 40, 43
Oral Diseases, 34, 38, 46, 49, 54
Oral Health, 33-39, 41-54, 176, 184

P
Periodontal Disease, 36, 38-39, 45-47, 49, 51
Periodontitis, 38, 41, 54
Placenta, 5, 134, 178, 181
Policymakers, 180, 183, 212
Polymorphisms, 130, 161
Postpartum, 8, 77-78, 83, 89, 138, 183
Postpartum Depression, 77
Preeclampsia, 12, 95, 124, 137
Pregnancy, 5-9, 11-14, 24-28, 31-32, 39, 49, 70, 77, 91, 95, 102-103, 110, 115-116, 121, 125-126, 129, 134, 136, 138-141, 153, 174-175, 187, 234, 239
Prenatal Period, 35, 51, 73, 148, 150
Preterm Delivery, 102, 185, 225, 228
Preterm Infants, 26, 90-91, 96, 100, 103-104, 110-111, 113, 115-116, 137, 238
Psychopathology, 56, 77-78, 80, 82-84, 89, 116, 142, 173, 207, 210, 212

R
Research Questions, 161

S
Sensitive Periods, 5, 33, 51, 72-73, 93, 120-121, 147, 153, 163, 170, 193, 206
Sex Differences, 132, 165, 186
Sleep Duration, 75, 79, 89
Social Influences, 45, 79
Social Stratification, 52
Social Support, 51, 70, 75, 109, 126, 140, 202

W
Working Memory, 62, 67, 80, 98-99, 193, 196, 200, 203-204, 209

Y
Young Adults, 67, 69, 79-83, 85, 88, 107, 135, 149, 154-155, 163, 214, 237

www.ingramcontent.com/pod-product-compliance
Lightning Source LLC
LaVergne TN
LVHW080607210926
848485LV00003B/115